Topics in Industrial Microbiology

Topics in Industrial Microbiology

Novel Microbial Products for Medicine and Agriculture

Editors

A.L. Demain

Massachusetts Institute of Technology, Cambridge, MA, U.S.A.

G.A. Somkuti

Agricultural Research Service, USDA, Peoria, IL, U.S.A.

J.C. Hunter-Cevera

Cetus Corporation, Palo Alto, CA, U.S.A.

H.W. Rossmoore

Wayne State University, Detroit, MI, U.S.A.

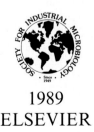

1989
ELSEVIER

Published by Elsevier Science Publishers
on behalf of the Society for Industrial Microbiology

ISBN 0-444-81066-8
ISSN 0923-2303

This book is printed on acid-free paper.

Published by:

Elsevier Science Publishers B.V. (Biomedical Division)
P.O. Box 211
1000 AE Amsterdam
The Netherlands

Sole distributors for the USA and Canada:
Elsevier Science Publishing Company, Inc.
655 Avenue of the Americas
New York, NY 10010
U.S.A.

Library of Congress Cataloging in Publication Data
Novel microbial products for medicine and agriculture / editors, A.L.
   Demain ... [et al.].
       p.   cm. –– (Topics in industrial microbiology, ISSN 0923-2303)
   Papers presented at the First International Conference on the
Biotechnology of Microbial Products, held Mar. 13-16, 1988, in San
Diego, Calif., under the sponsorship of the Society for Industrial
Microbiology.
   Includes bibliographies and index.
   ISBN 0-444-81066-8 (U.S.)
   1. Microbial products––Testing––Congresses.   2. Pharmaceutical
microbiology––Congresses.   I. Demain, A. L. (Arnold L.), 1927-
II. International Conference on the Biotechnology of Microbial
Products (1st : 1988 : San Diego, Calif.) III. Society for
Industrial Microbiology (U.S.) IV. Series.
   [DNLM: 1. Biological Products––congresses. 2. Industrial
Microbiology––methods––congresses.   QW 800 N937 1988]
QR53. N58   1989
660'.62––dc20
DNLM/DLC
for Library of Congress   89-1420
                                                       CIP

Printed in The Netherlands

Foreword

With this publication, the Society for Industrial Microbiology enters a new arena in service to the applied microbiological community. Future contributions will continue to focus on areas of topical interest to that community, bringing together wherever and whenever possible the interdisciplinary flavor so necessary to successfully treat the subject encompassed by our charter.

This volume and the conference that preceded it owe their genesis and nurturing to the tireless efforts and dedication of George Somkuti, Chair of the Society for Industrial Microbiology Conference Committee, and the members of the Program Committee: A.L. Demain (Chair), T. Beppu, R. Hamill, J.C. Hunter-Cevera, R. Monaghan, S. Ōmura, G.A. Somkuti, and M. Weinstein.

I hope that subsequent 'Topics in Industrial Microbiology' are favored with individuals of equal devotion, for this – above all – is a requirement for a successful venture.

Harold W. Rossmoore
Chairman
Society for Industrial Microbiology Publications Committee

Preface

The material in this volume was presented at the *'First International Conference on the Biotechnology of Microbial Products'*, held March 13–16, 1988, in San Diego, California, under the sponsorship of the Society for Industrial Microbiology, U.S.A. Attended by many of the scientific world's foremost authorities in the subject areas covered, the conference was dedicated to the memory of the late Professor Hamao Umezawa, the internationally recognized and respected investigator of bioactive microbial metabolites.

The establishment of this special and much-needed conference series reflects a rapidly increasing level of scientific inquiry worldwide in the search for useful microbial metabolites with other than antiinfective activities. The cases of confirmed applications and the anticipated impact of such microbial products in medicine and agriculture appear to signal the unfolding of an exciting and promising era in microbiological research that we are privileged to witness.

The new conference series, that will no doubt grow in recognition and stature, also represents the reaffirmation of the Society for Industrial Microbiology's mission, which is the *'advancement of the applied microbiological sciences'*.

George A. Somkuti, Chairman, SIM Conference Committee
Agricultural Research Service
United States Department of Agriculture
Philadelphia, PA 19118, U.S.A.

List of Contributors

Acebal, C., PharmaMar SA, Madrid, Spain.

Aharonowitz, Y., Department of Microbiology, Tel Aviv University, The George S. Wise Faculty of Life Sciences, Ramat Aviv 69978, Israel.

Andoh, T., Research Laboratories, Fujisawa Pharmaceutical Co., Ltd., 1-6-2 Chome, Kashima, Yodogawa-ku, Osaka 532, Japan.

Aoki, H., Exploratory Research Laboratories, Fujisawa Pharmaceutical Co., Ltd., 5-2-3 Tokodai, Tsukuba, Ibaragi 300-26, Japan.

Aoyagi, T., Institute of Microbial Chemistry, 3-14-23 Kamiosaki, Shinagawa-ku, Tokyo 141, Japan.

Aranha, H.G., Department of Biological Sciences, Mississippi State University, Mississippi State, MS, U.S.A.

Arnett, K.L., Martek Corporation, Columbia, MD, U.S.A.

Asahi, A., Medicinal Research Laboratory, Toyo Jozo Co., Ltd., Ohito, Shizuoka 410-23, Japan.

Asano, M., Exploratory Research Laboratories, Fujisawa Pharmaceutical Co., Ltd., 5-2-3 Tokodai, Tsukuba, Ibaragi 300-26, Japan.

Barash, I., Department of Botany, Tel Aviv University, The George S. Wise Faculty of Life Sciences, Ramat Aviv 69978, Israel.

Bauer, S., Department of Microbiology, Tel Aviv University. The George S. Wise Faculty of Life Sciences, Ramat Aviv 69978, Israel.

Behrens, P.W., Martek Corporation, Columbia, MD, U.S.A.

Beppu, T., Department of Agricultural Chemistry, The University of Tokyo, Yakoi, 1-1-1, Bunkyo-ku, Tokyo 113, Japan.

Billich, A., Institut für Biochemie und Molekulaire Biologie, Technische Universität Berlin, Franklinstrasse 29, D-1000 Berlin 10 (West), Germany

Brown, L.R., Department of Biological Sciences, Mississippi State University, Mississippi State, MS, U.S.A.

Buckland, B., Merck, Sharp & Dohme Research Laboratories, Rahway, NJ 07065, U.S.A.

Burrascano, M., Mycogen Corporation, 5451 Oberlin Drive, San Diego, CA 92121, U.S.A.

Carter, G.T., American Cyanamid Company, Medical Research Division, Lederle Laboratories, Pearl River, NY, U.S.A.

Clement, J.J., Research Laboratories, SeaPharm, 5602 Old Dixie Highway, Fort Pierce, FL, U.S.A.

Cole, M.S., Martek Corporation, Columbia, MD, U.S.A.

Dolce, G.J., Boyce Thompson Institute for Plan Research, Ithaca, NY, 14853, U.S.A.

Doyle, T.W., Bristol-Myers Company, Pharmaceutical Research and Development Division, P.O. Box 5100, Wallingford, CT 06492, U.S.A.

Dybas, R.A., Merck, Sharp & Dohme Research Laboratories, Three Bridges, NJ 08887, U.S.A.

Eskola, P., Merck, Sharp & Dohme Research Laboratories, Rahway, NJ 07065, U.S.A.

Espinosa, O., Mycogen Corporation, 5451 Oberlin Drive, San Diego, CA 92121, U.S.A.

Everich, R., Mycogen Corporation, 5451 Oberlin Drive, San Diego, Ca 92121, U.S.A.

Fisher, M.H., Merck, Sharp & Dohme Research Laboratories, Rahway, NJ 07065, U.S.A.

Forenza, S., Bristol-Myers Company, Pharmaceutical Research and Development Division, P.O. Box 5100, Wallingford, CT 06492, U.S.A.

Furumai, T., Department of Microbiology and Chemistry, Nippon Roche Research Center, 200 Kajiwara, Kamakura City, Kanagawa 247, Japan.

Gbewonyo, K., Merck, Sharp & Dohme Research Laboratories, Rahway, NJ 07065, U.S.A.

G :nick, D.L., Department of Microbiology, Tel Aviv University, The George S. Wise Faculty of Life Sciences, Ramat Aviv 69978, Israel.

Hallada, T., Merck, Sharp & Dohme Research Laboratories, Rahway, NJ 07065, U.S.A.

Hashizume, K., Tokyo Research Laboratories, Kyowa Hakko Kogyo Co., Ltd., Machida-shi, Tokyo 194, Japan.

Hayashi, M., Medicinal Research Laboratory, Toyo Jozo Co., Ltd., Ohito, Shizuoka 410-23, Japan.

Health, B., Mycogen Corporation, 5451 Oberlin Drive, San Diego, CA 92121, U.S.A.

Heubner, T.A., Martek Corporation, Columbia, MD, U.S.A.

Hilton, N.J., Merck, Sharp & Dohme Research Laboratories, Rahway, NJ 07065, U.S.A.

Hoeksema, S.D., Martek Corporation, Columbia, MD, U.S.A.

Hori, M., Showa College of Pharmaceutical Sciences, 5-1-8 Tsurumaki, Setagaya-ku, Tokyo 154, Japan.

Iida, T., Tokyo Research Laboratories, Kyowa Hakko Kogyo Co., Ltd., Machida-shi, Tokyo 194, Japan.

Imanaka, H., Exploratory Research Laboratories, Fujisawa Pharmaceutical Co., Ltd., 5-2-3 Tokodai, Tsukuba, Ibaragi 300-26, Japan.

Inouye, S., Central Research Laboratories, Meiji Seika Kaisha, Ltd., Yokohama 222, Japan.

Inouye, Y., Institute of Pharmaceutical Sciences, Hiroshima 734, Japan.

Iwasaki, S., Institute of Applied Microbiology, The University of Tokyo, Bunkyo-ku, Tokyo 113, Japan.

Jensen, P.R., Research Laboratories, SeaPharm, 5602 Old Dixie Highway, Fort Pierce, FL, U.S.A.

Kanamaru, T., Applied Microbiology Laboratories, Central Research Division, Takeda Chemical Industries, Ltd., Juso, Yodogawa-ku, Osaka 532, Japan.

Kaplan, L., Merck, Sharp & Dohme Research Laboratories, Rahway, NJ 07065, U.S.A.

Kase, H., Tokyo Research Laboratories, Kyowa Hakko Kogyo Co., Ltd., Machida-shi, Tokyo 194, Japan.

Kida, T., Central Research Laboratories, Ajinomoto Co., Inc., 1-1 Suzuki-cho, Kawasaki 210, Japan.

Kitamura, S., Tokyo Research Laboratories, Kyowa Hakko Kogyo Co., Ltd., Machia-shi, Tokyo 194, Japan.

Kleinkauf, H., Institut für Biochemie und Molekulaire Biologie, Technische Universität Berlin, Franklinstrasse 29, D-1000 Berlin 10 (West), Germany.

Kohsaka, M., Exploratory Research Laboratories, Fujisawa Pharmaceutical Co., Ltd., 5-2-3 Tokodai, Tsukuba, Ibaragi 300-26, Japan.

Kondo, S., Central Research Laboratories, Meiji Seika Kaisha, Ltd., Yokohama 222, Japan.

K. ipal, L.R., Department of Fermentation Microbiology, Merck, Sharp & Dohme Research Laboratories, Rahway, NJ 07065, U.S.A.

Kyle, D.J., Martek Corporation, Columbia, MD, U.S.A.

Lam, K.S., Bristol-Myers Company, Pharmaceutical Research and Development Division, P.O. Box 5100, Wallingford, CT 06492, U.S.A.

Lawen, A., Institut für Biochemie und Molekulare Biologie, Technische Universität Berlin, Franklinstrasse 29, D-1000 Berlin 10 (West), Germany.

Masurekar, P., Merck, Sharp & Dohme Research Laboratories, Rahway, NJ 07065, U.S.A.

Mizuno, K., Medicinal Research Laboratory, Toyo Jozo Co., Ltd., Ohito, Shizuoka 410-23, Japan.

Monaghan, R.L., Department of Fermentation Microbiology, Merck, Sharp & Dohme Research Laboratories, Rahway, NJ 07065, U.S.A.

Mrozik, H., Merck, Sharp & Dohme Research Laboratories, Rahway, NJ 07065, U.S.A.

Mueller, L., EP Corporate Project Management, Bayer AG, D-5090 Leverkusen, F.R.G.

Nakamura, S., Institute of Pharmaceutical Sciences, Hiroshima University School of Medicine, 1-2-3 Kasumi, Minami-ku, Hiroshima 734, Japan.

Newman, D.J. Research Laboratories, 2026 14th Place, Vero Beach, FL 32960, U.S.A.

Ohmori, K., Pharmaceutical Research Laboratory, Kyowa Hakko Kogyo Co., Ltd., Nagaizumi-cyo, Shuzuoka, Japan.

Okami, Y., Institute of Microbial Chemistry, 3-14-23 Kamiosaki, Shinagawa-ku, Tokyo 141, Japan.

Okazaki, H., Applied Microbiology Laboratories, Central Research Division, Takeda Chemical Industries, Ltd., Juso, Yodogawa-ku, Osaka 532, Japan.

Ōmura, S., The Kitasato Institute, Minato-ku, Tokyo 108, Japan.

Payne, J., Mycogen Corporation, 5451 Oberlin Drive, San Diego, CA 92121, U.S.A.

Pearce, C.J., School of Pharmacy, University of Connecticut, Storrs, CT 06268, U.S.A.

Peeters, H., Institut für Biochemie und Molekulare Biologie, Technische Universität Berlin, Franklinstrasse 29, D-1000 Berlin 10 (West), Germany.

Pirson, W., Department of PF/DO, F. Hoffmann-La Roche & Co., Ltd., CH-4002 Basel, Switzerland.

Preiser, F.A., Merck, Sharp & Dohme Research Laboratories, Rahway, NJ 07065, U.S.A.

Rutten, J.M., Martek Corporation, Columbia, MD, U.S.A.

Schreiber, R., Department of Microbiology, Tel Aviv University, The George S. Wise Faculty of Life Sciences, Ramat Aviv 69978, Israel.

Schroeder, D.R., Bristol-Myers Company, Pharmaceutical Research and Development Division, P.O. Box 5100, Wallingford, CT 06492, U.S.A.

Shih, T.L., Merck, Sharp & Dohme Research Laboratories, Rahway, NJ 07065, U.S.A.

Shutter, R., Mycogen Corporation, 5451 Oberlin Drive, San Diego, CA 92121, U.S.A.

Soares, G., Mycogen Corporation, 5451 Oberlin Drive, San Diego, CA 92121, U.S.A.

Stowell, L.J., Pace Consulting, 1267 Diamond, San Diego, CA 92109, U.S.A.

Suhara, Y., Department of Microbiology and Chemistry, Nippon Roche Research Center, 200 Kajiwara, Kamakura City, Kanagawa 247, Japan.

Takada, M., Medicinal Research Laboratory, Toyo Jozo Co., Ltd., Ohito, Shizuoka 410-23, Japan.

Takeuchi, T., Institute of Microbial Chemistry, 3-14-23 Kamiosaki, Shinagawa-ku, Tokyo 141, Japan.

Talbot, H.W., Mycogen Corporation, 5451 Oberlin Drive, San Diego, CA 92121, U.S.A.

Tanaka, H. School of Pharmaceutical Sciences, Kitasato University, Minato-ku, Tokyo 108, Japan.

Tomoda, H., The Kitasato Institute, Minato-ku, Tokyo 108, Japan.

Tsujino, M., Medicinal Research Laboratory, Toyo Jozo Co., Ltd., Ohito, Shizuoka 410-23, Japan.

Umezawa, K., Institute of Microbial Chemistry, 3-14-23 Kamiosaki, Shinagawa-ku, Tokyo 141, Japan.

Von Döhren, H., Institut für Biochemie und Molekulare Biologie, Technische Universität Berlin, Franklinstrasse 29, D-1000 Berlin 10 (West), Germany.

Yaginuma, S., Medicinal Research Laboratory, Toyo Jozo Co., Ltd., Ohito, Shizuoka 410-23, Japan.

Yokose, K., Department of Microbiology and Chemistry, Nippon Roche Research Center, 200 Kakiwara, Kamakura City, Kanagawa 247, Japan.

Yoshida, K., Research Laboratories, Fujisawa Pharmaceutical Co., Ltd., 1-6-2 Chome, Kashima, Yodogawa-ku, Osaka 532, Japan.

Yoshida, M., Department of Agricultural Chemistry, The University of Tokyo, Yayoi 1-1-1, Bunkyo-ku, Tokyo 113, Japan.

Zocher, R., Institut für Biochemie und Molekulare Biologie, Technische Universität Berlin, Franklinstrasse 29, D-1000 Berlin 10 (West), Germany.

The contribution of the following organizations in the support of the conference and this publication is gratefully acknowledged:

Abbott Laboratories
Ajinomoto Company, Inc.
Allied-Signal Engineered Materials Research
American Cyanamid Company
AMGen
Bection Dickinson Microbiology Systems
Boehringer Ingelheim Pharmaceuticals, Inc.
Bristol Myers Company Industrial Division
Cetus Corporation
Eastman Kodak Company
Fujisawa Pharmaceutical Company, Inc.
Genencor, Inc.
Hoffmann-LaRoche, Inc.
Kerin Brewery Compary, Ltd.
Kyowa Hakko Kogyo Company, Ltd.
Lab-Line Instruments, Inc.
Lilly Research Laboratories
Marcor Development Corporation
Meiji Seika Kaisha, Ltd.
Merck Sharp & Dohme Research Laboratories
Novo Laboratories, Inc.
Pfizer, Inc.
Pioneer Hi-Bred International, Inc.
Pitman-Moore, Inc.
Praxis Biologics, Inc.
Sankyo Company, Ltd.
Schering-Plough Corporation
Takeda Chemical Industries, Ltd.
Toyo Jozo Company, Ltd.
U.S. Department of Agriculture-Agricultural Research Service
The Upjohn Company
Xenova, Ltd.

Contents

Foreword. V
Preface. VII
List of Contributors. IX
Introduction. XXV

1. Hamao Umezawa, the man and his dream 1
   Y. Okami (Tokyo, Japan)

2. Use of the Plackett & Burman technique in a discovery program for new natural products 25
   R.L. Monaghan and L.R. Koupoal (Rahway, NJ, U.S.A.)
   Summary. 25
   Introduction 25
   Materials and Methods 25
   Results 26
       Formulation of screening media 26
       Fermentations containing multiple activities 27
       Similarity between complex fermentation ingredients. 28
       Use to increase titers 29
       Production of the same products by different microorganisms 30
   Discussion 31
   Acknowledgements 31
   References 31

3. Screening of cardiovascular agents 33
   T. Andoh and K. Yoshida (Osaka, Japan)
   Summary. 33
   Introduction 33
   Materials and Methods 34
       Aorta-superfusion method 34
       ACE assay. 34
       Platelet aggregation assay 34
       Blood pressure and heart rate measurement. 34
       Antihypertensive action in conscious spontaneously hypertensive rats (SHR). 34
   Results and Discussion 34
       WS-1228A and B 34
       Amauromine 35
       WF-10129 37
       FR-900452 38

Vinigrol 40
Conclusion 42
Acknowledgement 42
References 42

4. Screening of immunomodulating agents 45
   M. Asano, M. Kohsaka, H. Aoki and H. Imanaka (Ibaragi, Japan)
   Summary 45
   Introduction 45
   Materials and Methods 45
      Screening systems 45
   Results 46
      Structures 46
      Biological Properties 46
      FK-506 47
   Conclusion 48
   References 48

5. Enzymic synthesis of immunomodulators 49
   H. Kleinkauf, H. von Döhren, A. Billich, A. Lawen, H. Peeters and R. Zochner (Berlin, Fed. Rep.
   Germany)
   Introduction 49
   Peptide biosynthesis 49
   Immunomodulators and their pathways 49
   References 54

6. Microbial secondary metabolites inhibiting oncogene functions 57
   K. Umezawa, M. Hori and T. Takeuchi (Tokyo, Japan)
   Summary 57
   Introduction 57
   Erbstatin, a tyrosine kinase inhibitor 58
   Herbimycin inhibits src oncogene expression 59
   Oxanosine, an inhibitor of ras oncogene functions 59
   Inhibitors of phosphatidylinositol turnover 60
   References 61

7. Biosynthesis of rebeccamycin, a novel antitumor agent 63
   K.S. Lam, S. Forenza, D.R. Schroeder, T.W. Doyle and C.J. Pearce (Wallingford, CT, U.S.A.)
   Summary 63
   Introduction 63
   Materials and Methods 63
      Microorganism 63
      Media and culture conditions 64
      Preparation of rebeccamycin 64
      Antitumor assay 64
      Results and Discussion 64

Physiology of rebeccamycin production 64
Purification and biological activity. 64
Labeled precursor experiments 64
Conclusion 66
References 66

8. New adenosine deaminase inhibitors, adechlorin and adecypenol 67
   H. Tanaka and S. Omura (Tokyo, Japan)
   Summary 67
   Introduction 67
   Screening 68
   Isolation and structure of adechlorin 68
   ADA-inhibiting and biological activities of adechlorin 68
   Isolation and structure of adecypenol 69
   ADA-inhibiting and biological activities of adecypenol 70
   Discussion 71
   References 71

9. Trichostatin and leptomycin: specific inhibitors of the G1 and G2 phases of the eukaryotic cell
   cycle 73
   T. Beppu and M. Yoshida (Tokyo, Japan)
   Summary 73
   Introduction 73
   Trichostatins 74
   Leptomycins 75
   Discussion 76
   References 77

10. Rhizoxin, an inhibitor of tubulin assembly 79
    S. Iwasaki (Tokyo, Japan)
    Summary 79
    Introduction 79
    Materials and Methods, Results 79
    Effects of RZX and its homologs (*1a 3b*) on rice seedling roots 79
    Antifungal activity of RZX 79
    Antitumor activity of RZX and its homologs 81
    Morphological changes and cell cycle analysis of tumor cells 83
    Effects of RZX on cleavage of fertilized sea urchin eggs 84
    Effects of RZX on the polymerization of tubulin and on polymerized microtubule proteins . . 84
    Comparison of the effects of RZX, VLB, P-3 and CLC on tubulin polymerization 85
    Effect of RZX homologs and derivatives on the polymerization of tubulin 86
    Determination of RZX binding to tubulin 86
    Determination of the RZX binding site on tubulin 87
    Differential effect of RZX and benomyl on mutant strains of Aspergillus nidulans 87
    Discussion 88
    Acknowledgements 88
    References 88

11. Reverse transcriptase inhibitors 91
   S. Nakamura and Y. Inouye (Hiroshima, Japan)
   Summary. 91
   Materials and Methods 91
      Assay methods for enzyme activities 91
      Determination of cytotoxicity toward L5178Y cells. 92
      The in vitro replication of HIV. 92
      The in vivo replication of FLV 92
   Results and discussion. 92
      Screening for AMV-RTase inhibitors 92
      Inhibition of AMV-RTase by known antibiotics 93
      Cytotoxicity of AMV-RTase inhibitors 93
      Effect on the in vitro replication of HIV. 93
      Effect on the in vitro replication of FLV. 95
      Biological properties of STN derivatives. 95
      Inhibition of AMV-RTase by the quinones 97
   References 99

12. Low molecular weight enzyme inhibitors produced by microorganisms 101
   T. Aoyagi and T. Takeuchi (Tokyo, Japan)
   Summary. 101
   Introduction 101
   Discussion 102
      Endopeptidase inhibitors 102
      Inhibitors of cell surface enzymes 103
      Therapeutics applications of enzyme inhibitors 105
   Acknowledgements 105
   References 106

13. Chemistry, biochemistry and therapeutic potential of microbial α-glucosidase inhibitors 109
   L. Mueller (Leverkusen, Fed. Rep. Germany)
   Summary. 109
   Introduction 109
   Acarbose and homologs. 110
   Other pseudo-oligosaccharide inhibitors 113
   Tendamistat 113
   Monosaccharide inhibitors 114
   α-Glucosidase inhibition as a new therapeutic principle. 114
   References 115

14. Trestatin: α-amylase inhibitor 117
   K. Yokose, T. Furumai, Y. Suhara and W. Pirson (Kanagawa, Japan and Basel, Switzerland)
   Summary. 117
   Introduction 117
   Taxonomic studies on the producing organism 118
   Fermentation 118

Isolation of trestatin. 118
    Isolation of trestatin complex (Ro 09-0154). 118
    Isolation of trestatins A, B and C 119
    Isolation of minor components (Ro-09766, Ro 09-767 and Ro 09-0768) 119
Physicochemical properties of trestatins A, B and C, Ro 09-0766, Ro 09-0767 and Ro 09-0768 . 119
Structure determination of trestatins, A, B and C. 120
    Structure of trestatin B 120
    Structure of trestatins A and C. 121
Structure determination of Ro 09-0766, Ro 09-0767 and Ro 09-0768 122
Structure determination of Ro 09-0765, Ro 09-0896 and Ro 09-0897 123
Biological properties. 123
    Toxicity 124
Antidiabetic properties of trestatin (Ro 09-0154) 124
    Animal studies 124
    Healthy volunteer studies. 124
    Patient studies. 125
Acknowledgements 125
References 125

15. Aldostatin, a novel aldose reductase inhibitor 127
    S. Yaginuma, A. Asahi, M. Takada, M. Hayashi, M. Tsujino and K. Mizuno (Shizuoka, Japan)
    Summary. 127
    Introduction 127
    Materials and Methods 127
        Materials 127
        Microorganism 128
        Aldose reductase preparation 128
        Enzymatic activity 128
        Rat lens preparation and incubation. 128
        Determination of sorbitol content in lesn 128
        Production of aldostatin 128
        Assay of aldostatin 129
        Hydrolysis of aldostatin 129
        Preparation of LL-bityrosine 129
    Results 129
        Production 129
        Isolation procedure 129
        Physico-chemical properties 129
        Biological properties 129
    Discussion 131
    References 133

16. Emeriamine: a new inhibitor of long chain fatty acid oxidation and its antidiabetic activity. 135
    T. Kanamaru and H. Okazaki (Osaka, Japan)
    Summary. 135
    Introduction 135

Materials and Methods 136
    Materials 136
    Microorganisms. 136
    Assay of mitochondrial oxidation of long chain fatty acids. 136
    Assay of carnitine palmitoyltransferase I 136
    Assay of carnitine acetyltransferase 136
    Measurements of hypoglycemic and antiketogenic activities in rats 136
    Determination of protein. 137
    Statistics. 137
Results 137
    Screening for inhibitors of long chain fatty acid oxidation in culture filtrates of
    microorganisms. 137
    Fermentation, isolation, and structures of emericedins A, B and C 137
    Inhibition of long chain fatty acid oxidation in rat liver mitochondria by emeriamine and the
    inhibition site 139
    Effect of emeriamine, acetylemeriamine and palmitoylemeriamine on carnitine acetyltrans-
    ferase and carnitine palmitoyltransferase 139
    Effect of emeriamine on glucoeogenesis in hepatocytes. 141
    In vivo hypoglycemic and antiketogenic activity of emeriamaine 141
    Tissue specificity of inhibition of fatty acid oxidation by emeriamine 142
Discussion 143
Acknowledgements 143
References 143

17. Lipoxygenase inhibitors 145
    S. Kitamura, K. Hashizume, T. Iida, K. Ohmori and H. Kase (Shuzuoka, Japan)
    Summary. 145
    Introduction 145
    Materials and Methods 146
        5-Lipoxygenase inhibitors from microbial metabolites 146
        Characterization of 5-lipoxygenase inhibitors. 146
        12-Lipoxygenase inhibitors from microbial metabolites 149
    Discussion 149
    References 149

18. A Specific bacterial inhibitor of the extracellular polygalacturonase of Geotrichum candidum . . . 151
    Y. Aharonowitz, S. Bauer, S. Loya, R. Schreiber, I. Barash and D.L. Gutnick (Ramat Aviv, Israel)
    Summary. 151
    Introduction 151
    Materials and Methods 152
        Microbial strains 152
        Media 152
        Culture conditions 152
        Preparation of polygalacturonase from G. candidum culture broth 152
        Phosphate determination. 153
        Reducing group determination. 153

    Tissue maceration assay 153
  Results 153
    In vitro assay for polygalacturonase inhibitor 153
    Growth and production of polygalacturonase inhibitor by *S. satsumaensis* 154
    Purification of inhibitory activity 154
    Polyphosphate composition of the polygalacaturonase inhibitor from *S. satsumaensis* 155
    The tissue maceration assay 155
    Inhibition of enzyme-mediated tissue maceration 156
    Inhibition of spore-mediated maceration 157
  Discussion 157
  Acknowledgements 158
  References 159

19. Production of lovastatin, an inhibitor of cholesterol accumulation in humans 161
    B. Buckland, K. Gbewonyo, T. Hallada, L. Kaplan and P. Masurekar (Rahway, NJ, U.S.A.)
  Summary 161
  Introduction 161
  Materials and Methods 162
    Organism 162
    Media and fermentation conditions 162
    Fermentor studies 162
    Analysis 163
  Results and discussion 163
    Reisolation of the culture 163
    Medium optimization 163
    Kinetics of fermentation 163
    Effect of additional glucose 164
    Effect of pH control 164
    Effect of alternate carbon sources 164
    Kinetics of fermentation of reisolate 46-7 165
    Effect of shot addition to the glycerol medium 165
    Effect of buffers in glycerol 165
    Scale-up studies 165
    Cascade control strategy 166
    Effectiveness of Prochem impellers 166
    Kinetics of fermentation in fermentors 167
    Biosynthesis of lovastlatin 168
  References 169

20. Triacsins, acyl-CoA synthetase inhibitors and F244, a hydroxymethylglutaryl-CoA synthase inhibitor 171
    H. Tomoda and S. Omura (Tokyo, Japan)
  Summary 171
  Introduction 171
  Results and discussion 172
    Triacsins 172

Assay of acyl-CoA synthetase 172
Inhibition of acyl-CoA synthetase by triacsins 172
Steady-state kinetics of the inhibition of acyl CoA synthetase by triacsins. 173
Inhibition of Raji cell growth by triacsins 173
Proposed mechanism of selective toxicity of triacsins to animal cells. 173
F-244 174
Effect of F-244 on Vero cell growth 175
Effect of F-244 on the incorporation of ^{14}C-labeled precursors into digitonin-precipitable
sterols in a rat liver enzyme system. 175
Inhibition of HMG-CoA synthase by F-244. 175
Effects of F-244 and its derivatives on HMG-CoA synthase and Vero cell growth 175
Acknowledgements 176
References 176

21. Amicoumacin and SF-2370, pharmacologically active agents of microbial origin 179
S. Inouye and S. Kondo (Yokohama, Japan)
Summary. 179
Anicoumacin A, a potent antiinflammatory and anticulcer agent. 179
Introduction. 179
Isolation of amicoumacins 179
Antiinflammatory and anticulcer activity of amicoumacin A. 181
Isolation and evaluation of AI-77s. 184
SF-2370 and its derivatives, potent hypotensive agents 185
Introduction. 185
Isolation of SF-2370
Hypotensive activity of SF-2370 and NA derivatives 187
Effects of SF-2370 and NA derivatives on aortic contraction. 189
Acknowledgement. 191
References 191

22. Screening of microbial products affecting plant metabolism. 195
T. Kida (Kawasaki, Japan)
Summary. 195
Introduction 195
Materials and Methods 196
Microbial strains 196
Culture media. 196
Plants 196
Antimicrobial assay. 196
Detection of the greening of dark-grown S. obliquus C-2A'. 196
Detection of de novo starch synthesis 196
Detection of oxygen evolution from the algal cells 196
Assay of herbicidal activity. 197
Results and discussion. 197
Structures and biological activity of new antibiotics, pereniporins A and B 197
7-Deoxy-D-glucero D-glucoheptose, as an inhibitor of the greening of dark-grown

  S. obliquus C-2A′ 198
  A new assay method to detect photosynthesis inhibitors by examining de novo starch
  synthesis 199
  Active compounds as inhibitors of de novo starch synthesis in excised leaf segments
  of barnyard millet 200
  Acknowledgements 202
  References 202

23. Novel second-generaton avermectin insecticides and miticides for crop protection 203
  R.A. Dybas, N.J. Hilton, M.H. Fisher, H. Mrozik, F.A. Preiser, P. Eskola, T.L. Shih and G.J.
  Dolce (Ithaca, NY, U.S.A.)
  Summary 203
  Introduction 203
  Materials and Methods 205
    Avermectin formulations 205
    Insecticide formulations 205
    Insect bioassays 205
    Spider mite bioassays 205
  Results and discussion 206
    Insecticidal activities 206
    Miticidal activities 209
  References 211

24. Unique strains of *Bacillus thuringiensis* with activity against Coleoptera 213
  H.W. Talbot, M. Burrascano, O. Espinosa, R. Everich, K. Nette, J. Payne and G. Soares (San
  Diego, U.S.A.)
  Summary 213
  Introduction 213
  Materials and Methods 214
    Primary screen of *B. thuringiensis* isolates for activity against Coleoptera 214
    Secondary screen of *B. thuringiensis* isolates for activity against the CPB 214
    Electron micrographs 214
    Serotyping of B. thuringiensis strains 214
  Results and discussion 214
  References 217

25. Fermentation alternatives for commercial production of a mycoherbicide 219
  L.J. Stowell, K. Nette, N. Heath and R. Shutter (San Diego, CA, U.S.A.)
  Summary 219
  Introduction 219
  Propagule production using submerged fermentation 221
    Mycelia production using submerged fermentation 221
    Spore production using submerged fermentation 221
  Propagule production on artificial surfaces 222
    Mathematical model of sporulation from a solid surface 222
  Spore production on living plant surface 225

Discussion 225
References 226

26. New anthelmintic and growth promoting agents from actinomycetes 229
   G.T. Carter (Pearl River, NY, U.S.A.)
   Introduction 229
   LL-F28249 anthelmintic agents 229
   LL-E19020 growth-promotants 233
   References 236

27. Novel activities from marine-derived microorganisms 239
   D.J. Newman, P.R. Jensen, J.J. Clement and C. Acebal (Fort Pierce, FL, U.S.A.)
   Summary 239
   Introduction 239
   Sources of organisms 240
   Microbe isolation, purification and storage 240
   Media used 241
   Taxonomic identification 242
      Bacteria 242
      Actinomycetes and fungi 242
   Growth and extraction of metabolites 242
      Small-scale and seed growths (10-15 ml) 242
      Larger scale (up to 15 liters) 242
   Biological assays used 243
      Antitumor assays 243
      Antiviral assays 243
      Antimicrobial assays 243
      Immunomodulation assays 244
   Results of antitumor, antiviral and antimicrobial studies 244
   General comments on summary tables 244
   Modulation of the immune system 245
   Physico-chemical separation of activities from selected organisms 247
   SOB055: antitumor and immunomodulation activities 247
   SOC142: antitumor and antiviral activities 248
   Slow-growing marine fungi 249
   Closing comments 251
   Acknowledgements 251
   References 251

28 Eicosapentaenoic acid from microalgae 253
   P.W. Behrens, S.D. Hoeksema, K.L. Arnett, M.S. Cole, T.A. Heubner, J.M. Rutten and D.J. Kyle (Columbia, MD, U.S.A.)
   Summary 253
   Introduction 253
   Materials and Methods 254
   Results 255

Discussion 257
Acknowledgement 258
References 258

29. Use of a double-sided plate to screen for microorganisms producing methionine 261
    H.G. Aranha and L.R. Brown (Mississippi State, MS, U.S.A.)
    Summary 261
    Introduction 261
    Materials and Methods 262
    Results 263
    Discussion 264
    References 266

Introduction

Hamao Umezawa and the Second Coming of Microbial Secondary Metabolites

Arnold L. Demain

Fermentation Microbiology Laboratory, Biology Department, Massachusetts
Institute of Technology, Cambridge, MA, 02139 U.S.A.

With great vision, Hamao Umezawa began in the 1960's his pioneering efforts to broaden the scope of industrial microbiology to low molecular weight secondary metabolites which had activities other than, or in addition to, antibacterial, antifungal and antitumor potency. He and his colleagues at the Institute of Microbial Chemistry focused on enzyme inhibitors and over the years have discovered, isolated, purified and studied the *in vitro* and *in vivo* activity of many of these novel compounds. We are fortunate that a number of antibiotic companies, research institutes and academic laboratories throughout the world interpreted this effort in a positive way and began similar programs. Today we see on the market microbial metabolites with activities such as β-lactamase inhibition, immunostimulation, immunodepression, hypocholesteremic, anthelmintic, insecticidal, herbicidal, coccidiostatal, plant growth stimulation and animal growth promotion.

The above successes came about in two ways: (1) broad screening of known compounds with antibiotic and/or toxic activities and (2) screening of unknown compounds in fermentation broths for enzyme inhibition or inhibition of a target pest. Both strategies had one important concept in common, i.e. that microbial metabolites have activities other than, or in addition to, inhibition of other microbes. The outmoded concept that microbial products could only be used for curing microbial diseases was very popular during the early days of the antibiotic era and it has taken a long time to discredit this narrow view. One reason for its unfortunate perpetuation was the hesitancy of pharmacologists to inject crude (dark and ugly? microbial broths into their animal model systems. Fortunately some enlightened (and adventurous) companies and laboratories refused to take the narrow path and broadly screened known antibiotics (which had failed as commercially important products) and mycotoxins for new activities. This led to the development of ergot alkaloids for various medical uses, monensin as a coccidiostat, gibberellin as a plant growth stimulator, zearelanone as an animal growth promotant, phosphinothricins as herbicides, and cyclosporin as an immunodepressant, the last-named virtually revolutionizing the practice of organ transplantation in medicine. The testing of inknown compounds as enzyme inhibitors in Tokyo and other places complemented the above efforts and soon resulted in the discovery of many potent inhibitors. Enzyme inhibitors which have been well accepted include those for research (antipain, pepstatin, leupeptin, cerulenin), medicine (clavulanic acid, lovastatin) and agriculture (polyoxins, phosphinothricins). Direct *in vivo* screening of fermentation broths against nematodes led to the major discovery of the potent activity of the avermectins against helminths causing disease in animals and humans.

The above successes have brought about a major change in our concepts of the potential of the microbe for the improvement of human welfare. Realization of this development led the Society for Industrial Microbiology to organize the *First International Conference on the Biotechnology of Microbial Products: 'Novel Pharmacological and Agrobiological Activities'* Indeed, it was the first special conference organized by the Society for Industrial Microbiology in recent times and most of the credit goes to the foresight, enthusiasm and energy of former President and Conference Committee Chairman, George A. Somkuti.

This book offers to the reader the flavor of the field today as an ever-increasing number of companies pursue the activities of a virtually limitless feast of secondary metabolites from microorganims. Today's screens are searching for better immunomodulating agents, anticholesterol compounds, antitumor agents, insecticides, anthelmintics, herbicides, plant and animal growth regulators as well as receptor antagonists and agonists, antiviral agents, antiinflammatory drugs, carbohydrase, inhibitors, cardiovascular drugs, lipoxygenase inhibitors, antiulcer agents, aldose reductase inhibitors, antidiabetes agents and adenosine deaminase inhibitors, among others.

I know that the visions of Hamao Umezawa and other pioneers in this worldwide effort are reaching fruition and will continue to provide products of benefit to humankind. I know that fermentation research and development will continue to expand beyond its previous narrow focus, aided by new technologies of molecular biology and genetic engineering. I regret that Hamao Umezawa passed away before he could see the fruits of his ideas come together in San Diego in 1988. However, I am pleased that his work was presented at the Conference by his colleagues and his son and that his concepts will be advanced and spread throughout the world by publication of this volume.

Novel Microbial Products for Medicine and Agriculture
Editors: A.L. Demain, G.A. Somkuti, J.C. Hunter-Cevera and H.W. Rossmoore
© 1989, Society for Industrial Microbiology

1

CHAPTER 1

Hamao Umezawa, the man and his dream

Yoshiro Okami

Institute of Microbial Chemistry, Tokyo, Japan

SUMMARY

Professor Hamao Umezawa passed away on December 25th, 1986, at the age of 72. Few scientists have achieved as much success as he had in both academe and industry. In high school he was greatly influenced by a chemistry teacher. In medical school his primary interest was immunochemistry, as well as biochemistry and microbiology. During World War II, his humanitarian and medical interests led him to join a penicillin research group, to work on that magnificent drug which cured distressing diseases in post-war Japan. He studied and worked hard both day and night in the laboratory. His humanistic character and broad scientific knowledge resulted in his great influence on the industrialization of the production of antibiotics. His discovery and the subsequent development of kanamycin was followed by hundreds of discoveries of new antibiotics and their efficient development in industry. Based on the royalties of his inventions, he was successful in establishing a basic research institute. He effectively promoted the microbe's talent to provide useful antibiotics and non-antibiotic substances beneficial for mankind. He believed that original and creative results could be obtained from clear goals, and he always committed himself completely to his work.

There is a Roman proverb which says that one who runs after two hares at one time will not catch either. Professor Hamao Umezawa (Fig. 1) was an exception, successful in both academe and industry. A genius in many areas, he was not only a bright man but also a man of great endeavor.

Healthy throughout his life, in 1985 he unexpectedly suffered a stroke. Recovering with some minor after-effects, he attempted to return to his normal schedule, including travel overseas to give lectures. One year later he was stricken by pneumonia and hospitalized, the first of several repeated hospitalizations.

On November 5th, 1986, Professor Umezawa was called from the hospital to the Imperial Palace of Japan, to be decorated by Emperor Hirohito.

One and a half months later, on December 25th, he passed away at the age of 72, leaving his colleagues in deep sorrow.

Hamao Umezawa was born in 1914, the second son of Dr. Junichi Umezawa, the medical director of the principal hospital in the city of Obama, Fukui Prefecture. Located north of Kyoto near the Sea of Japan, Obama is situated in an agricultural area of beautiful rice fields. Umezawa often remarked that he enjoyed his early childhood in that rural area, bountiful with nature.

The family moved several times, eventually settling in Tokyo. One of six sons, Umezawa and his brothers were all educated in natural science or medicine, continuing a family tradition. Umezawa's grandfather had been a physician, and Ume-

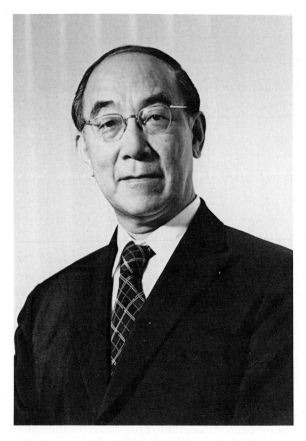

Fig. 1. Hamao Umezawa.

A book by R. Dubos greatly influenced him, and he later cited it as an inspiration for his antibiotic investigations. 'I was studying viruses and immunology from a chemical aspect, but after I read an interesting paper by Dr. Dubos on the isolation of an antibacterial compound of soil bacteria, I was attracted by his work ', Umezawa said.

Returning from the Army in 1943, Umezawa was asked by the Japanese Army Medical School to develop the large-scale production of penicillin. His medical and humanitarian concerns led him to work on the project, with a goal of curing diseases causing misery in soldiers and citizens. Working day and night, with the assistance of Dr. J.W. Foster of Texas, he continued until the successful postwar production of penicillin was initiated.

Further work by Umezawa to find antibacterial compounds led to the discovery of tyrothricin, actinomycin, streptothricin, chloramphenicol, aureomycin and streptomycin (Table 1). The production and use of streptomycin contributed greatly to curing the dreaded disease tuberculosis during a difficult period in the history of Japan.

Widespread and long-term use of streptomycin led to the development of organisms resistant to the antibiotic. Working to overcome this problem, Umezawa searched for agents effective against the resistant organisms. He discovered kanamycin, from a soil actinomycete, in 1957, at the National Institute of Health in Tokyo. That discovery and the subsequent worldwide production of kanamycin brought him international fame, opening the gate to his brilliant future.

Using royalties from kanamycin, Umezawa established the nonprofit Microbial Chemistry Research Foundation in 1956, followed by the founding of the research-oriented Institute of Microbial Chemistry in 1962. Today, about 150 people work at the Institute, including approximately 40 senior scientists from both academe and industry.

Umezawa was appointed director of the Institute and, at the same time, named Professor at both the Institute of Applied Microbiology and the Institute of Medical Science at the University of Tokyo. Additionally, he was the head of the antibiotics division of the National Institutes of Health. In all, he

zawa himself had two sons, both of whom also studied science and now work at the Institute of Microbial Chemistry, founded by their father. Few families have enriched science with the distinguished brilliance of four generations as has Umezawa's family.

Prior to entering medical school at the University of Tokyo, young Hamao Umezawa was educated at Musashi High School, a private school emphasizing natural science and languages. He was greatly influenced in science philosophy by a chemistry teacher, Dr. Bunichi Tamamushi. In addition, his language education gave him the background to later becoming a prolific reader of thousands of papers in science and other fields, from throughout the world.

During his university studies Umezawa became interested in biochemistry and immunochemistry.

Table 1

Antibacterial, antifungal, antiviral, antiprotozoal, and anti-tumor compounds discovered by Hamao Umezawa up to 1962

Antibacterial	streptothricins (neomycins) ('48), aureothricin ('49), griseoluteins ('50), nitrosporin ('51), actinomycin J ('51), exfoliatin ('52), thiazolidine antibiotic ('53), pyridomycin ('53), phthiomycin ('53), seligomycin ('54), mesenterin ('55), kanamycin ('57), althiomycin ('57), alboverticillin ('58), mikamycin ('59), nitromycin ('60), amidinomycin ('60)
Antifungal	moldin ('50), mediocidin ('54), tertiomycins ('55), blastmycin ('57), variotin ('59), unamycin ('60), emimycin ('60), ilamycins ('60), cytomycin ('61), griseococcin ('62)
Antiviral	abikoviromycin ('52), achromoviromycin ('53)
Antiprotozoal	azomycin ('53), aureothin ('54), antitoxoplasmic substance ('55)
Antitumor	No. 289 substance ('53), caryomycin ('53), sarkomycin ('53), actinoleukin ('54), ractiomycin ('55), pluramycin ('56), raromycin ('57), phleomycin ('57), peptiomycin ('61)

was responsible for directing nearly 250 researchers.

Before setting up the Institute of Microbial Chemistry, Umezawa had already discovered 50 antibiotics, including antiviral agents (Table 1). He recognized that most viruses are at their zenith when symptoms first appear in the patient, and are difficult to cure by medication. That recognition changed the course of his research interest from the study of viruses to cancer. He thought that microbial products might exhibit selectivity for malignant cells.

Umezawa had initiated the study of antitumor antibiotics as early as 1951, and demonstrated in one of his original studies that antitumor principles can be found by testing microbial cultures against experimental animal tumors. By 1962 he had found 10 antitumor compounds (Table 1), with sarkomycin being the first to be put into industrial produc-

tion. Sarkomycin production soon ceased, however, because of its instability.

Phleomycin (Fig. 2), discovered in 1957, exhibited strong antitumor action against some experimental animal tumors, but also displayed strong renal toxicity. Umezawa searched for a phleomycin-like substance with less renal toxicity, discovering bleomycin (Fig. 2) in 1965. After elucidating its chemical structure he discovered that bleomycin was primarily active against squamous cell carcinomas of the skin, with much less effect on normal cells.

The inactivation of bleomycin was rapid in normal organs and tissues but slow in skin and lung. Umezawa showed that this was due to an enzyme which hydrolyzes the carboxamide bond of the bleomycin molecule. The presence of this enzyme was low in squamous cell carcinoma, but not in sarcomas of mouse skin. Based on these results, Umezawa stated that an antitumor agent might be therapeutically effective against specific, limited types of human tumors. Therefore, the selective distribution of antitumor substances in animal organs, tissues or tumor cells may be useful for predicting the sensitivity of human tumors to chemotherapy.

This new line of approach for finding antitumor compounds for the treatment of certain human cancers was an original concept. Using it, Umezawa continued his search for new antitumor agents, and strove to initiate their production on an industrial scale.

In collaboration with scientists from Nippon Kayaku Co., a Japanese pharmaceutical company, the actinomycete which produced bleomycin was found to also produce various types of bleomycin-related compounds (Fig. 2). The chemical structure of each of these bleomycins was elucidated and it was discovered that the compounds differ from one another in the terminal amine moiety. Addition of an amine into the culture medium increased the production of the bleomycin containing that particular amine. Methods for the preparation of bleomycinic acid by enzymatic hydrolysis of bleomycin B2, or by chemical cleavage of bleomycin demethyl-A2, have been established and more than 400 semi-synthetic bleomycins have been prepared.

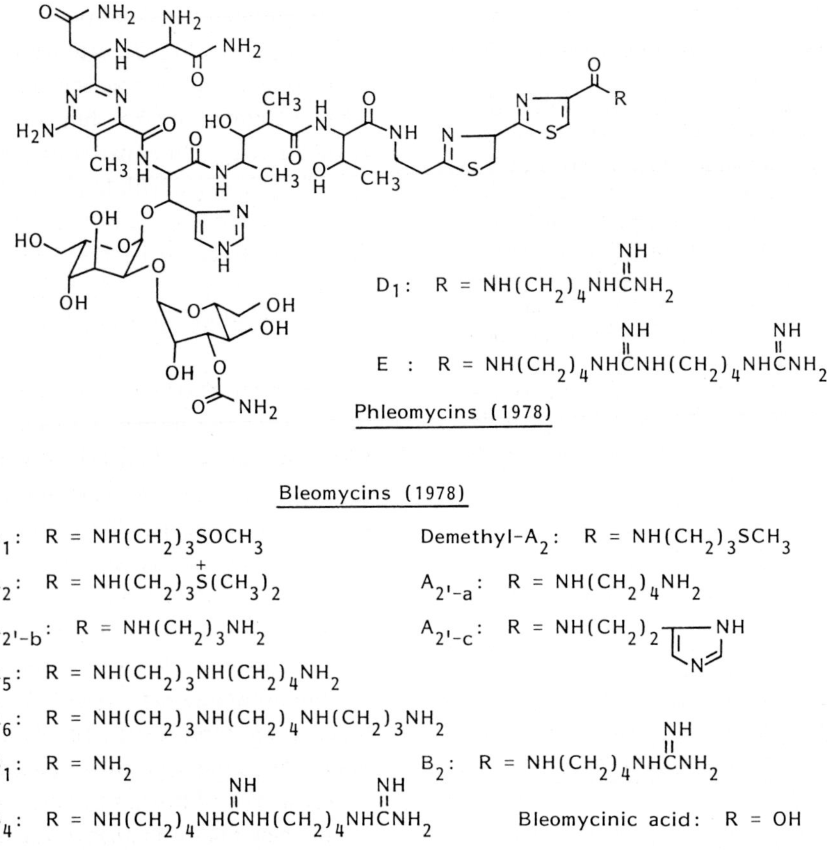

4

D_1 : R = $NH(CH_2)_4NH\overset{\overset{NH}{\|}}{C}NH_2$

E : R = $NH(CH_2)_4NH\overset{\overset{NH}{\|}}{C}NH(CH_2)_4NH\overset{\overset{NH}{\|}}{C}NH_2$

Phleomycins (1978)

Bleomycins (1978)

A_1 : R = $NH(CH_2)_3SOCH_3$ Demethyl-A_2 : R = $NH(CH_2)_3SCH_3$

A_2 : R = $NH(CH_2)_3\overset{+}{S}(CH_3)_2$ $A_{2'-a}$: R = $NH(CH_2)_4NH_2$

$A_{2'-b}$: R = $NH(CH_2)_3NH_2$ $A_{2'-c}$: R = $NH(CH_2)_2$-imidazole

A_5 : R = $NH(CH_2)_3NH(CH_2)_4NH_2$

A_6 : R = $NH(CH_2)_3NH(CH_2)_4NH(CH_2)_3NH_2$

B_1 : R = NH_2 B_2 : R = $NH(CH_2)_4NH\overset{\overset{NH}{\|}}{C}NH_2$

B_4 : R = $NH(CH_2)_4NH\overset{\overset{NH}{\|}}{C}NH(CH_2)_4NH\overset{\overset{NH}{\|}}{C}NH_2$ Bleomycinic acid: R = OH

Fig. 2. Phleomycins and bleomycins.

Peplomycin (Fig. 3), one of the artificial bleomycins, was selected as a second-generation bleomycin with less pulmonary toxicity and a broad antitumor spectrum. Peplomycin has been used clinically since 1981 for the treatment of squamous cell carcinoma, Hodgkin's disease, testis tumors and prostatic carcinoma. However, the pulmonary toxicity of peplomycin still requires it to be dose-limited.

Among 227 newly prepared derivatives, liblomycin, containing a bulky lipophilic terminal amine (Fig. 3), was selected as a candidate for clinical studies. It showed distinctly stronger activity than peplomycin. Currently in phase I clinical studies, liblomycin is expected to become a useful agent.

The syntheses of pyrimidoblamic acid (1980), of deglycobleomycin A2 (1981) and of the disaccharide moiety of bleomycin (1981) were completed, and total synthesis of bleomycin was achieved in 1981, followed by the synthesis of several bleomycin analogs.

It was discovered that the bithiazole moiety of bleomycin intercalates between bases of double-stranded DNA. The terminal amine is involved in the binding (Fig. 4). The bleomycin-DNA complex thus formed results in doubled-stranded scission. Bleomycin-$Fe^{3+}O^{2-}$ has been suggested to be the active form.

Bleomycin also forms an equimolar complex with cupric ion (Fig. 5). The bleomycin-metal complex is taken up by lung tumors in particular, and can be used as a diagnostic tool for lung cancer.

In screening for new antitumor substances, Umezawa found aclacinomycin, an anthracycline (Fig. 6), in 1975. Active against tumors resistant to adria-

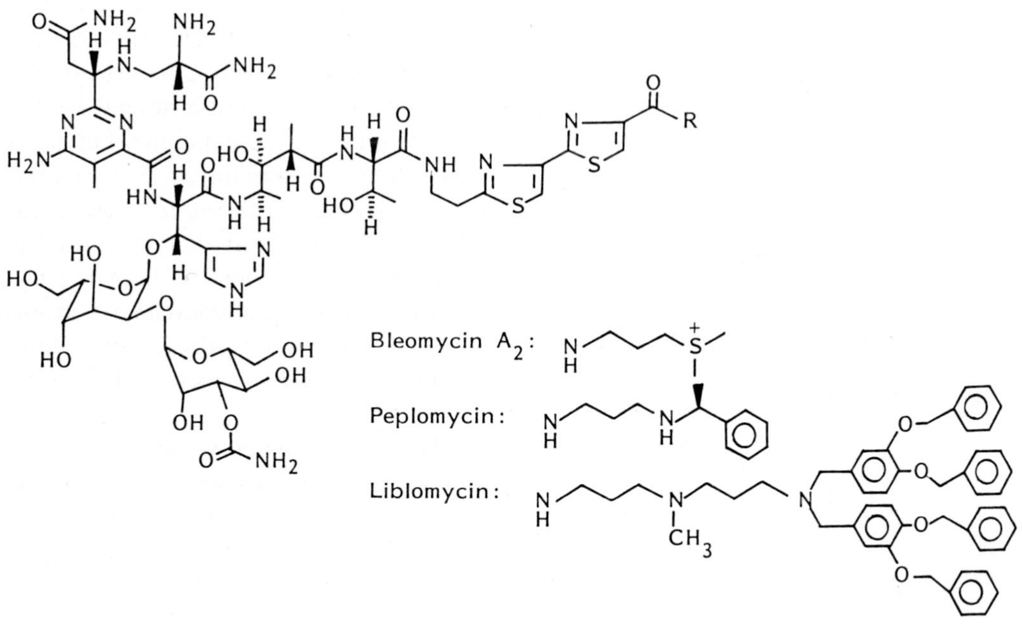

Fig. 3. Peplomycin and liblomycin.

mycin, it also possessed lower cardiac toxicity.

Clinical studies of aclacinomycin were conducted, in collaboration with the Sanraku Co. of Japan and Professor G. Mathe of France. Aclacinomycin gave a good therapeutic response in leukemia, and had low cardiac toxicity. Aclacinomycin was thus launched.

Umezawa found baumycins (Fig. 7), other anthracycline compounds, in 1977. Baumycins are 4'-O-acetal derivatives of daunomycin. They showed weak cardiac toxicity in hamster. Synthetic studies of 4'-O-acetal derivatives of daunomycin and adriamycin were conducted and 50 derivatives synthesized. Among them, 4'-O-tetrahydropyranyl (THP)-adriamycin (Fig. 7) showed stronger inhibition than adriamycin in almost all mouse tumors.

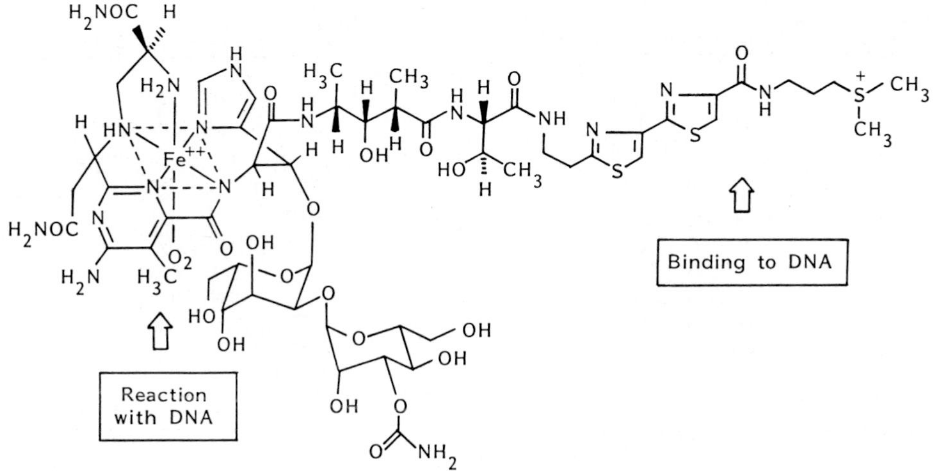

Fig. 4. Mechanism of bleomycin action.

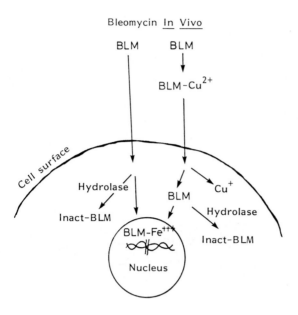

Fig. 5. The mode of action of the bleomycin-cupric complex.

The clinical effects of THP have been studied, and no cardiac toxicity and little vomiting or alopecia have been observed. Complete or partial regression has been observed in several kinds of tumors. Leucopenia was dose-limiting, but was reversible. Thus, this THP-adriamycin (Fig. 7) was launched.

Continuing to screen for new anthracyclines, Umezawa discovered that ditrisarubicin (Fig. 8) contains trisaccharides at both the C-7 and the C-10 positions of anthracycline. It strongly inhibits adriamycin-resistant cells *in vitro*, with its DNA-binding being the strongest of all known anthracyclines.

Decilorubicin (Fig. 8) was a new antitumor antibiotic with two nitro sugars (decilonitrose).

Oxaunomycin (Fig. 8) also has strong cytotoxic action – the concentration producing 50% inhibition against L1210 cells is 300 pg/ml.

Umezawa always stressed the importance of

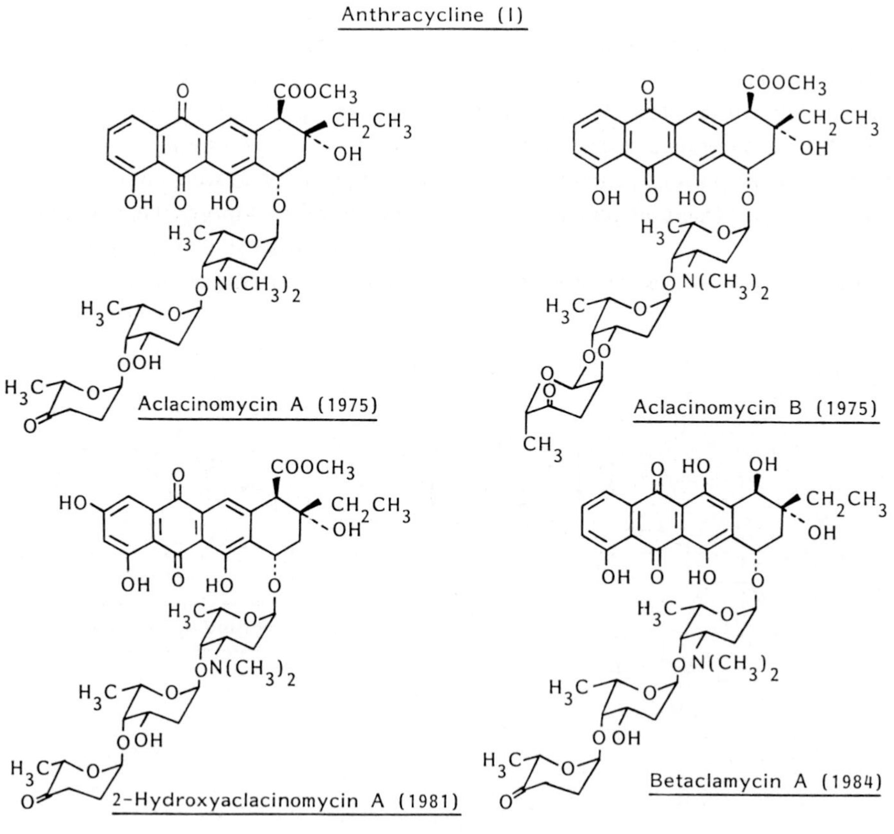

Anthracycline (I)

Aclacinomycin A (1975)

Aclacinomycin B (1975)

2-Hydroxyaclacinomycin A (1981)

Betaclamycin A (1984)

Fig. 6. Antitumor anthracyclines: aclacinomycin A, aclacinomycin B, 2-hydroxyaclacinomycin A, betaclamycin A.

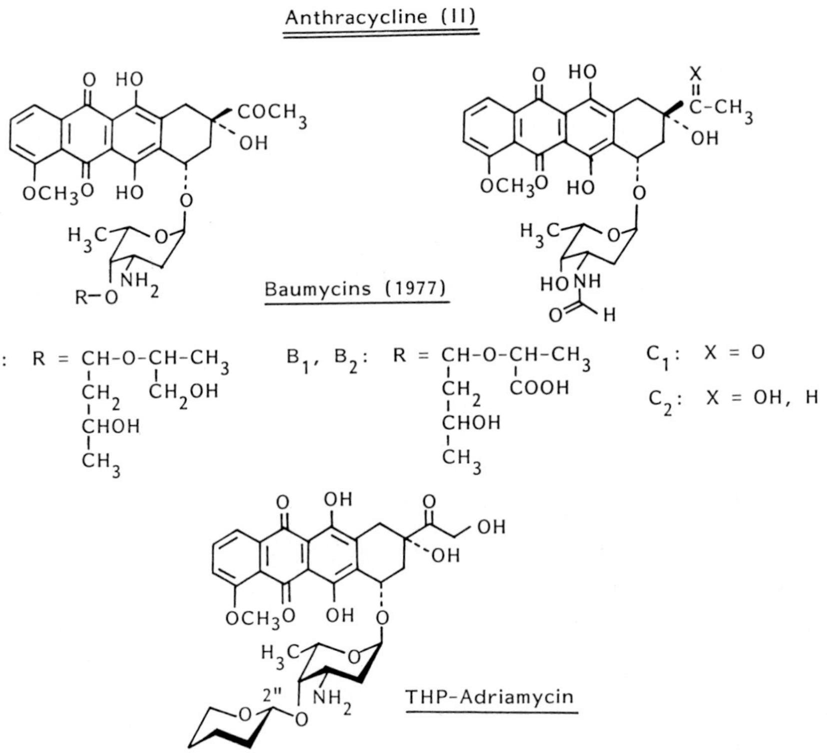

Anthracycline (II)

Fig. 7. Antitumor anthracyclines: baumycins, THP-adriamycin.

assay systems in his research. While searching for cytotoxic antitumor agents he designed a new assay system to find antitumor activity. Spergualin (Fig. 9) was isolated from the culture broth of a bacillus, based on the inhibition of focus formation of chick embryo fibroblasts with Rous sarcoma virus. Its structure contained spermidine and guanidine. Spergualin inhibited both gram-positive and gram-negative bacteria at concentrations ranging from 6.25 to 100 μg/ml. It showed chemotherapeutic effects in mice with various leukemias, rat hepatoma and fibrosarcoma. Spergualin was especially effective against L1210 (IMC) tumors, which were completely cured at appropriate doses of the drug. It was of interest that the cured mice rejected the second challenge of L1210 (IMC), indicating the induction of specific immunity. Thus, the antitumor activity of spergualin was suggested to be due to both its cytotoxic activity and its induction of specific immunity.

In collaboration with Takara Co. and Nippon Kayaku Co., about 150 analogs of spergualin were synthesized. Among them, 15-deoxyspergualin (Fig. 9) had the strongest antitumor activity against mouse leukemia. Clinical studies on 15-deoxyspergualin are currently in progress in the United States and in Japan.

It is of interest that spergualins in high doses suppress delayed-type hypersensitivity without secondary effects, indicating their possible usefulness in organ transplants or in the therapy of autoimmune diseases.

Continuously screening for antitumor compounds, Umezawa found many other biologically and chemically interesting compounds. Coriolins (1969) were found in a cultured mushroom, *Coriolus consors*. Diketocoriolin B was shown to inhibit Na^+/K^+-ATPase and increase the number of antibody-forming cells.

Formycin, formycin B, and oxoformycin B (Fig.

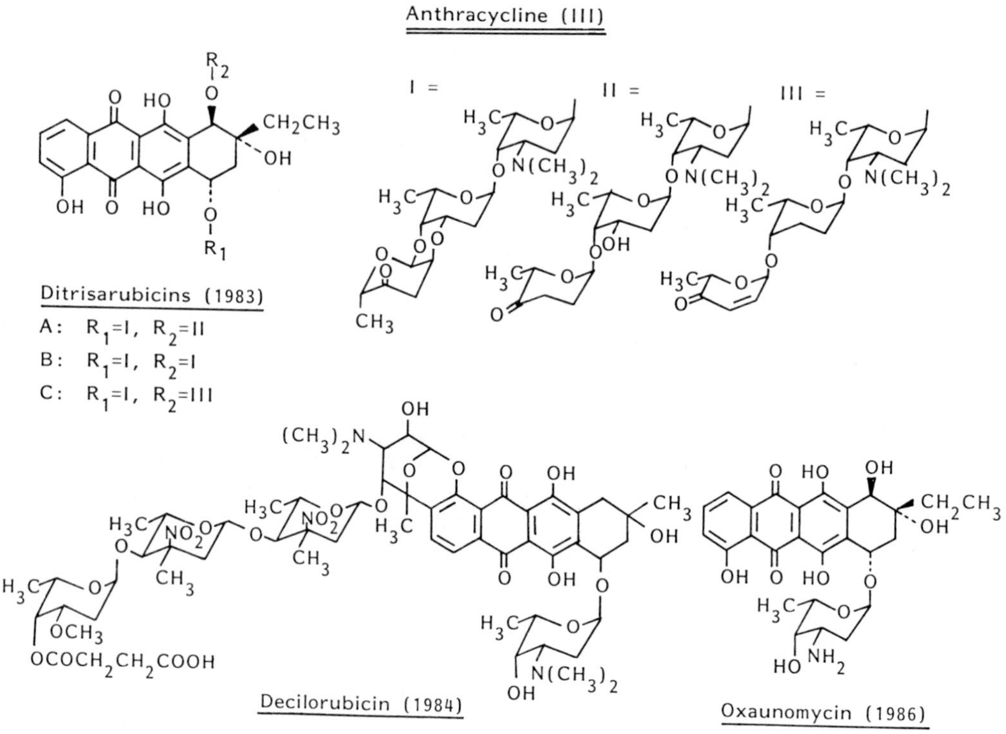

Anthracycline (III)

Ditrisarubicins (1983)

A: R_1=I, R_2=II
B: R_1=I, R_2=I
C: R_1=I, R_2=III

Decilorubicin (1984)

Oxaunomycin (1986)

Fig. 8. Antitumor anthracyclines: ditrisarubicins, decilorubicin, oxaunomycin.

10) from *Streptomyces* sp. were unique nucleosides. Coformycin (Fig. 10) strongly inhibits adenosine deaminase and enhances the antitumor activity of formycin.

Pluramycins and the less toxic neopluramycin (Fig. 11) are anthraquinone antibiotics.

Saquayamycins (Fig. 12) are glycosides of aquayamycin.

Neothramycin and mazethramycin are benzodiazepines from actinomycetes.

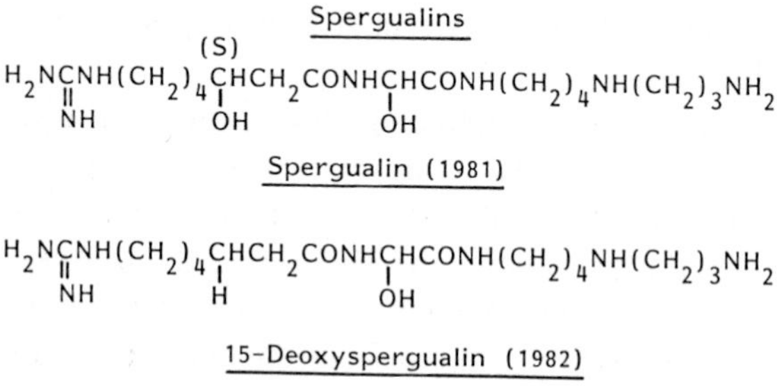

Bactobolin (Fig. 13), a chlorine-containing antibiotic, was found in the culture of a *Pseudomonas* sp. bacterium. It is structurally related to actinobolin, of streptomycete origin.

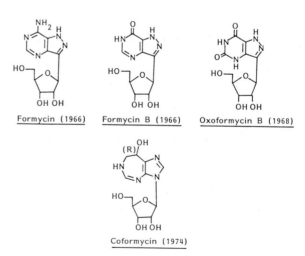

Formycin (1966) Formycin B (1966) Oxoformycin B (1968)

Coformycin (1974)

Fig. 10. Antitumor agents: formycin, formycin B, oxoformycin B, coformycin.

Spergualins

(S)
H₂NCNH(CH₂)₄CHCH₂CONHCHCONH(CH₂)₄NH(CH₂)₃NH₂
‖ | |
NH   OH   OH

Spergualin (1981)

H₂NCNH(CH₂)₄CHCH₂CONHCHCONH(CH₂)₄NH(CH₂)₃NH₂
‖ | |
NH   H   OH

15-Deoxyspergualin (1982)

Fig. 9. Antitumor agents: spergualin, 15-deoxyspergualin.

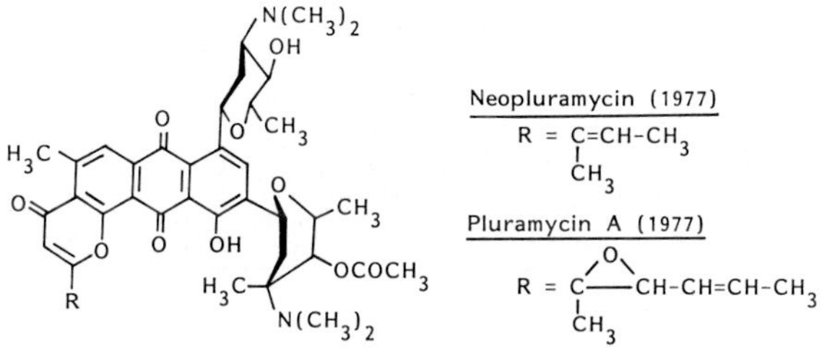

Fig. 11. Antitumor agents: neopluramycin, pluramycin A.

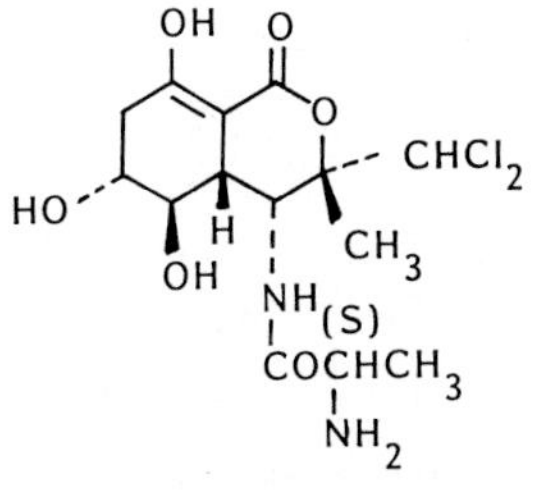

Bactobolin (1979)

Fig. 13. Antitumor agents: bactobolin.

Terpentecin (Fig. 14) was isolated from a culture broth of *kitasatospora* sp.

Valanimycin (Fig. 14) was isolated by a growth inhibition assay against *recA⁻ Escherichia coli*. It

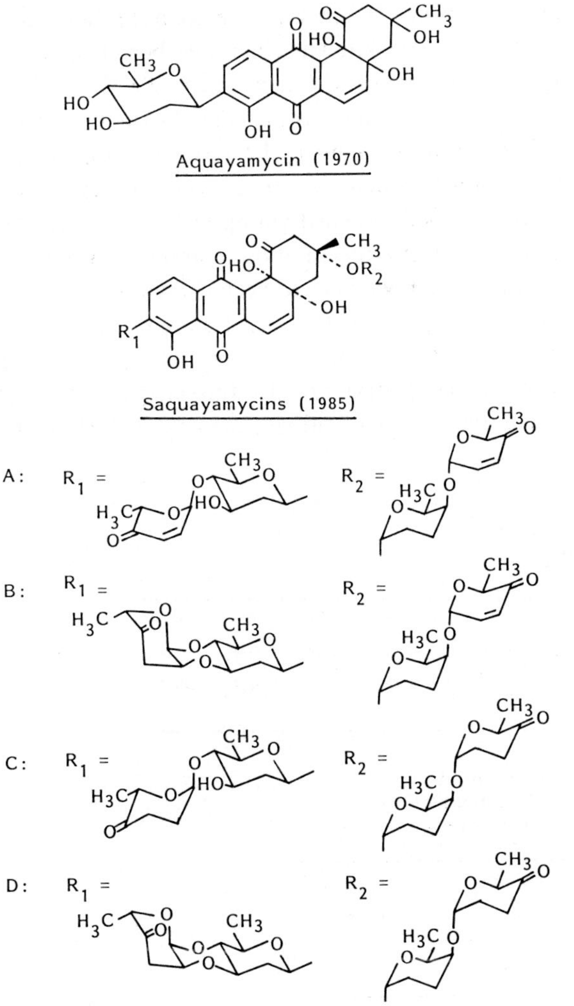

Fig. 12. Antitumor agents: aquayamycin, saquayamycins.

exhibited medium activity against gram-positive and gram-negative bacteria, but caused significant lengthening of the life span of tumor-bearing mice.

Umezawa's research activities were not only wide-ranging and varied, but his work was also very rapid. When problems needed to be solved urgently he organized his work very quickly to find the solution.

When the Institute of Microbial Chemistry was first established in 1962, a new compound was urgently needed to combat rice diseases caused by *Pyricularia oryzae*. Phenyl mercuric compounds had been widely used, but were a hazard because of their accumulation in soil.

Umezawa organized a screening system in collaboration with Hokko Chemical Co., an agricultural drug company. The system tested for antifungal activity on rice grown in pots. Culture filtrates of actinomycetes were sprayed on infected rice plants. A strain was selected and classified as *S. kasugaensis*. Its culture filtrate showed activity on rice in pots,

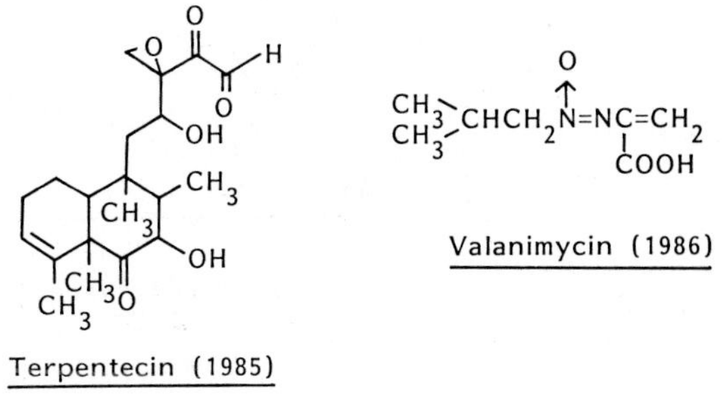

Fig. 14. Antitumor agents: terpentecin, valanimycin.

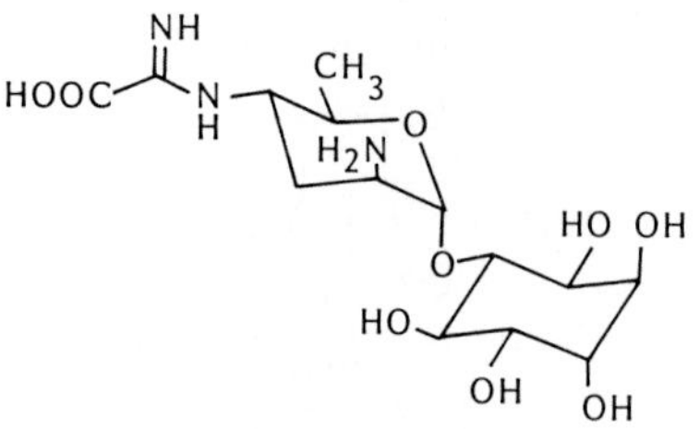

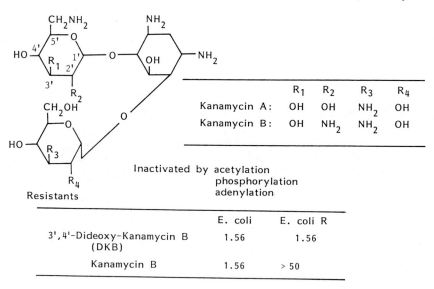

Kasugamycin (1966)

Fig. 15. Antibacterial: kasugamycin.

Josamycin

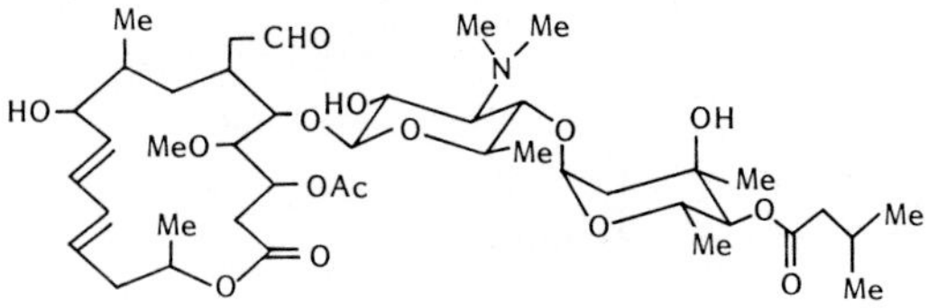

Fig. 17. Antibacterial: josamycin.

but showed no inhibition of the fungus using ordinary medium *in vitro*. Umezawa obtained information about the inner pH of the rice plant from a botanist, and adjusted the pH of the assay medium to acidic, or added rice plant extract to the assay medium. Strong inhibition was observed in both the acidic medium and the medium with rice plant extract. The active compound, kasugamycin (Fig. 15), was extracted and purified. It strongly inhibited *Py. oryzae*, and some *Pseudomonas* sp. Its structure was elucidated and chemical synthesis completed in 1968.

Umezawa improved the kasugamycin strain to yield high production from fermentation. Used to protect rice plants, over 100 tons per year of kasugamycin is now produced by fermentation for agricultural use.

The discovery and initiation of the industrial production of kasugamycin were accomplished within 5 years, because of Umezawa's rapid research.

Work on overcoming the resistance of kanamycin (Fig. 16) is another example of the speed of his research. When the chemical resistance of kanamycin first became known, Umezawa began basic research to determine the mechanism of resistance.

Umezawa predicted the chemical structure which would be active against the resistants and which would not be inactivated by enzymes, based on the mechanism of the inactivating enzymes. Since the inactivating enzyme of most common strains resistant to kanamycins had been shown to phosphorylate the 3'-hydroxyl group of kanamycin, he synthesized many derivatives of kanamycin that resisted phosphorylation by this enzyme. Among the derivatives, 3',4'-dideoxykanamycin B (Fig. 16)

	R₁	R₂	R₃	R₄
Kanamycin A:	OH	OH	NH₂	OH
Kanamycin B:	OH	NH₂	NH₂	OH

Inactivated by acetylation
phosphorylation
adenylation

	E. coli	E. coli R
3',4'-Dideoxy-Kanamycin B (DKB)	1.56	1.56
Kanamycin B	1.56	> 50

Fig. 16. Kanamycin A and B.

(dibekacin) has been marketed since 1975 as a chemotherapeutic agent useful in the treatment of infections caused by resistant bacteria.

This research was rapidly completed in about 5 years, in collaboration with Meiji Seika Co. The use of this reaction mechanism method to solve the resistance problem was a new area of research, begun by Umezawa.

Umezawa found many other new compounds and clarified their biological or physico-chemical properties.

Josamycin (Fig. 17), a new member of the macrolide antibiotics group, was discovered in 1967 in collaboration with the Research Institute of the Yamanouchi Pharmaceutical Co. In contrast to other macrolides, it showed no induction of resistance and caused no irritation of the stomach. It was put into clinical use.

Negamycin (Fig. 18) from a *Streptomyces* sp. is an interesting antibiotic in structure and activity. It caused inhibition of *Ps. aeruginosa* and of gramnegative bacteria both *in vitro* and *in vivo*. Negamycin inhibited the protein synthesis of bacterial ribosomes but not that of mammalian ribosomes. It caused miscoding in protein synthesis, inhibiting the termination step. The structure of negamycin was determined and its total synthesis completed. Among biologically active negamycin derivatives, deoxynegamycin (Fig. 18) and *O*-methylnegamycin

were found to be the most stable in aqueous solution.

Cyclamidomycin (Fig. 18) from a *Streptomyces* sp. broth inhibited bacteria and had relatively low toxicity. It inhibited adenosine diphosphate kinase of bacteria, but not of mammalian cells.

Laspartomycin (1968) from *Streptomyces* sp. is an acidic peptide.

Pepthiomycins (1968) from a *Streptomyces* sp. are new peptide antibiotics which contain sulfur. They exhibited therapeutic effects on staphylococcal infections *in vivo*.

Deoxynybomycin (Fig. 19) from a *Streptomyces* sp. showed much stronger activity than nybomycin.

Requinomycin (1972) was isolated from a *Streptomyces* sp. by testing for antiphage activity. It inhibited the reproduction of phage f2 in *E. coli* S-26, and the transfer of R factors between *E. coli* strains.

Spinamycin (Fig. 19) from a *Streptomyces* sp. inhibited the growth of Yoshida rat sarcoma cells and the growth of fungi and mycobacteria.

Calvatic acid (Fig. 19), active against gram-positive and some gram-negative bacteria, was isolated from the culture filtrate of a mushroom *Calvatia*. Total synthesis was completed. It inhibited the growth of L1210 cells and of Yoshida sarcoma.

Minosaminomycin (Fig. 19) from a *Streptomyces* sp. was active against mycobacteria and inhibited initiation of protein synthesis in a cell-free system of *E. coli*.

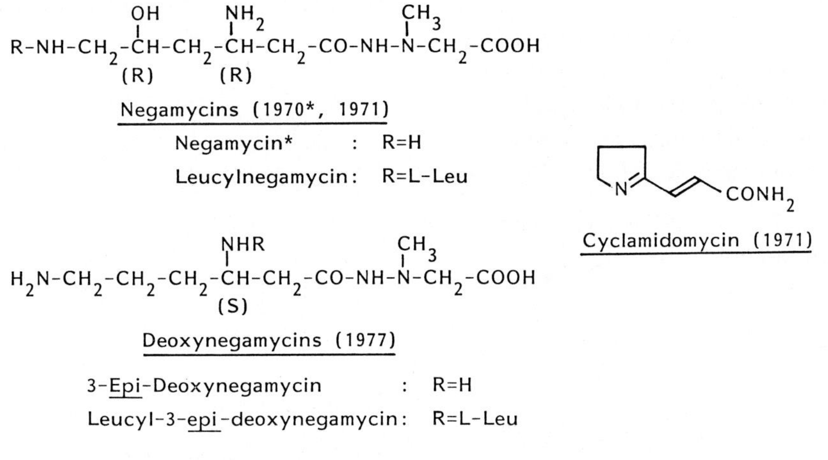

Fig. 18. Antibacterials: negamycins, deoxynegamycins, cyclamidomycin.

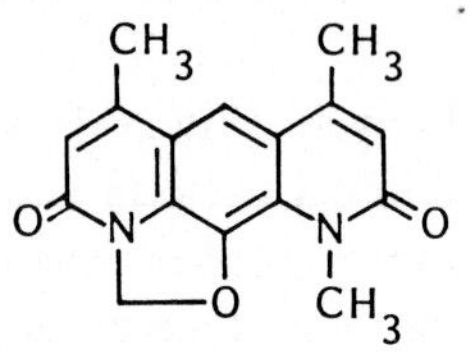

12

Deoxynybomycin (1970)

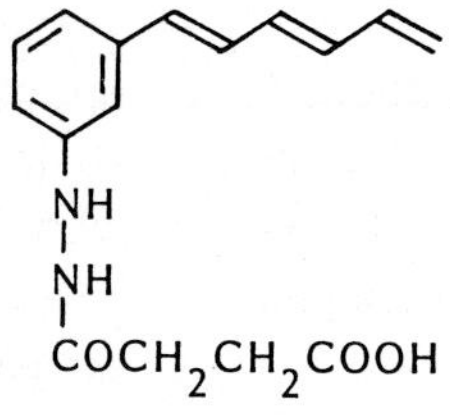

Spinamycin (1968)

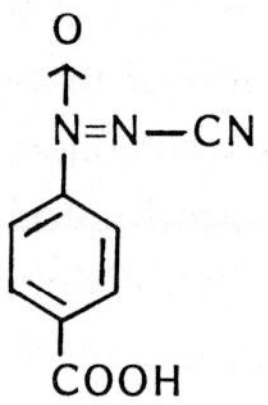

COCH₂CH₂COOH

Calvatic acid (1975)

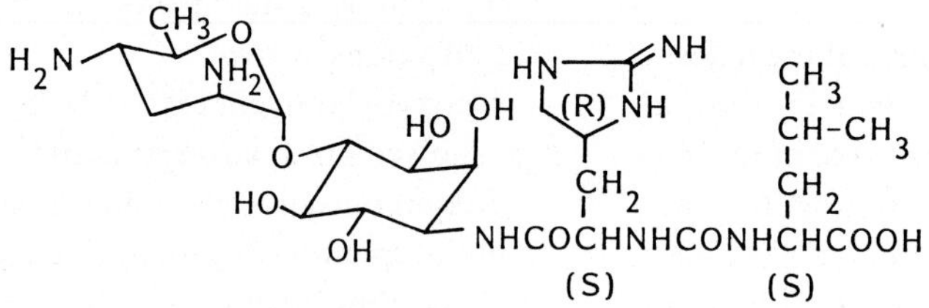

Minosaminomycin (1975)

Fig. 19. Antibacterials: deoxynybomycin, spinamycin, calvatic acid, minosaminomycin.

Amiclenomycin (Fig. 20), a new amino acid antibiotic active against mycobacteria, was isolated from a *Streptomyces* sp. It inhibited KAPA-DAPA aminotransferase in the biosynthetic pathway of biotin, but showed noncompetitive binding in terms of the ping-pong bi-bi mechanism.

Gougeroxymycin (1969) from a *Streptomyces* sp. inhibited *Trichophyton* and *Candida albicans*. Relatively low in toxicity to mice, it is a new antifungal antibiotic.

Oryzoxymycin (Fig. 20) from a *Streptomyces* sp. inhibited *Xanthomonas oryzae, in vitro,* but not in tests of potted rice plants. It was labile to light.

New metabolites of actinomycetes, sphydrofuran, arglecin, argvalin, and KD16-U1 (Fig. 21),

were found in actinomycetes, by color reaction screening.

Oxanosine (Fig. 22), a novel nucleoside, was isolated from a *Streptomyces* sp. It strongly inhibited the growth of *src*-integrated rat kidney cells when the *src* gene was expressed; inhibition was weak when the *src* gene was not expressed.

Two chlorine-containing antibiotics, clazamycins A and B (Fig. 22) from a *Streptomyces* sp., both showed antibacterial and antitumor activity.

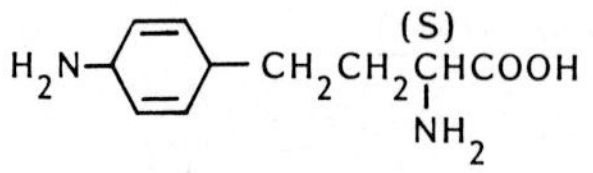

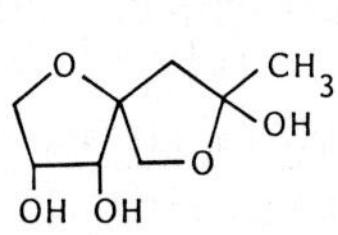

Sphydrofuran (1971)

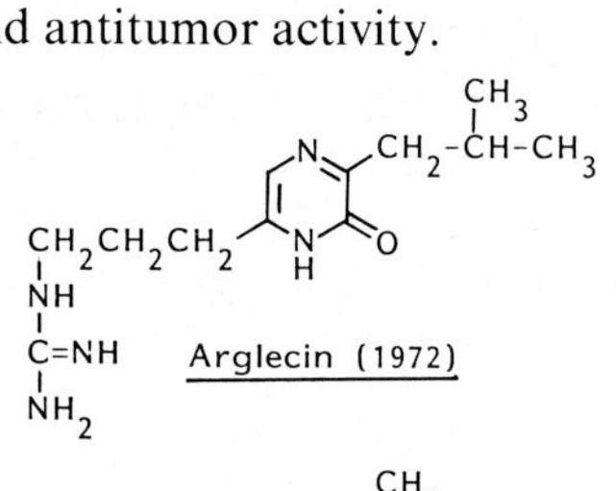

Arglecin (1972)

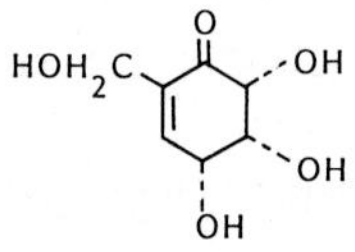

Argvalin (1973)

KD16-U1 (1974)

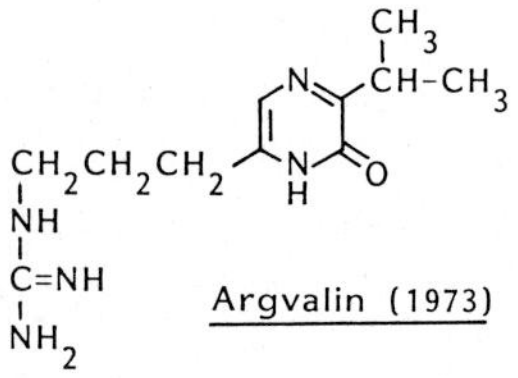

Fig. 21. New metabolites of actinomycetes: sphydrofuran, arglecin, KD16-U1, argvalin.

Amiclenomycin (1974)

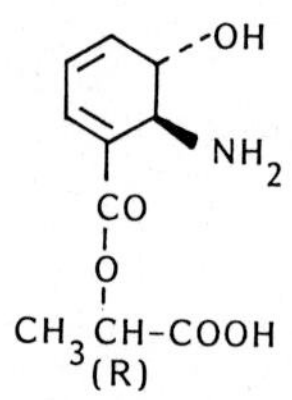

Oryzoxymycin (1972)

Fig. 20. Antibacterials: amiclenomycin, oryzoxymycin.

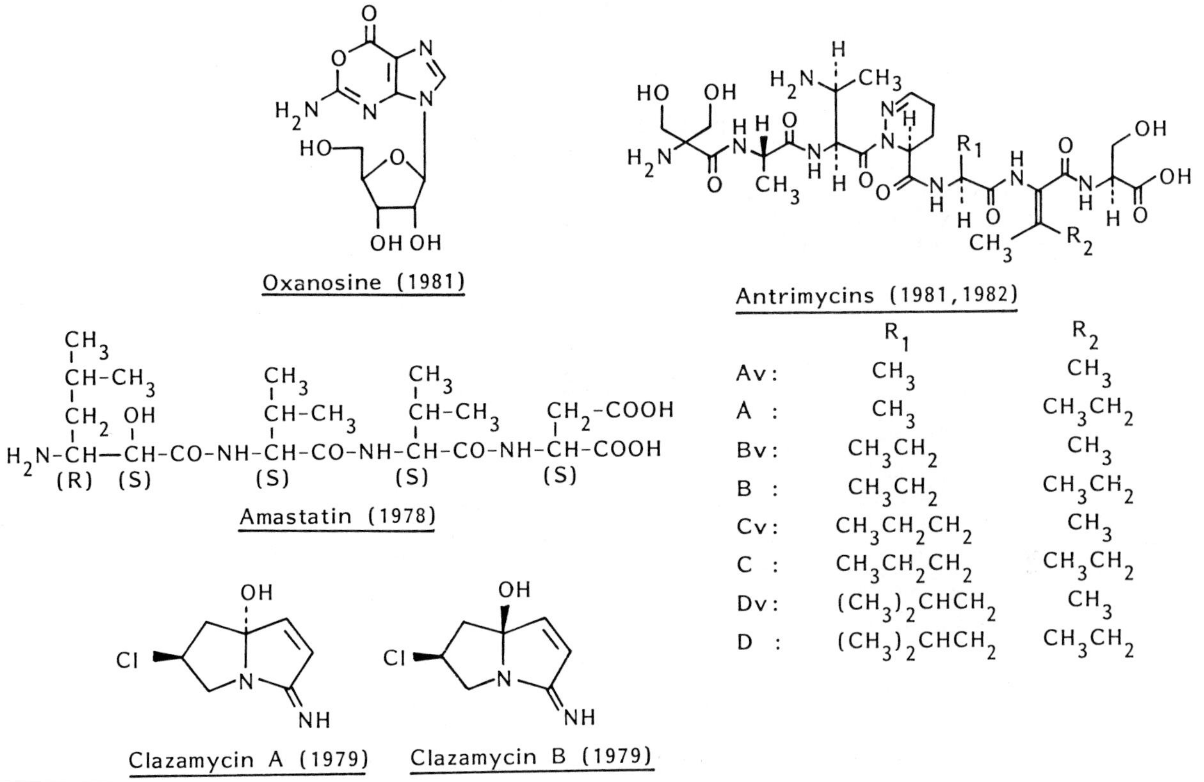

Fig. 22. Antibacterials: oxanosine, amastatin, clazamycin A and B, antrimycins.

Antrimycin (Fig. 22) from a *Streptomyces* sp. is a new peptide antibiotic which contains novel amino acids. It inhibits *Mycobacterium* sp.

Dihydroxyindoxazene (Fig. 23), a new antibiotic active against gram-negative bacteria, was found in a *Chromobacterium* sp.

Glycocinnasperimicin D (Fig. 23), a broad anti-bacterial, was produced from a *Nocardia* sp.

Dotriacolide (Fig. 24), a new inhibitor from a *Micromonospora* sp., was found by Umezawa in 1981, while screening for inhibitors of β-lactamase, by UV spectrophotometric methods.

2-Hydroxy-5-iminoazacyclopent-3-ene (Fig. 24) was isolated in 1979 from a *Streptoverticillium* sp. It caused cell elongation of bacteria.

L-2-Amino-5-methyl-5-hexenoic acid (Fig. 24) was isolated from a *Streptomyces* sp. by inhibition against the induction of (*his*⁻) revertant from *Salmonella typhimurium* (*his*⁻).

Basidalin (Fig. 24), from a culture of basidiomy-cetes, inhibited gram-positive bacteria.

D-β-Lysylmethanediamine (Fig. 24), a new amine with a unique open chain aldoaminal structure, was isolated from a *Streptomyces* sp. in 1986. It exhibit-ed weak antibacterial activity.

Napyradiomycins (Fig. 25) were isolated from a *Chainia* sp. by activity against gram-positive bacteria having multi-drug resistance. These compounds possess a chromophore containing straight aliphatic side chains in the A type napyradiomycin, a 6-member ring in the B type, and a 14-member ring rejoined to the chromophore in the C type.

Dioxapyrrolomycin (Fig. 26) from a *Streptomyces* sp. showed strong activity against gram-positive bacteria.

Saphenamycin (Fig. 26), which contains a phenazine nucleus, was produced by a *Streptomyces* sp. It was strongly active against gram-positive bacteria, especially against *rec*⁻ strains.

Indisocin (Fig. 26) was produced by a *Nocardia*

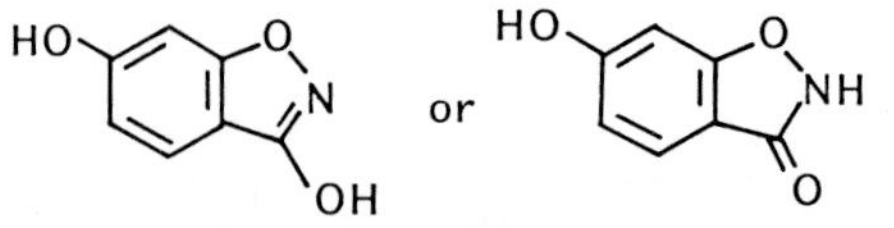

14

3,6-Dihydroxyindoxazene (1983)

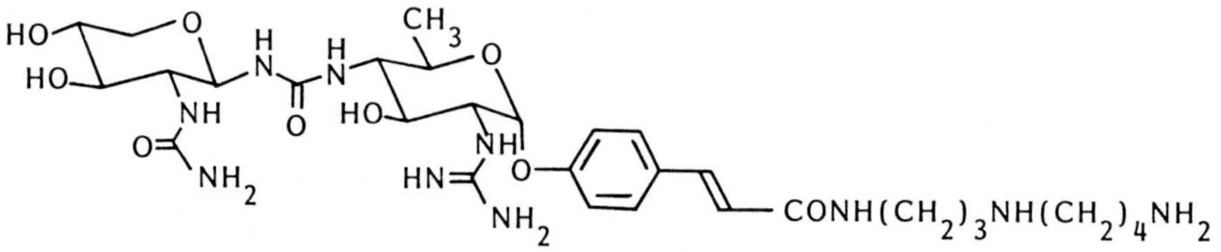

Glycocinnasperimicin D (1985)

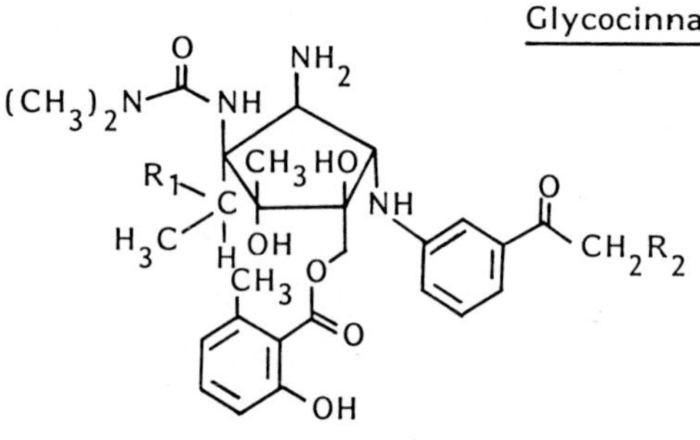

8"-Hydroxypactamycin: R_1=OH, R_2=OH

7-Deoxypactamycin : R_1=H, R_2=H

Pactamycin analogues (1986)

Fig. 23. Antibacterials: 3,6-dihydroxyindoxazene, glycocinnasperimicin D, pactamycin analogs.

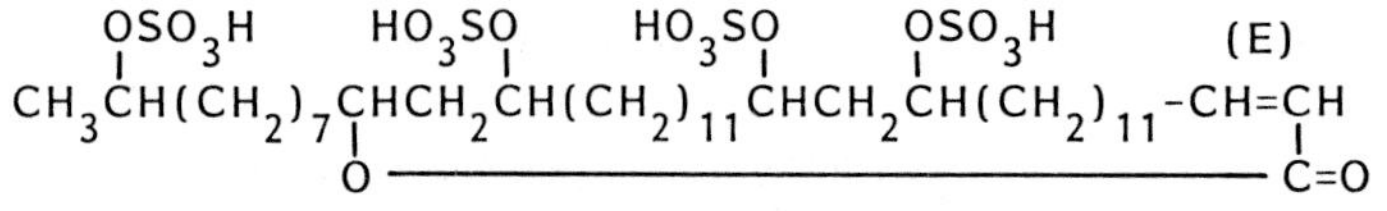

Dotriacolide (1981)

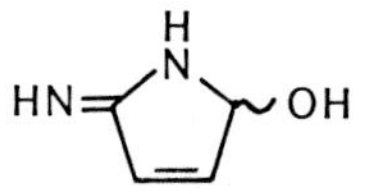

2-Hydroxy-5-iminoazacyclopent-3-ene (1979)

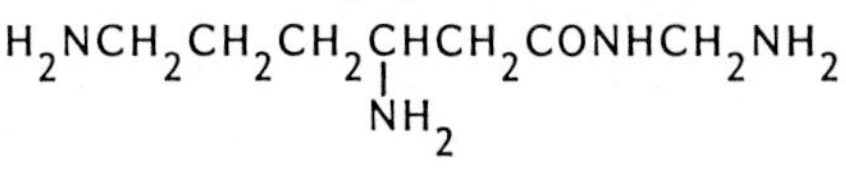

D-β-Lysylmethanediamine (1986)

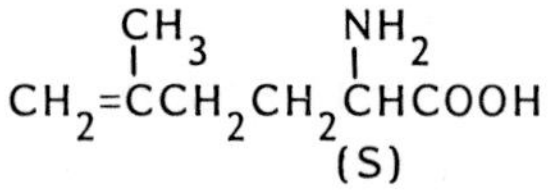

L-2-Amino-5-methyl-5-hexenoic acid (1979)

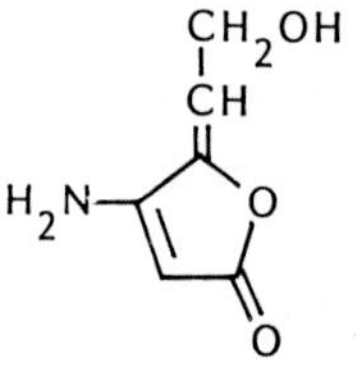

Basidalin (1983)

Fig. 24. Antibacterials: dotriacolide, D-β-lysylmethanediamine, 2-hydroxy-5-iminoazacyclopent-3-ene, L-2-amino-5-methyl-5-hexenoic acid, basidalin.

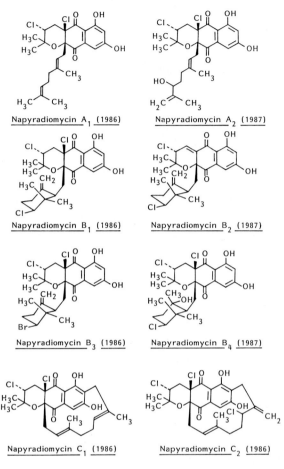

Napyradiomycin A₁ (1986)

Napyradiomycin A₂ (1987)

Napyradiomycin B₁ (1986)

Napyradiomycin B₂ (1987)

Napyradiomycin B₃ (1986)

Napyradiomycin B₄ (1987)

Napyradiomycin C₁ (1986)

Napyradiomycin C₂ (1986)

Fig. 25. Antibacterials: napyradiomycins.

sp. in a diluted medium. The structure is unique, having oxindole and isonitrile groups. Indisocin is strongly active against both gram-positive and gram-negative bacteria, and also against fungi.

Istamycins (Fig. 27), new aminoglycoside antibi-

otics containing diaminocyclitol, were isolated from a new *Streptomyces* sp. in sea mud. They strongly inhibit resistants to other known aminoglycoside antibiotics. Istamycin B has the strongest activity of the istamycins.

The total synthesis of istamycin A (Fig. 27) was achieved in 1979. 3-*O*-Demethyl and 3-demethoxy derivatives of istamycin B showed excellent activity against *Pseudomonas* strains.

Dopsisamine, a novel polyamine-type antibiotic with broad antimicrobial activity, was produced by *Nocardiopsis*, a new actinomycete, in 1986.

Bagougeramines (Figs. 27, 28) exhibited broad antimicrobial activity, and specific activity against mite.

Umezawa's research interests extended beyond antimicrobial and antitumor antibiotics, and included non-antibiotic substances of microbial origin. In 1965, he began new research searching for enzyme inhibitors of microbial origin.

About 70 enzyme inhibitors were found, indicating that microorganisms are capable of producing inhibitors of various enzymes involved in both microbial function and physiology. This is a rational approach to finding pharmacologically active agents. For example, inhibitors of enzymes involved in norepinephrine metabolism exhibit hypotensive action.

Enzymes of norepinephrine metabolism were studied in relation to their vascular and neural functions. Umezawa thought their inhibitors might be valuable for the control of catecholamine function. In collaboration with Professor T. Nagatsu of the University of Nagoya, he selected tyrosine

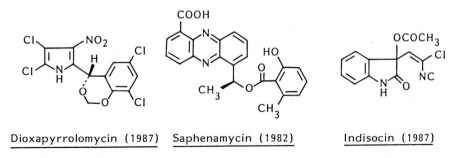

Dioxapyrrolomycin (1987)   Saphenamycin (1982)   Indisocin (1987)

Fig. 26. Antibacterials: dioxapyrrolomycin, saphenamycin, indisocin.

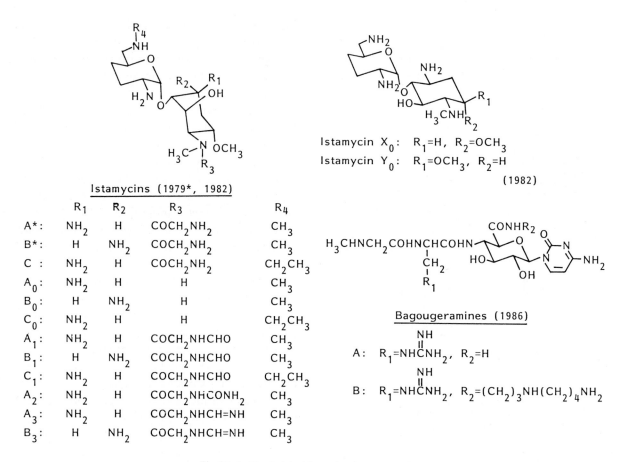

Istamycin X_0: R_1=H, R_2=OCH$_3$
Istamycin Y_0: R_1=OCH$_3$, R_2=H

(1982)

Bagougeramines (1986)

A: R_1=NHĊNH$_2$, R_2=H

B: R_1=NHĊNH$_2$, R_2=(CH$_2$)$_3$NH(CH$_2$)$_4$NH$_2$

Istamycins (1979*, 1982)

	R_1	R_2	R_3	R_4
A*:	NH$_2$	H	COCH$_2$NH$_2$	CH$_3$
B*:	H	NH$_2$	COCH$_2$NH$_2$	CH$_3$
C :	NH$_2$	H	COCH$_2$NH$_2$	CH$_2$CH$_3$
A$_0$:	NH$_2$	H	H	CH$_3$
B$_0$:	H	NH$_2$	H	CH$_3$
C$_0$:	NH$_2$	H	H	CH$_2$CH$_3$
A$_1$:	NH$_2$	H	COCH$_2$NHCHO	CH$_3$
B$_1$:	H	NH$_2$	COCH$_2$NHCHO	CH$_3$
C$_1$:	NH$_2$	H	COCH$_2$NHCHO	CH$_2$CH$_3$
A$_2$:	NH$_2$	H	COCH$_2$NHCONH$_2$	CH$_3$
A$_3$:	NH$_2$	H	COCH$_2$NHCH=NH	CH$_3$
B$_3$:	H	NH$_2$	COCH$_2$NHCH=NH	CH$_3$

Fig. 27. Antibacterials: istamycins, bagougeramines.

Bagougeramine A: R_1=NHĊNH$_2$, R_2=H

Bagougeramine B: R_1=NHĊNH$_2$

R_2=CH$_2$CH$_2$CH$_2$NHCH$_2$CH$_2$CH$_2$CH$_2$NH$_2$

Fig. 28. Antibacterial and miticidal bagougeramines.

hydroxylase and dopamine β-hydroxylase, both involved in the biosynthesis of norepinephrine. Later, tryptophan hydroxylase, catechol *O*-methyltransferase and histidine decarboxylase were also selected.

Oudenone (Fig. 29), a specific tyrosine hydroxylase inhibitor, was found in the culture filtrate of the mushroom *Oudemansiella*. It exhibited hypotensive effects in spontaneously hypertensive rats.

Fusaric acid (Fig. 29), an inhibitor of dopamine hydroxylase exhibiting strong hypotensive effects, was found in *Fusarium*. Dopastin (Fig. 29), another inhibitor, was found in a *Pseudomonas* sp. It exhibited strong hypotensive effects.

Isoflavone compounds (Fig. 30) inhibited catechol *O*-methyltransferase and histidine decarboxylase *in vitro*. They did not show hypotensive effects.

In screening for catechol *O*-methyltransferase inhibitors, methylspinazarin and dihydromethylspinazarin (Fig. 30) were found in actinomycetes. Two spinochromes (Fig. 30) were found in culture filtrates of fungi. Dehydrodicaffeic acid dilactone (Fig. 30) was found in a cultured mushroom.

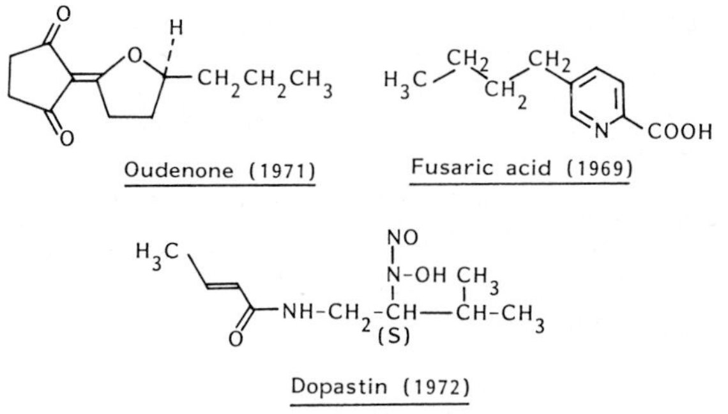

Fig. 29. Enzyme inhibitors: oudenone, fusaric acid, dopastin.

Inhibitors of histidine decarboxylase and trypta-
mine N-methyltransferase were found in a fungus.
Identified as lecanoric acid in 1974, they had previously been obtained from a lichen. Tetrahydropy-
ridylpentadiene, another inhibitor of these enzymes, was found in actinomycetes, also in 1974.

More information about inhibitors was obtained

from screening proteinase inhibitors.

Leupeptins and antipain (Fig. 31) containing
L-argininal inhibited trypsin, plasmin, papain, cathepsin B, etc. Chymostatin (Fig. 31) containing
L-phenylalaninal inhibited chymotrypsins. Elastatinal (Fig. 31) containing L-alaninal inhibited pancreatic elastase. These inhibitors were isolated from
culture filtrates of *Streptomyces* sp. They contain
aldehyde groups at the C-terminal. If the aldehyde
groups are oxidized or reduced to an acid or alcohol, the compounds lose their activity, indicating
that α-acylamino aldehydes are the active sites.

Pepstatin and related compounds (Fig. 32) were
found to be inhibitors of pepsin. In addition, they
inhibited cathepsin D, chymosin, renin, etc.

Phosphoramidon (Fig. 32), an inhibitor of metalloproteinases, was obtained from a *Streptomyces*
sp.

These proteinase inhibitors have all been widely
used for the identification of proteinases, the study

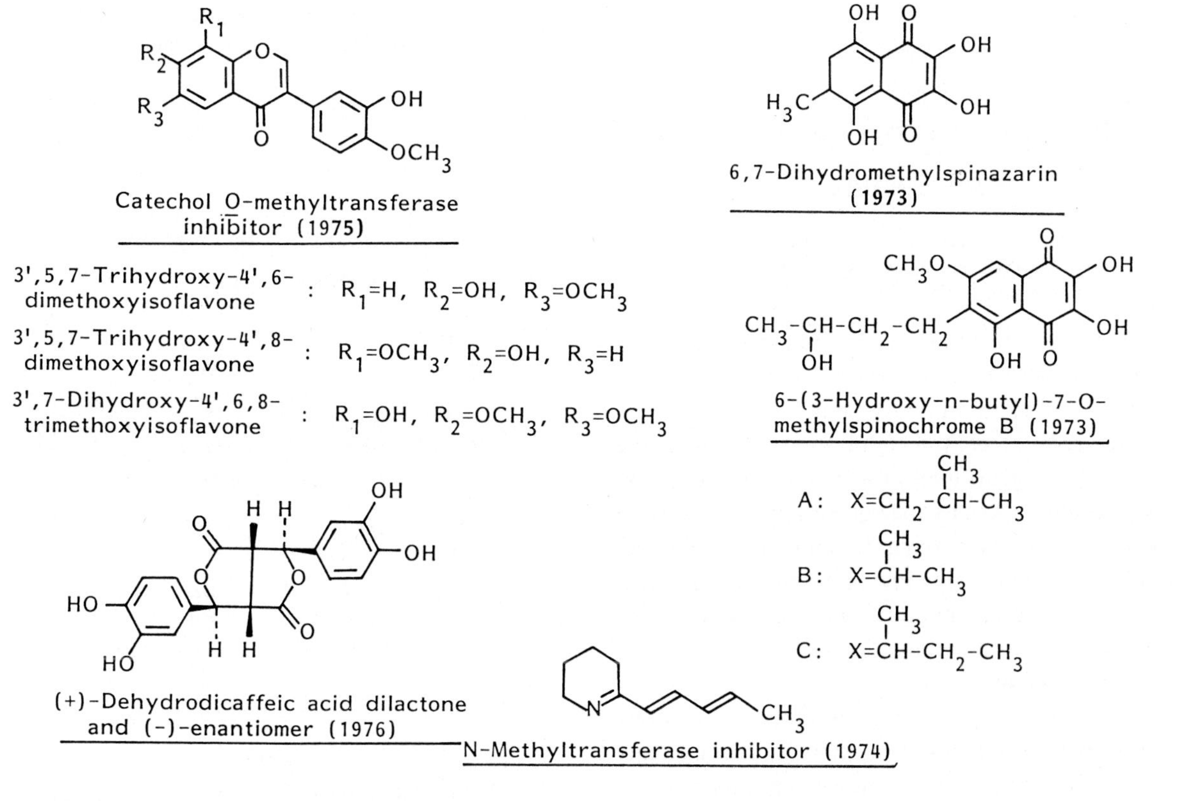

Fig. 30. Enzyme inhibitors – epinephrine enzymes.

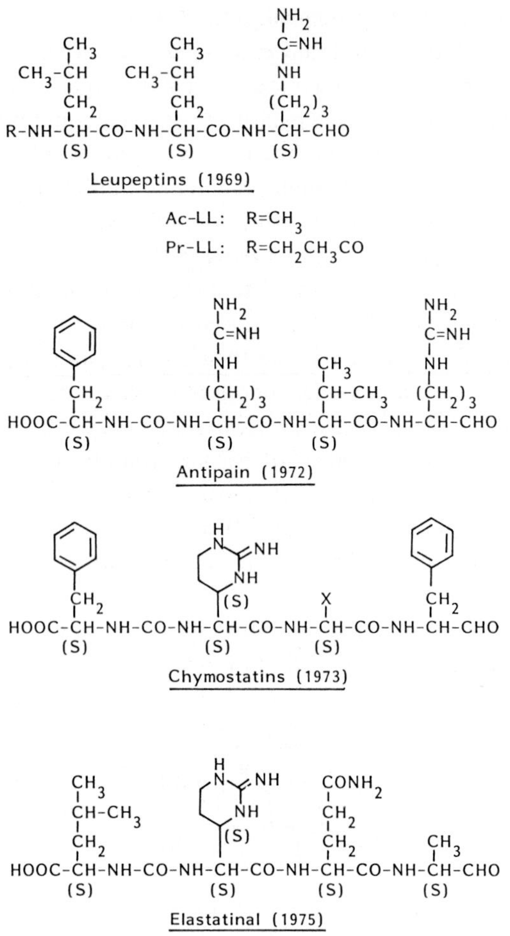

18

Fig. 31. Enzyme inhibitors – proteinases, peptidases: leupeptins, antipain, chymostatins, elastatinal.

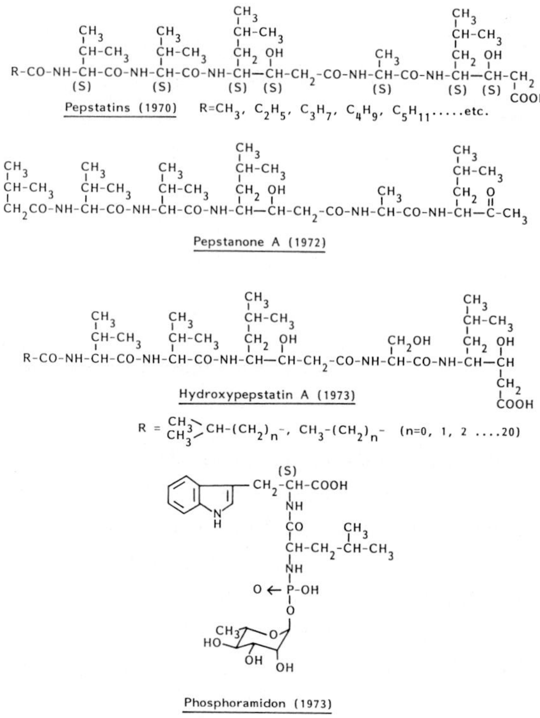

Fig. 32. Enzyme inhibitors: pepstatins, pepstanone A, hydroxy-pepstatin A, phosphoramidon.

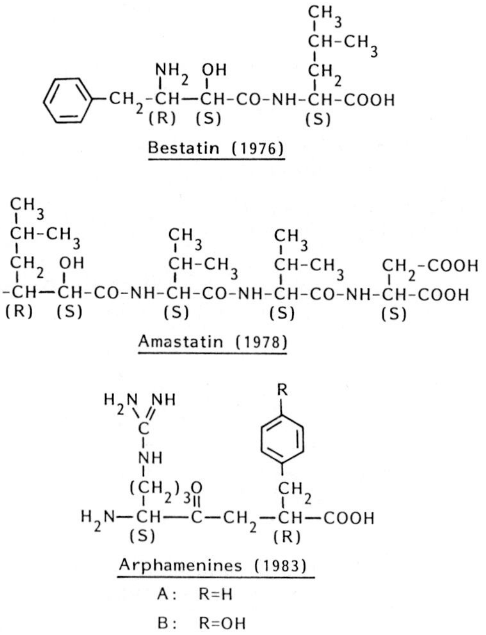

Fig. 33. Enzyme inhibitors – peptidases: bestatin, amastatin, arphamenines.

of proteinase functions, the inhibition of proteolysis during the extraction process, and as functional groups in affinity chromatography.

The study of enzyme inhibitors resulted in the discovery of agents useful for enhancing or decreasing immunity. Agents increasing immunity can be used in the treatment of cancer and microbial infections in patients having low immunity. Those causing a decrease in immunity may be useful in the treatment of autoimmune diseases, or in tissue or organ transplants.

During his study of enzyme inhibitors, Umezawa noted that the inhibitors of many animal cell surface enzymes enhanced or reduced immunity.

Inhibitors of exopeptidases were found in culture

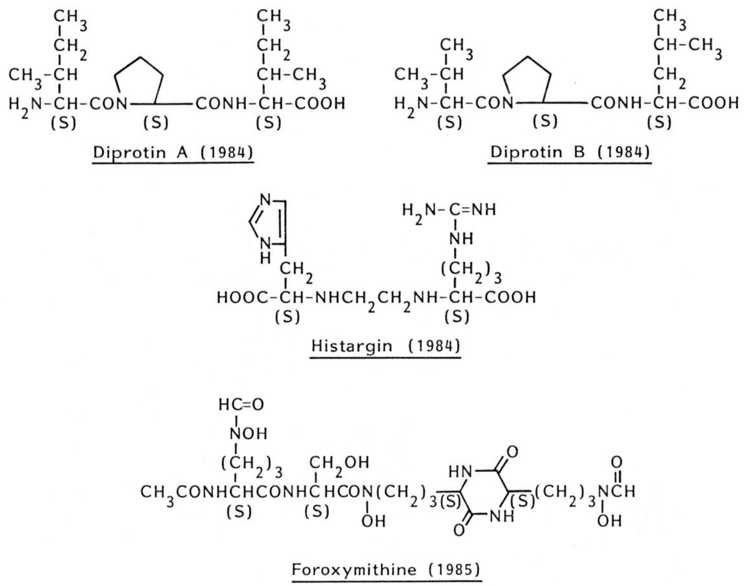

Fig. 34. Enzyme inhibitors – aminopeptidases: diprotin A, diprotin B, histargin, foroxymithine.

filtrates of *Streptomyces* sp. Bestatin (Fig. 33), and other inhibitors of aminopeptidases, enhanced immune responses significantly, stimulating the study of inhibitors of these enzymes in relation to the immune response.

Bestatin (Fig. 33) inhibited aminopeptidase B. In tumor-bearing hosts, antitumor agents such as macrophages, T cells and NK cells are activated by bestatin. Bestatin augments the production of cytokines, such as interleukin 1 and 2, the colony stimulating factor, etc. There has been random study of bestatin in cancer patients, and its therapeutic activity against acute nonlymphatic leukemia and other tumors has been confirmed. Bestatin is now clinically used in Japan for suppression of leukemia.

Another peptide, amastatin (Fig. 33) inhibits aminopeptidase A.

Arphamenines (Fig. 33) inhibit aminopeptidase B very strongly. Unlike bestatin, they do not inhibit aminopeptidase A and leucine aminopeptidase. Arphamenines have unique structures in which the peptide bond is replaced by a methylene ketone bond.

Actinonin, an inhibitor of aminopeptidase M, also inhibited leucine aminopeptidase. Diprotins

(Fig. 34) are inhibitors of dipeptidyl aminopeptidase IV.

Benzylmalic acid is a specific inhibitor of carboxypeptidase A, although it weakly inhibits carboxypeptidase B.

Histargin (Fig. 34), a specific inhibitor of carboxypeptidase B, inhibited angiotensin-converting enzyme. Foroxymithine (Fig. 34) is another angiotensin-converting enzyme inhibitor.

Interesting compounds having β-lactone structures were found and named ebelactones and esterastin (Fig. 35). They strongly inhibited pancreatic esterase and some of the cholesterol esterases.

Panosialin (Fig. 35) was found by screening sialidase inhibitors. It also inhibited proteinases.

Siastatins (Fig. 35), found in an actinomycete, inhibit sialidase. Bacterial sialidases were strongly inhibited, but sialidases of mammalian cells were only weakly inhibited.

Pyridindolol and dihydroxyisoflavone-rhamnopyranoside (Fig. 35) were two new β-galactosidase inhibitors.

A xanthine oxidase inhibitor was identified in 1972 as formyluracil.

Six inhibitors of cAMP phosphodiesterase were found in actinomycetes. One was identified as reti-

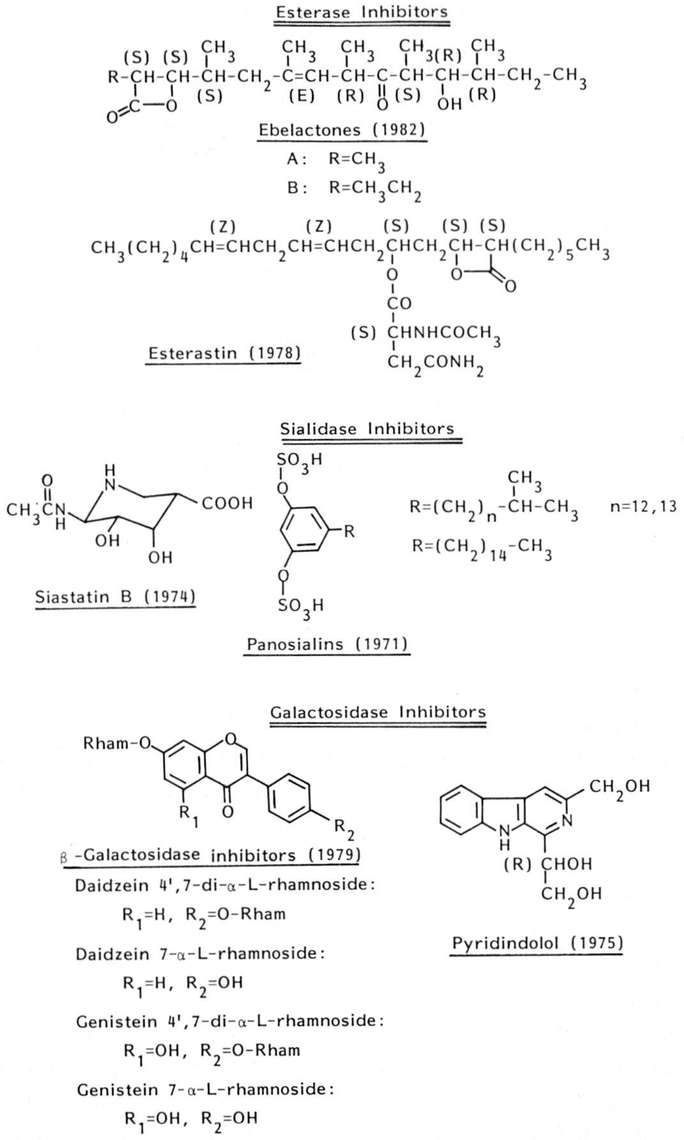

Esterase Inhibitors

(S) (S) CH_3 CH_3 CH_3 $CH_3(R)$ CH_3
R-CH-CH-CH-CH$_2$-C=CH-CH-C-CH-CH-CH-CH$_2$-CH$_3$
O=C—O (S) (E) (R) O (S) OH (R)

Ebelactones (1982)

A: R=CH$_3$

B: R=CH$_3$CH$_2$

(Z) (Z) (S) (S) (S)
CH$_3$(CH$_2$)$_4$CH=CHCH$_2$CH=CHCH$_2$CHCH$_2$CH-CH(CH$_2$)$_5$CH$_3$
O O—CO
CO
(S) CHNHCOCH$_3$
CH$_2$CONH$_2$

Esterastin (1978)

Sialidase Inhibitors

CH$_3$CN—N—COOH
O OH OH

Siastatin B (1974)

SO$_3$H
O
R=(CH$_2$)$_n$-CH-CH$_3$ n=12,13
CH$_3$
R=(CH$_2$)$_{14}$-CH$_3$
O
SO$_3$H

Panosialins (1971)

Galactosidase Inhibitors

Rham-O
R$_1$ O
R$_2$

β-Galactosidase inhibitors (1979)

Daidzein 4',7-di-α-L-rhamnoside:
R$_1$=H, R$_2$=O-Rham

Daidzein 7-α-L-rhamnoside:
R$_1$=H, R$_2$=OH

Genistein 4',7-di-α-L-rhamnoside:
R$_1$=OH, R$_2$=O-Rham

Genistein 7-α-L-rhamnoside:
R$_1$=OH, R$_2$=OH

CH$_2$OH
N
(R) CHOH
CH$_2$OH

Pyridindolol (1975)

Fig. 35. Esterase inhibitors: ebelactones, esterastin; sialidase inhibitors: siastatin B, panosialins; galactosidase inhibitors: β-galactosidase, pyridindolol.

culol (Fig. 36). Two others, phosphodiesterases I and II (Fig. 36), had interesting new structures and showed stronger effects than reticulol and papaverine, a known phosphodiesterase inhibitor.

Forphenicine (Fig. 37) strongly inhibited alkaline phosphatase from chicken intestine, but only weakly inhibited that enzyme from other sources. The immunomodulating effect was exhibited on injection only, not following oral administration.

Forphenicinol, a derivative of forphenicine, was orally active. Forphenicinol exhibits weak inhibition of alkaline phosphatase but augments immune responses. It inhibited the growth of murine transplanted tumors, and exhibited a protective effect against microbial infections through activation of macrophages/granulocytes. Forphenicinol enhanced production of cytokines, such as tumor necrosis factors, interferons and activating factors of

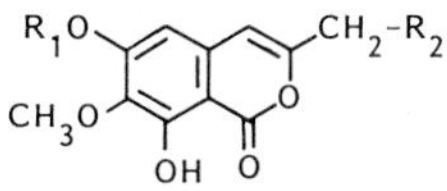

cAMP phosphodiesterase
inhibitors (1977)

Reticulol: R_1=H, R_2=H
8-Hydroxy-6,7-dimethoxy-3-
 hydroxymethylisocoumarin:
   R_1=CH$_3$, R_2=OH
6,8-Dihydroxy-7-methoxy-3-
 hydroxymethylisocoumarin:
   R_1=H, R_2=OH

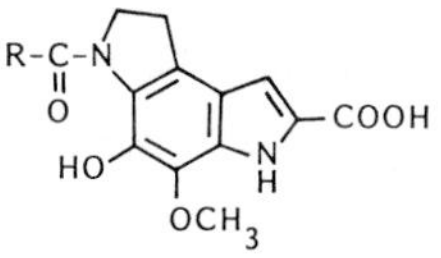

PDE-I : R=NH$_2$
PDE-II: R=CH$_3$

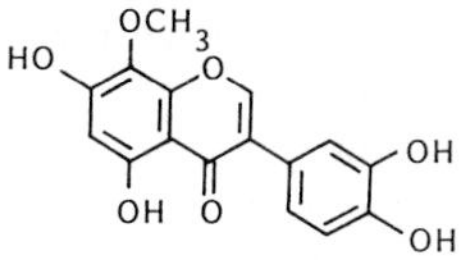

Dopa decarboxylase
inhibitor (1975)

Fig. 36. cAMP kinase inhibitors.

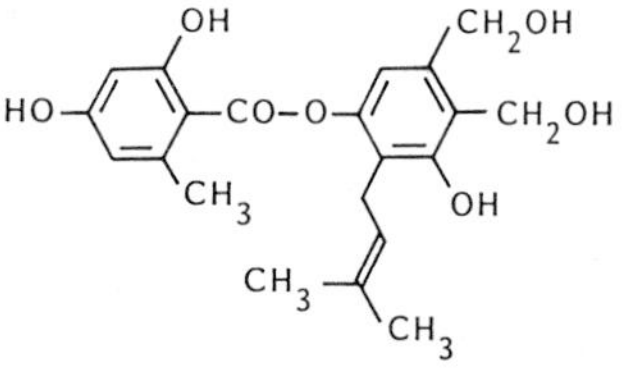

Glyo-I (1975)

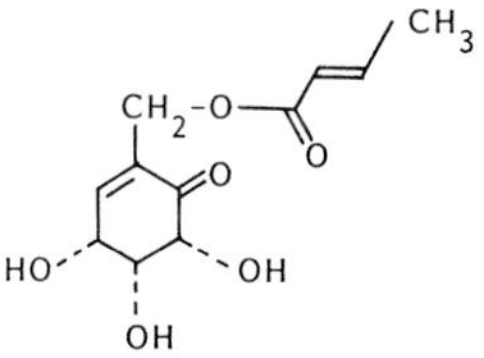

Glyo-II (1975)

Fig. 38. Glyoxalase inhibitors: glyo-I and glyo-II.

Various oncogenes, such as *src, erb B* and others, are known to act through tyrosine kinase activity. An inhibitor of tyrosine kinase on the epidermal

macrophages and/or granulocytes in mice. Forphenicinol is now being studied clinically.

Glyoxalase consists of two enzymes, I and II. An inhibitor, named glyo-I (Fig. 38), was found in a cultured mushroom in 1975. Another inhibitor, named glyo-II (Fig. 38), was found in an actinomycete, also in 1975. However, these compounds did not exhibit remarkable tumor inhibition *in vivo*.

A strong inhibitor of reverse transcriptase of the murine leukemia virus was found in an actinomycete. It was named revistin (Fig. 39).

An inhibitor of rat liver phenylalanine hydroxylase was isolated from a fungal culture and its structure determined to be 3,4-dihydroxystyrene. The inhibitor of guanine deaminase, found in a streptomycete, was named azepinomycin (Fig. 39).

Vanoxonin (Fig. 39), a thymidylate synthetase inhibitor, was found in an actinomycete. Intraperitoneal administration of a vanoxonin-vanadium complex showed weak activity against L1210 mouse leukemia and Ehrlich ascites carcinoma.

Plipastatins (Fig. 39), inhibitors of phospholipase A2, were found in 1986.

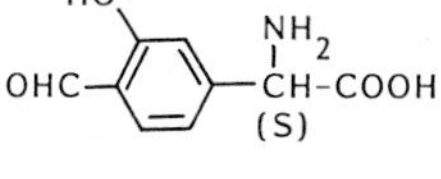

Reverse Transcriptase Inhibitor

Revistin

Phenylalanine hydroxylase inhibitor

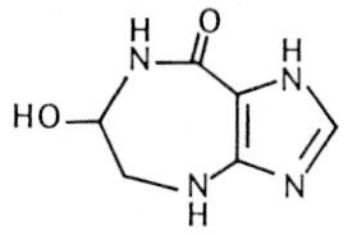

Azepinomycin (1987)

Thymidylate synthetase inhibitor

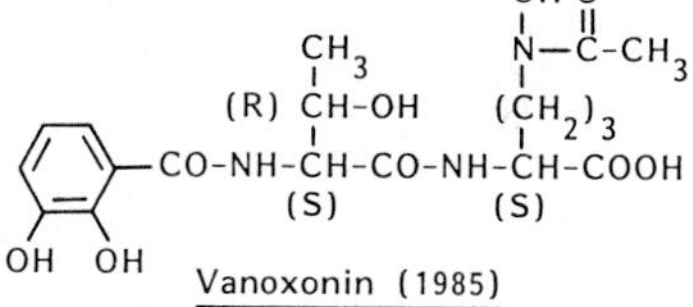

Vanoxonin (1985)

Phospholipase Inhibitor

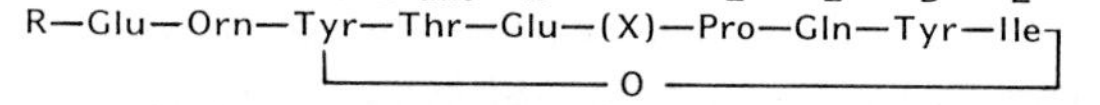

$$\begin{array}{c}\text{L} \quad \text{D} \quad \text{L} \;\; \text{D-allo} \;\; \text{L} \qquad \text{L} \quad \text{L} \quad \text{D} \quad \text{L}\\ \text{R—Glu—Orn—Tyr—Thr—Glu—(X)—Pro—Gln—Tyr—Ile}\\ \text{O}\end{array}$$

Plipastatins (1986)

	R	(X)
A_1:	(R) CH$_3$(CH$_2$)$_{12}$CHCH$_2$CO– OH	D-Ala
A_2:	(S) (R) CH$_3$CH$_2$CH(CH$_2$)$_{10}$CHCH$_2$CO– CH$_3$ OH	D-Ala
B_1:	(R) CH$_3$(CH$_2$)$_{12}$CHCH$_2$CO– OH	D-Val
B_2:	(S) (R) CH$_3$CH$_2$CH(CH$_2$)$_{10}$CHCH$_2$CO– CH$_3$ OH	D-Val

Forphenicine (1978)

Fig. 37. Alkaline phosphatase inhibitor: forphenicine.

Fig. 39. Revistin, azepinomycin, vanoxonin, plipastatins.

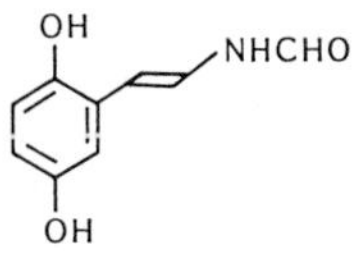

Erbstatin (1986)

Fig. 40. Tyrosine kinase inhibitor: erbstatin.

growth factor (EGF) receptor was found in a *Strep-tomyces* sp. It was isolated and named erbstatin (Fig. 40).

Erbstatin inhibited the phosphorylation and internalization of the EGF receptor, but not the binding of EGF to the receptor. It reduced the phosphorylation of pp60^{src} in Rous sarcoma virus-transformed cells of the rat kidney. It exhibited cytotoxicity against A431, ts-*src*/NRK and L1210 *in vitro*. Administration of erbstatin or foroxymithine (Fig. 34) caused antitumor effects in L1210-bearing mice.

More than 250 new compounds (Tables 1, 2) were discovered under Umezawa's direction. He directed the research on their mode of action, biosynthesis, yield improvement, preclinical studies *in vitro* and *in vivo*, and was a leader in developing them for industry.

His research was often conducted in cooperation with members of other research institutes and pharmaceutical firms. This type of research, requiring mutual communication and stimulation, was possible under the strong leadership of Umezawa.

Umezawa published more than 1200 professional papers throughout his career. His papers were important for researchers worldwide and there were frequent and numerous citations of his work in the scientific literature.

One month before his death, in a magazine interview, Umezawa said: 'Decide the target, continue the effort, and the results will be the creation'. It was his philosophy throughout his professional life.

Except for a few days off at the beginning of each new year, Umezawa worked in his office each day, reading a stack of literature, usually two feet high, and meeting with researchers and with visitors. When he was young, he took time off on the after-

Table 2

Antibiotics found and developed by Hamao Umezawa at the Institute of Microbial Chemistry

	Found	Launched
I. Antimicrobial antibiotics		
fradiomycin (neomycin)	1948	1954
aureothricin	1949	1953
kanamycin	1957	1958
kanamycin B	1957	1968
variotin	1959	1959
blasticidin S	1958	1961
mikamycin	1959	1962
kasugamycin	1965	1965
josamycin	1967	1970
O-propionyljosamycin	1973	1975
dibekacin (3′,4′-dideoxykanamy-cin B)	1971	1975
macarbomycin	1970	1972
arbekacin (derivative of dibeka-cin)	1973	
II. Antitumor antibiotics		
sarkomycin	1953	1954
bleomycin	1965	1969
aclarubicin (aclacinomycin A)	1975	1981
peplomycin (derivative of bleo-mycin)	1978	1981
bestatin	1975	1987
THP-adriamycin	1980	
oxanosin	1981	
spergualin	1981	
marinactan	1983	
III. Enzyme inhibitors		
coformycin (as a reagent)	1967	1978
fusaric acid	1969	
leupeptin (as a reagent)	1969	1976
pepstatin A (as a reagent)	1970	1975
chymostatin (as a reagent)	1970	1976
antipain (as a reagent)	1972	1976
dopastin (as a reagent)	1972	1983
phosphoramidon (as a reagent)	1973	1978
elastatinal (as a reagent)	1975	1977
bestatin (as a reagent)	1975	1980
forphenicine	1978	
esterastin	1978	
forphenicinol	1980	
ebelactones	1980	
ribocitrin	1980	
arphamenines	1983	

noon of his wedding, but was back at work that same evening. His assistants did not know that he had left for that special occasion.

His memory was very clear, even recalling the page number, volume and issue number of papers in the scientific literature. Visitors were often astonished that he could remember the date, place, and often even the time of a previous meeting years ago. The face of workers under him would often become blue when he inquired about the remaining 95 mg of a compound obtained 10 years ago, of which 5 mg had been used.

He had an excellent memory, not only in science, but also in politics, economics, the stock market, sports, art and many other areas. Although he did not actively participate in sports, he was able to name the pitcher in a past baseball game, and also who won the game. At home he enjoyed painting, crafts and music, and he loved his pet dog. He selected paintings for the walls of his office, which was also equipped with an audio system for music.

He treated his friends, both in Japan and in other countries, warmly and courteously. The range of his friendships was broad, including many Nobel Prize laureates and sports writers. He kept up a long-lasting friendship with Dr. A.R. Menotti of the Bristol Co., beginning with the development of kanamycin in 1948. He liked to greet visitors to his laboratories, regardless of his schedule. Always very gracious, he treated his guests as cordially as his friends.

I had the honor to accompany him when Professors S.A. Waksman, V. Prelog, E. Chain, D. Barton, J. Axelrod, U.S. von Euler, S.K. Bergstrom and B.I. Samuelson visited him. He maintained long-lasting friendships with distinguished scientists in many countries, including Professors J.C. Sheehan, B. Davis, D. Gottlieb, A. Demain and others from the United States, and Professors E.A. Abraham, G. Mathe, G. Skryabin and others from Europe.

He had good relations with experts outside his own field of expertise. He met frequently with Professor Sackler, famous for restoring artifacts from the Aswan Dam area in Egypt. Umezawa said: 'It is a basic truth that a man cannot have a good life without good friends. I admire the individual who can truly appreciate and understand the essence of great literature and arts, including paintings and antiquities'. Thus, he paid respect both to eminent friends and also to experts in various fields.

He adsorbed information and ideas very quickly and clearly; not just scientific information and data, but financial information and budgets were memorized without notes. His ability to calculate seemed to be beyond that of machines. Experts in real estate and the stock market were amazed at the speed and precision of his calculations.

Because of his business sense, the nonprofit foundation which he founded 25 years ago has been able to financially support many research activities.

From the time he was in medical school, Umezawa had been interested in the chemical aspects of immunology. Even after extensive antibiotic research, he continued his interest in the specificity of immunological reactions, attracted to the biological selectivity of chemotherapeutic agents. He believed

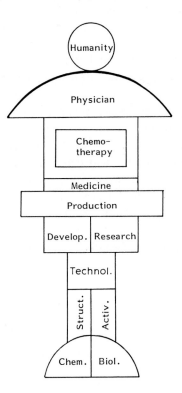

Fig. 41. The interrelationships of the philosophy and work of Hamao Umezawa.

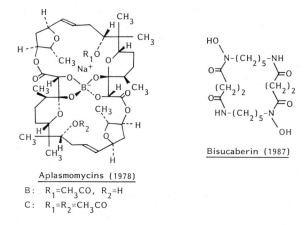

Aplasmomycins (1978)

B: R₁=CH₃CO, R₂=H
C: R₁=R₂=CH₃CO

Bisucaberin (1987)

Fig. 42. Aplasmomycins and bisucaberin, inhibitory substances of marine origin.

selectivity to be one of the most important criteria in the search to find new and useful compounds for medicine and for humanity (Fig. 41). This belief led to the discovery and consequent development of many selective agents for chemotherapy.

For his antibiotic research, Umezawa collected his own soil samples, extending his research interests to include the ecology, taxonomy, and classification of organisms, and fermentation, chemical and physical regulation, biochemical aspects of biosynthesis, genetics, including plasmid involvement in secondary metabolism, advanced methods of extraction and purification, structure determination using methods such as NMR, MS and X-ray crystallography, new chemical synthesis, computerized drug design, etc. He would study with specialists to understand each field, learning the most current research techniques and procedures.

At the same time, he employed and directed young specialists, often discussing their work with them and encouraging them. I, myself, was encouraged by him to continue work seeking biologically active agents in soil and marine microbes, including aplasmomycin and bisucaberin (Fig. 42), unusual and interesting substances of marine origin. Aplasmomycin is inhibitory to *Plasmodium*, the cause of malaria. Bisucaberin sensitizes tumor cells, to be lysed by a macrophage.

Umezawa encouraged coworkers who were interested in the genetic approach to antibiotic resistance, and in the antibiotic production mechanism. He himself became interested in plasmid involvement in secondary metabolism.

Chemists, biologists, and experts from other fields, such as medicine, pharmacology and veterinary science, worked under him. He knew the details of all experiments undertaken in his laboratories, and was very strict about the research and about ambiguities in experimental data. He read all papers written by his workers, and was very concerned that their work should be of high quality.

In contrast to his discipline, he was a warm person who encouraged his students and had great patience with them.

With tremendous effort and patience, Hamao Umezawa discovered large numbers of new and useful agents which have contributed to science and to humanity (Table 2).

Umezawa always dreamed about future achievements, even after he had made all his great contributions. He believed in the potential of the microbe to provide beneficial substances for mankind, and said: 'Once a clear goal is decided and the best effort has been made, original and creative achievements can be accomplished from research on microbial chemistry'.

Novel Microbial Products for Medicine and Agriculture
Editors: A.L. Demain, G.A. Somkuti, J.C. Hunter-Cevera and H.W. Rossmoore

CHAPTER 2

Use of the Plackett & Burman technique in a discovery program for new natural products

Richard L. Monaghan and Lawrence R. Koupal

Department of Fermentation Microbiology, Merck Sharp & Dohme Research Laboratories, Rahway, NJ, U.S.A.

SUMMARY

The Plackett & Burman experimental design was used to find conditions to increase the detection of antibiotic production from fungi isolated from nature. The technique determined important fermentation parameters for a mevinolin fermentation that resulted in titers of > 1 g/l in two experimental steps. The procedure also allowed a comparison between complex fermentation ingredients. Analysis of fermentation variables using the Plackett & Burman technique has successfully predicted whether multiple screening activities are due to one or more components in the fermentation broth. An analysis of the production of thienamycin by three microorganisms showed that the most significant fermentation variables for the three microorganisms were not the same.

INTRODUCTION

In the search for new natural products from micro-organisms, the selection of proper fermentation conditions is of critical importance, especially when that natural product is a secondary metabolite. Our experience and a survey of the literature both reveal that fermentation media containing complex ingredients yield more activities in screens and higher fermentation titers than media containing defined nutrients. The selection of ingredients and optimal conditions for a particular fermentation has in the past relied upon experience, luck and economics. This paper describes results obtained with the Plackett & Burman technique [2]. It has aided us substantially in quickly selecting fermentation media and conditions in a search for new natural products.

MATERIALS AND METHODS

The Plackett & Burman design is a fractional method that allows the testing of multiple independent variables within a single experiment. Experimental designs for 8, 12, 16 and up to 100 variables in multiples of 4 may be selected using a series of arrays constructed for this purpose [5]. Table 1 illustrates an array for $n = 8$ trials that will test $n - 1$ independent variables. Each row represents one trial (fermentation medium) and each column represents a single variable (medium component). The + and − elements represent the two different levels of each variable present within each trial. All variables tested by this method have the following characteristics: Each is present at a high level in half of the trials and at low levels or not at all in the other half. The interaction between any two variables is such that both are present in one quarter of the trials,

Table 1

Plackett & Burman matrix for $n = 8$

Medium	Variable						
	A	B	C	D	E	F	G
I	+	+	+	−	+	−	−
II	+	+	−	+	−	−	+
III	+	−	+	−	−	+	+
IV	−	+	−	−	+	+	+
V	+	−	−	+	+	+	−
VI	−	−	+	+	+	−	+
VII	−	+	+	+	−	+	−
VIII	−	−	−	−	−	−	−

both are absent in one quarter of the trials and only one of the two is present in the remainder of the trials. After the independent variables and their corresponding levels have been selected, the trials are performed and the responses, such as productivity, are measured. The effect of each variable upon the measured response is determined by the difference between the average of the + and − responses. The calculated effect can be positive, negative or neutral depending upon the overall influence of the variable upon the measured response. Experimental error is estimated from the dummy variables and represents the degree of expected variability within the experiment. The variance of effect (V_{eff}) is calculated by:

$$V_{eff} = (E_d)^2 / n$$

where E_d is each calculated dummy effect and n is the number of dummy variables used in the experiment. The standard error (S.E.) is determined by taking the square root of the variance:

$$S.E. = \sqrt{V_{eff}}$$

The significance level of each variable effect (E_x) is determined by Student's t test:

$$t = E_x / S.E.$$

In this report the sign of each calculated effect was applied to its significance level merely to depict direction of effect.

RESULTS

Formulation of screening media

Merck and Company has had a tradition of finding secondary metabolites from the actinomycetes, and a battery of fermentation media has been empirically formulated which supports good growth and production of secondary metabolites from actinomycetes. These same media also supported good growth of filamentous fungi but unfortunately did not support comparable levels of biosynthesis of their secondary metabolites. Rather than to randomly screen the media found in the literature or single variations of our current media, we chose to use the Plackett & Burman experimental protocol. This procedure allowed us to approach the design of general screening media on a more rational basis. The data analysis presented in Tables 2 and 3 was the start of that process.

Table 2

Production of antibiotic activity by fungi – I

Variable	High value[a]	Low value[a]	% Significance
Time (days)	14	7	93
Yeast extract (g)	0.5	0	87
Glycerol (ml) +	1.0	0	−50
Corn oil (ml)	0.1	0	
KH$_2$PO$_4$ (g)	0.1	0	−79
H$_2$O (ml)	30.0	0	−87
Agitation (rpm) (1st 7 days)	220	0	−91

[a]All values per 250 ml Erlenmeyer flask which contains 10.0 g corn and 15 ml of base solution which contains 0.1 g/l MgSO$_4$·7H$_2$O, 0.1 g/l sodium tartrate, 0.01 g/l FeSO$_4$·7H$_2$O, 0.01 g/l ZnSO$_4$·7H$_2$O. Incubation at 25°C at 220 rpm unless otherwise specified.

Since we were looking for secondary metabolite synthesis by fungi we chose a base medium that contained corn and a salts solution consisting of $MgSO_4 \cdot 7H_2O$, sodium tartrate, $FeSO_4 \cdot 7H_2O$ and $ZnSO_4 \cdot 7H_2O$. Incubation was at 25°C. Using the Plackett & Burman experimental design, media were formulated to test the effect of variables upon production of antibiotic activity by naturally occurring isolates. The analysis reported in Table 2 indicated that for general production of antibiotic activity incubation for 14 days was preferred to 7 days and supplementation with yeast extract was beneficial. Growing these fungi in a liquid medium with agitation resulted in a very strong tendency to limit antibiotic production, as did supplementing the medium with KH_2PO_4. Adding glycerol and corn oil had what was described as a neutral effect upon antibiotic production.

One of the attractions of this experimental protocol in the formulation of screening media is that one can build upon the experience of a previous experiment. Using the results from Table 2, cultures were again grown on corn but in this case the corn was supplemented only with a solution of yeast extract. The fermentation was carried out for 14 days at 25°C. In this experiment we again looked at the effect of six variables upon antibiotic production (Table 3). Two of the variables, supplementing the fermentation with water after 7 days of incubation and supplementing with $FeSO_4 \cdot 7H_2O$, resulted in

Table 3

Production of antibiotic activity by fungi – II

Variable	High value[a]	Low value[a]	% Significance
H_2O at 7 days (ml)	20	0	94
$FeSO_4 \cdot 7H_2O$ (g)	0.01	0	84
$MgSO_4 \cdot 7H_2O$ (g)	0.10	0	−50
Sodium tartrate (g)	0.10	0	−70
$ZnSO_4 \cdot 7H_2O$ (g)	0.01	0	−80
Agitation (rpm)	220	0	−84

[a] All values per 250 ml Erlenmeyer flask which contains 10.0 g corn and 15.0 ml of a 33 g/l solution of yeast extract. Incubation for 14 days at 25°C.

more fungal isolates producing antibiotic activity than when they were not included in the medium. Agitation again appeared to inhibit general antibiotic synthesis. Supplementation with $ZnSO_4 \cdot 7H_2O$, sodium tartrate and $MgSO_4 \cdot 7H_2O$ had negative effects upon general antibiotic synthesis. At this point it was instructive to compare the extremes of our results. Cultures grown in these experiments under an optimal set of conditions described above, that is with yeast extract and $FeSO_4 \cdot 7H_2O$, supplementation after 7 days with water and incubation for a total of 14 days without agitation, produced 17 times more antibiotic activity than cultures grown under a less than optimal set of conditions, of added $ZnSO_4 \cdot 7H_2O$ and sodium tartrate, and incubation with agitation for 7 days in a liquid medium.

Fermentations containing multiple activities

In a screen for secondary metabolites that involves testing fermentation broths for many types of activity it is not unusual for a fermentation broth to be reported as positive by more than one screening assay. It is also not uncommon for a fermentation broth to contain more than one active chemical compound. The challenge at the screening stage of a project is not to spend time on characterization of the fermentation that contains a single compound with multiple nonspecific activities. The Plackett & Burman protocol can be used to help in the early determination of whether a fermentation contains one compound with multiple activities or more than one compound responsible for different activities.

In one of our cultures, two activities were detected in the first fermentation of the culture. An experiment was run to see whether we could find a relationship between these activities using the Placket & Burman experimental design. We reasoned that if the two activities were due to the same (or a very similar) compound then the analysis of variables would exhibit a very close similarity. On the other hand, if the two activities were due to different compounds, the analysis would not be expected to show a strong similarity. The data outlined in Table 4 very strongly suggested that for this culture the two activities were caused by the same

Table 4

Search for mixtures in a fermentation containing antifungal activity

Variable	% Significance	
	antifungal effect 1	antifungal effect 2
Polyglycol		
P2000	98	96
Ardamine pH	96	96
Glycerol	86	82
Lard water	78	82
Dextrose	75	82
Corn meal	73	82
Sodium citrate	65	82
$CoCl_2 \cdot 6H_2O$	81	0
Tomato paste	48	0
Glycine	40	0
Corn steep	29	0
Soybean meal	24	0
Pectin	16	0
KH_2PO_4	−21	−82
Cod liver oil	−89	−82
$(NH_4)_2SO_4$	−99	−98

Table 5

Production of two antibiotics by *S. cattleya*

Variable	% Significance	
	Thienamycin	L-681,217
$(NH_4)_2SO_4$	99	−99
Glycerol	99	99
Lard water	95	99
Peptonized milk	94	95
Ardamine pH	94	99
Dextrose	93	98
Corn steep	80	−73
$CoCl_2 \cdot 6H_2O$	32	−34
Pectin	−12	99
Peanut meal	−15	−23
Glycine	−15	17
Tomato paste	−39	−24
KH_2PO_4	−57	96
Soy flour	−78	−94
Cod liver oil	−96	−99
Distillers solubles	−97	64

compound. With the exception of one variable out of 16 tested, the variables' significance levels of the two activities were parallel when listed in order of significance. Subsequent isolation of the active compound confirmed the presumption that both activities were due to one compound.

An analysis of the production of thienamycin [3] and the antibiotic L-681,217 [4] is an example of what occurs when two detected activities are due to two compounds (Table 5). In this case, there is an overall similarity of response for many of the variables; however, for five variables there is an opposite response and for two others a markedly different response depending upon whether the analysis is done using a measure of thienamycin activity or a measure of L-681,217 activity. $(NH_4)_2SO_4$, corn steep liquor, pectin, KH_2PO_4 and distillers solubles affected the synthesis of thienamycin and L-681,217 in opposite ways in this study.

Similarity between complex fermentation ingredients

All fermentation microbiologists have the problem of having available to them hundreds of complex medium ingredients to evaluate in formulating their particular fermentation media. Often, one will be asked by a manufacturer to see whether their latest product is a worthwhile medium component substitute. In most cases, the fermentation microbiologist evaluates the source of the complex ingredient and the compositional analysis provided by the manufacturer to determine whether a particular nutrient is likely to have a desirable characteristic. In the end, however, only a test of the ingredient determines suitability for a particular fermentation. This is often done empirically using one-for-one substitution in the current medium. We wondered whether the Plackett & Burman protocol would make such a testing process more efficient and whether it would perhaps tell us whether unrelated complex fermentation ingredients could give similar results in a particular fermentation. We decided to test 16 complex nitrogen sources in three different antibiotic fermentations where these nitrogen sources were added, according to the Plackett & Burman array, to a basal medium containing a carbon source. All 16 nitrogen sources used in these experiments were from samples supplied by Marcor Development Co., Hackensack, NJ. Five milk products were tested: whole milk, casein B, lactalbumin, acid casein and casein M. Of these only acid casein and casein M showed similar effects in all three fermentations (Table 6). Two unrelated nitrogen sources, soy peptone and gelatin, showed responses comparable to acid casein and casein M. For these three fermentations, they could be considered reasonable substitutes for each other. Interestingly, the response produced by pancreatic gelatin was comparable to that produced by gelatin in two of the three fermentations only. Results for soy flour and soy peptone were not close in these three fermentations. Three meat products were also tested in this experiment: meat peptone PS, meat peptone 4820 and liver nf. The peptones showed opposite responses. Liver had an overall response closer to meat peptone PS than meat peptone 4820. Alfalfa, whole egg and torula yeast were products with unique responses shown in these three fermentations. These experiments confirmed to us what we had suspected, that for most complex fermentation ingredients one can assume little. They all should be tested. The Plackett & Burman procedure may, however, make that process more efficient.

Use to increase titers

The Plackett & Burman technique was designed to allow the investigator to test the significance of a large number of variables in a relatively small number of experiments. We have used this technique most often to rapidly increase product titers of new fermentations. The procedure we follow uses a Plackett & Burman array to determine the significant fermentation variables and then combines these variables in an optimization protocol. The power of this two-phase procedure is best exemplified by the production of mevinolin [1]. The culture *Aspergillus terreus* (ATCC 20542) was grown in 20 fermentation media with 16 complex ingredient variables using a Plackett & Burman array. The results (Table 7) indicated that six variables had a strong positive effect upon titer and that five variables exerted a net negative effect. The

Table 6

Complex medium ingredients – substitution

Variable	% Significance		
	culture 1	culture 2	culture 3
Whole milk	91	75	−97
Casein B	−90	63	0
Lactalbumin	−53	91	69
Acid casein	75	63	69
Casein M	93	75	69
Soy peptone	59	99	69
Gelatin	59	75	91
Pancreatic gelatin	64	0	91
Soy flour (50% protein)	88	−25	−69
Alfalfa	−72	0	69
Corn grits	−92	−47	69
Meat peptone PS	89	−93	69
Meat peptone 4820	−92	47	0
Liver nf	53	−95	−91
Whole egg	−47	−82	0
Torula yeast	97	−25	0

Table 7

Mevinolin fermentation – Placket & Burman

Ingredient	% Significance
Tomato paste	99
Ardamine pH	94
Glycerol	94
KH_2PO_4	91
Dextrose	90
Cod liver oil	89
Dummy	−
Dummy	−
Glycine	4
Corn steep	−4
Soybean meal	−11
Lard water	−19
Sodium citrate	−47
Dummy	−
$(NH_4)_2SO_4$	−59
Polyglycol P2000	−75
Corn meal	−78
Pectin	−94
$CoCl_2 \cdot 6H_2O$	−96
Titer range (mg/l)	0 − 152

dummy or null variables in this experiment were as expected in a valid run, found in the middle of the list of variables listed in order of their significance. The titer range across this experiment of 20 fermentations was from 0 to 152 mg/l. The top six variables from this experiment were then combined with four other variables in an array outlined in Table 8. Titers in this experiment ranged from 96 to 1129 mg/l. Mean titer from experiment 1 to experiment 2 increased from 30 mg/l to 311 mg/l, a 10-fold increase!

Production of the same products by different micro-organisms

We compared three thienamycin producers for their response to 16 fermentation ingredients using the Plackett & Burman design. The cultures tested were: *Streptomyces cattleya* (NRRL 8057), the original soil isolate found to produce thienamycin [3]; *S. cattleya* (ATCC 39203), a culture isolated from nature found to produce thienamycin and the antibiotic L-681,217 [4]; and *S. penemifaciens* (ATCC 31599), a culture reported by Tanaka *et al.* to produce thienamycin [6]. The results of this comparison are outlined in Table 9.

At $P=0.1$ *S. cattleya* (NRRL 8057) had eight significant variables. Six of these were also significant variables for *S. cattleya* (ATCC 39203). Only

from nature found to produce thienamycin and the antibiotic L-681,217 [4]; and *S. penemifaciens* (ATCC 31599), a culture reported by Tanaka *et al.* to produce thienamycin [6]. The results of this comparison are outlined in Table 9.

At $P=0.1$ *S. cattleya* (NRRL 8057) had eight significant variables. Six of these were also significant variables for *S. cattleya* (ATCC 39203). Only one of the eight (dextrose) was a significant positive variable when *S. penemifaciens* was analyzed for its production of thienamycin. Three of the eight significant variables for *S. cattleya* (NRRL 8057) were not significant variables for the other two producers.

S. cattleya (ATCC 39203) had ten significant variables at $P=0.1$ for its production of thienamycin. Five variables were significant for both *S. cattleya* (ATCC 39203) and *S. penemifaciens*. Four different variables were significant for both *S. cattleya* (ATCC 39203) and *S. cattleya* (NRRL 8057). One variable (dextrose) was significant for all three cultures. Pectin was uniquely significant for *S. cattleya* (ATCC 39203). *S. penemifaciens* had six significant variables at $P=0.1$. $CoCl_2 \cdot 6H_2O$ was the only uniquely significant variable. Thus in this study it appeared that production of the same compound by different cultures was not optimized by the same production medium. Separate natural isolates of

Table 8

Mevinolin fermentation – optimization

| Ingredient | Medium | | | | | | | | | |
	S1	S2	S3	S4	S5	S6	S7	S8	S9	S10
Dextrose (g/l)	75	75	75	75	50	50	50	100	100	100
Ardamine pH (g/l)	4	8	12	16	4	8	12	16	12	8
Glycerol (ml/l)	5	5	5	5	7.5	7.5	7.5	2.5	2.5	0
KH_2PO_4 (g/l)	1	2	4	1	2	4	0	1	2	4
Cod liver oil (ml/l)	0	1	2	0	1	2	0	1	2	0
Tomato paste (g/l)	5	20	0	5	20	0	5	20	0	12
Sodium acetate (g/l)	1	2	1	2	0	1	2	0	2	0
Methyl oleate (ml/l)	2	1	0	2	1	0	2	1	0	0
$CuSO_4 \cdot 4H_2O$ (mg/l)	5	5	0	0	5	5	0	0	5	5
$FeSO_4 \cdot 7H_2O$ (mg/l)	5	5	5	0	0	5	5	0	0	5
Titer (mg/l)	96	618	1044	1129	154	823	881	450	764	275

Table 9

Thienamycin production

Variable	% Significance		
	S. cattleya (NRRL 8057)	S. cattleya (ATCC 39203)	S. penemifaciens (ATCC 31599)
$(NH_4)_2SO_4$	99	3	16
Glycerol	99	95	26
Lard water	95	95	−76
Peptonized milk	94	3	−48
Ardamine pH	94	−94	−94
Dextrose	93	97	96
Corn steep	80	89	−1
$CoCl_2 \cdot 6H_2O$	32	22	98
Pectin	−12	−97	−87
Peanut meal	−15	89	−36
Glycine	−15	−97	−93
Tomato paste	−39	99	99
KH_2PO_4	−57	94	98
Soy flour	−78	25	−55
Cod liver oil	−96	−94	−63
Distillers solubles	−97	−94	56

the same species produced different titers of identical secondary metabolites under the same fermentation conditions.

DISCUSSION

The Plackett & Burman experimental technique does not always appear to work. If none or only a few of the fermentations one attempts in an experiment produce the activity of interest then the experiment is not successful. When activity is produced in most fermentations, on occasion an analysis of significance can be disappointing. This may occur if the difference between the high and low level of each variable is not large enough to ensure a measurable response. Some sensitive variables on the other hand may have their high and low levels chosen such that the size of their differential response is so great as to mask the effect of other variables.

When variables have low significance and the dummy or null variables are scattered the results indicate to the investigator that significant uncontrolled variables exist. The following uncontrolled variables have been found to affect Plackett & Burman analysis results: a contaminated culture, loss of power to shaker machines, an unstable culture, production of an assay artifact and marked assay variability. Results such as these have also been seen when the variables tested truly do not have significant positive or negative effects upon the measure used. For example, we tested the effect of some trace metal ions upon a culture's secondary metabolite production and on the final pH of the culture broth after fermentation. Results were significant for production of the secondary metabolite but were not significant when final pH was the measure (data not shown).

The Plackett & Burman method can be prone to a 'compounding' of effects. That is, two variables when tested apart may manifest little or no effect on the response; however, when tested together a much larger effect may be seen. Analysis of these responses by this method may yield biased estimates of the effects. Further experimentation must be done to ensure that the observed effects are meaningful. Titer optimization protocols are a good way to confirm suspected compounding of effects.

Prior to using the Plackett & Burman experimental protocol for the design and early optimization of fermentation conditions, a fermentation scientist often relied upon the literature and personal experience exclusively to do this job. Using the Plackett & Burman experimental protocol has resulted in increased detection of antibiotic producers, optimization of fermentation titers, and an ability to predict the presence of mixtures and to select substitutes for complex medium ingredients.

ACKNOWLEDGEMENTS

The authors wish to acknowledge Dr. J.A. Bland for thienamycin assays, Dr. C.H. Hoffman and M. Lopez for mevinolin assays and A. Kempf for L-681,217 assays. We further wish to acknowledge

Dr. S. Hernandez and the CIBE group at Madrid, Spain for the fungal cultures screening data and Dr. E.O. Stapley for his counsel and enthusiastic support of this project.

REFERENCES

1 Alberts, A.W., J. Chen, G. Kurov, V. Hunt, J. Huff, C. Hoffman, J. Rothrock, M. Lopez, H. Joshua, E. Harris, A. Patchett, R. Monaghan, S. Currie, E. Stapley, G. Albers-Schonberg, O. Hensens, J. Hirschfield, K. Hoogsteen, J. Liesch and J. Springer. 1980. Mevinolin, a highly potent competitive inhibitor of HMG-CoA reductase and cholesterol lowering agent. Proc. Natl. Acad. Sci. USA 77:3957–3961.

2 Greasham, R. and E. Inamine. 1986. Nutritional improvement of processes. In: Manual of Industrial Microbiology and Biotechnology (Demain, A.L. and N.A. Solomon, eds.), pp. 41–48, American Society for Microbiology, Washington, DC.

3 Kahan, J.S., F.M. Kahan, R. Goegelman, S.A. Currie, M. Jackson, E.O. Stapley, T.W. Miller, A.K. Miller, D. Hendlin, S. Mochales, S. Hernandez, H.B. Woodruff and J. Birnbaum. 1979. Thienamycin, a new β-lactam antibiotic. I. Discovery, taxonomy, isolation and physical properties. J. Antibiot. 32: 1–12.

4 Kempf, A.J., K.E. Wilson, O.D. Hensens, R.L. Monaghan, S.B. Zimmerman and E.L. Dulaney. 1986. L-681,217, a new and novel member of efrotomycin family of antibiotics. J. Antibiot. 39: 1361–1367.

5 Stowe, R.A. and R.P. Mayer. 1966. Efficient screening of process variables. Ind. Eng. Chem. 58: 36–40.

6 Tanaka, K., N. Tsuji, E. Kondo and Y. Kawamura. 1983. Fermentation production of thienamycin using *Streptomyces penemifaciens*. U.S. Patent 4371617.

Novel Microbial Products for Medicine and Agriculture
Editors: A.L. Demain, G.A. Somkuti, J.C. Hunter-Cevera and H.W. Rossmoore
© 1989, Society for Industrial Microbiology

CHAPTER 3

Screening of cardiovascular agents

Takeshi Andoh and Keizo Yoshida

Research Laboratories, Fujisawa Pharmaceutical Co., Ltd., Osaka, Japan

SUMMARY

We report on our recent screening studies for cardiovascular agents of microbial origin. WS-1228A and B are new hypotensive vasodilators which have been isolated from the culture product of *Streptomyces aureofaciens* and have an *N*-hydroxytriazene moiety. Their vasodilatory activity is the same as that of nitroglycerine. Amauromine is a unique alkaloid with vasodilatory activity similar to that of calcium antagonists. It has two reversed prenyl groups in its molecule and is a product of *Amauroascus* sp. WF-10129 is an angiotensin converting enzyme (ACE) inhibitor resembling enalaprilat, and is a substituted *N*-carboxymethyl dipeptide obtained from *Doratomyces putredinis*. FR-900452 is a platelet activating factor (PAF) antagonist having an unusual vinylogous diketopiperazine moiety, 5-(2-oxocyclopent-3-en-1-ylidene)-2-oxopiperazine; it was isolated from the fermentation products of *S. phaeofaciens*. Vinigrol is a unique diterpenoid with antihypertensive and platelet aggregation inhibiting activities, and is the first example of the decahydro-1,5-butanonaphthalene structural type; it was obtained from *Virgaria nigra*. These non-antibiotic cardiovascular agents of microbial origin are particularly interesting in view of their potential usefulness in such cardiovascular diseases as hypertension, angina pectoris, heart failure, thrombosis and endotoxin shock. Some synthetic derivatives of these natural products are now in late-preclinical studies.

INTRODUCTION

In view of the impressive biosynthetic ingenuity of microorganisms, the natural products synthesized by microorganisms with widely divergent chemical structures would be expected to have a broad range of pharmacological activities. Among pharmacologically active non-antibiotic natural products, those which show hypotensive and platelet aggregation inhibitory effects are particularly interesting in view of their potential usefulness in hypertension, angina pectoris, heart failure, thrombosis and endotoxin shock. In this paper, we report on our recent screening studies in new and extended areas of non-antibiotic cardiovascular agents of microbial origin, that is, a nitro-compound-like vasodilator, WS-1228 [38], a calcium antagonist, amauromine [28], an angiotensin converting enzyme (ACE) inhibitor, WF-10129 [1], a platelet activating factor (PAF) antagonist, FR-900452 [21] and a unique diterpenoid with antihypertensive and platelet aggregation inhibitory activities, vinigrol [2].

MATERIALS AND METHODS

Aorta-superfusion method

Male Sprague-Dawley rats aged 8–10 weeks were

stunned and bled to death and the thoracic aorta was quickly removed. After removing the fatty tissues, spiral strips (2 mm wide and 40 mm long) were made from the aorta and suspended under a resting tension of 1 g in 30 ml organ baths containing warm (37°C), oxygenated (95% O_2/5% CO_2) Tyrode solution of the following composition: NaCl 137 mM, KCl 2.7 mM, $CaCl_2$ 1.8 mM, $MgCl_2$ 1.02 mM, $NaHCO_3$ 11.9 mM, NaH_2PO_4 0.42 mM and glucose 5.55 mM. The tissues were equilibrated for about 90 min and then superfused with Tyrode solution containing a low concentration of noradrenaline (150 nM) or KCl (30 mM), to increase the tension of the tissues by about 500 mg. Changes of tension of the tissues were measured isometrically by force displacement transducers connected to a polygraph. The intensity of relaxation activity was standardized with papaverine (100 μM) which produced 100% dilation.

ACE assay

The ACE activity was measured fluorimetrically according to the method of Carmel *et al.* [8] with slight modification. *O*-Aminobenzoylglycyl-*p*-nitro-L-phenylalanyl-L-proline (ABz-Gly-Phe(NO$_2$)-Pro) was used as a substrate and diluted guinea pig serum was used as an enzyme source. In the routine assay, 200 μl of substrate solution containing 0.58 mM of ABz-Gly-Phe(NO$_2$)-Pro, 1 M NaCl and 0.2 M Tris-HCl buffer, pH 8.2, was mixed with 10 μl of fermentation broth and 40 μl of diluted guinea pig serum.

Platelet aggregation assay

Rabbit blood was collected through a polyethylene catheter from the carotid artery of a male white Japanese rabbit into a plastic tube that contained one volume of 3.8% sodium citrate to nine volumes of blood. After obtaining the platelet-rich plasma by centrifugation, the platelet number was adjusted to 5×10^5 cells/mm^3 by adding platelet-poor plasma. Human blood was collected from the antecubital vein of healthy volunteers and the platelet number adjusted to 3×10^5 cells/mm^3. Platelet aggregation was measured turbidimetrically with a platelet aggregation tracer (Niko Bioscience, Inc.)

at 37°C. Platelet aggregation agents used in these experiments were epinephrine 0.4 mM plus ADP 0.4 μM, PAF 20 nM, ADP 2.5 μM, bovine thrombin 0.5 U/ml and collagen 10 μg/ml for rabbit platelet aggregation, and epinephrine 5 μM, PAF 1.5 μM and ADP 2.5 μM for the human platelet test.

Blood pressure and heart rate measurement

Male Sprague-Dawley rats weighing 350–400 g were anesthetized with urethane (1 g/kg, i.p.). Arterial blood pressure was measured with a pressure transducer via a polyethylene catheter (PE50) inserted into the femoral artery. Blood pressure was recorded on a polygraph. The pulse pressure signal was used to trigger a tachometer for measuring heart rate. The active compound present in a fermentation broth or in a preparation thereof was detected by its hypotensive effect. To confirm the antihypertensive activity, the test sample was injected intravenously through a polyethylene catheter inserted into a femoral vein.

Antihypertensive action in conscious spontaneously hypertensive rats (SHR)

Male SHR weighing 260–300 g were anesthetized with ether and a polyethylene catheter (PE10 connected to PE50) was inserted from the femoral artery into the abdominal aorta. The catheter was held in place by a ligature around the femoral artery. In addition, the catheter was sutured to the surrounding muscle and exteriorized on the dorsal surface of the neck. This surgery was performed 2 days before measuring blood pressure. The mean arterial blood pressure of conscious SHR was measured from the implanted catheter with a pressure transducer connected to a polygraph.

RESULTS AND DISCUSSION

WS-1228A and B

We screened culture filtrates of various microorganisms by the aorta-superfusion technique [11]. This method, which is frequently used in research on prostaglandins, allowed us to detect active compounds quantitatively in a short time. From the culture filtrate of an actinomycete classified as *Streptomyces aureofaciens* (ATCC 31442), new vasodilators named WS-1228A and B have been discovered [38]. The active compounds were purified by column chromatography with Diaion HP-20 and silica gel, and finally separated by HPLC. They were obtained as pale yellow crystals and their molecular formulae were both $C_{11}H_{17}N_3O$ (Table 1). The structure of WS-1228B was determined as 1-hydroxy-3-[(2*E*,4*E*,6*E*)-2,4,6-undecatrienylidene] triazene (Fig. 1), on the basis of spectral and chemical evidence and synthesis [30]. To our knowledge, WS-1228A and B are the first naturally occurring compounds possessing a triazene group. They showed strong vasodilatory activity on rat aorta contracted by norepinephrine (Table 2). The activity of WS-1228B was markedly stronger than that of WS-1228A, and its mechanism of relaxation would appear to be similar to that of nitro compounds. We developed chemical variations of this prototype

Table 1

Physico-chemical properties of WS-1228A and B

	WS-1228A	WS-1228B
Appearance	yellow needles	yellow needles
m.p. (°C)	100–102	135–138
Molecular formula	$C_{11}H_{17}N_3O$	$C_{11}H_{17}N_3O$
Molecular weight	207	207
Elemental analysis		
found	C 63.88	C 63.46
	H 8.28	H 8.23
	N 20.09	N 20.51
calcd.	C 63.74	C 63.74
	H 8.27	H 8.27
	N 20.27	N 20.27
UV λ_{max} nm (ε)	300 (44 000)	339 (43 000)
Color reaction	$FeCl_3$	$FeCl_3$

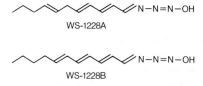

WS-1228A

WS-1228B

Fig. 1. Structures of WS-1228A and B.

Table 2

Relaxation of rat aorta superfused with Tyrode solution containing noradrenaline (NA; 150 nM) or KCl (30 mM)

Sample (μg/ml)	NA tone[a]		KCl tone[b]	
	relaxation (mg)	duration (min)	relaxation (mg)	duration (min)
WS 1228B				
0.1	420	10	200	20
0.05	190	10	n.t.	n.t.
Nifedipine				
0.15	150	45	n.t.	n.t.
0.075	n.t.[c]	n.t.	300	50

[a] The aorta was separated from a male Sprague-Dawley rat weighing 270 g and superfused with Tyrode solution containing noradrenaline (150 nM) which increased the tension of the tissue by 490 mg.

[b] The aorta was separated from a male Sprague-Dawley rat weighing 260 g and superfused with Tyrode solution containing KCl (30 mM) which increased the tension of the tissue by 510 mg.

[c] n.t. = not tested.

for optimal vasodilatory and platelet aggregation inhibiting activities and obtained a good candidate. It is now in late-preclinical study for angina pectoris. WS-1228B showed no antimicrobial activity at a concentration of 100 μg/ml against *Escherichia coli, Staphylococcus aureus*, or *Candida albicans*, and acute toxicity in ddy mice was above 250 mg/kg, i.p.

Amauromine

We also screened culture filtrates of fungi for vasodilatory activity on high-potassium depolarized rat aorta. This preparation was suitable for detecting calcium antagonists. From the culture broth of a fungus classified as *Amauroascus* sp. (ATCC 20595), a new alkaloid with vasodilatory activity, named amauromine, was isolated [28]. The active compound was purified by extraction with ethyl acetate, column chromatography with silica gel, and finally separated by recrystallization from ethanol. Amauromine was obtained as colorless prisms and its molecular formula was $C_{32}H_{36}N_4O_2$ (Table 3). Its structure was determined chemically and spectroscopically to be (5aS, 7aS, 8aR, 13aS, 15aS, 16aR)-8a,16a-bis-(1,1-dimethyl-2-propenyl)-5a,8,8a,13,13a,15a,16,16a-octahydropyrazino[1″, 2″:1,5;- 4″,5″:1′,5′]dipyrrolo-[2,3-b:2′,3′-b′]-diindole-7,15(5H,7aH)-dione [29] and it was fully synthesized [27] (Fig. 2). Amauromine is a unique dimeric alkaloid consisting of a hexahydropyrrolo indole skeleton and possessing a reversed prenyl group at position 3 of the indole nucleus. In tests on isolated vascular smooth muscle, amauromine relaxed rat aortic strips contracted with KCl (50 mM) with an IC_{50} of 2.3×10^{-8} M, but not norepinephrine-induced contractions (Fig. 3). According to the criteria proposed by Rahwan [24], amauromine can be classified as a novel calcium antagonist, about 4 times more potent than diltiazem, a standard calcium antagonist used clinically in hypertension and angina pectoris. As shown in Figs. 4 and 5, amauro-

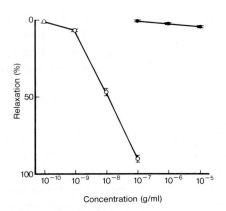

Fig. 3. Effect of amauromine on KCl- and norepinephrine-induced contraction of isolated rat aorta. ○, KCl; ●, norepinephrine.

mine produced clear antihypertensive effects in SHR at doses of 10 mg/kg, i.v. and 30 mg/kg, p.o. Further details of the pharmacological characteristics of amauromine indicating its unique profile as a novel calcium antagonist will be published in subsequent papers [12,13]. Amauromine showed no antimicrobial activity at a concentration of 1 mg/ml against *E. coli, Staph. aureus*, or *C. albicans*. Acute toxicity of amauromine in ddy mice was above 200 mg/kg, i.p.

WF-10129

Since the discovery and development of captopril

Table 3

Physico-chemical properties of amauromine

Appearance	colorless prisms
m.p. (°C)	156–158
$[\alpha]_D^{23}$ (c 1.0, CHCl$_3$)	$-583°$
UV (EtOH) λ_{max} nm (ε)	245 (11 000), 300 (4200)
IR (CHCl$_3$) cm^{-1}	3420, 2970, 1660, 1600, 1420, 1380, 1365, 920
Molecular formula	$C_{32}H_{36}N_4O_2$
Elemental analysis	
found	C 74.00, H 7.18, N 10.64
calcd. for $C_{32}H_{36}N_4O_2 \cdot \frac{1}{2}H_2O$	C 74.25, H 7.20, N 10.82
MS e/z	
obsd.	508.2825
calcd.	508.2840

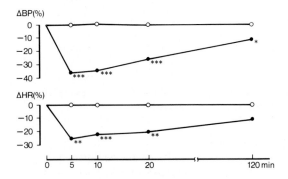

Fig. 4. Effect of intravenously administered amauromine on blood pressure and heart rate in conscious SHR. ○, vehicle control ($n=4$); ●, amauromine 10 mg/kg, i.v. ($n=4$). *, **, *** Significantly different from vehicle-treated group ($P<0.05$, $P<0.01$, $P<0.001$, respectively).

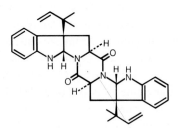

Fig. 2. Structure of amauromine.

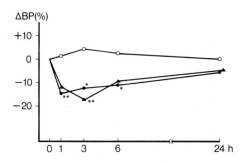

Fig. 5. Effect of orally administered amauromine on blood pressure in conscious SHR. ○, vehicle control ($n=4$); ●, amauromine 30 mg/kg, p.o. ($n=4$); ▲, amauromine 100 mg/kg, p.o. ($n=4$). *, ** Significantly different from vehicle-treated group ($P<0.05$, $P<0.01$, respectively).

as a clinically important antihypertensive drug, many research groups have screened for novel ACE inhibitors from microbial products [6,7,14–20,34, 37]. In our screening studies, we isolated WF-10129 from a fungus classified as *Doratomyces putredinis* (FERM P-7303). This compound showed strong inhibition of ACE [1]. Most of the currently reported ACE inhibitors of microbial origin were produced from strains of actinomycetes [6,7,14–18,20,34,37], only aspergillomarasmine [19] and WF-10129 originating from fungi. WF-10129 was purified from the cultured filtrate by successive ion exchange chromatography and HPLC as shown in Fig. 6. WF-10129 was obtained as colorless powder and its molecular formula was $C_{20}H_{28}N_2O_8$ (Table 4). Its structure was elucidated chemically and spectroscopically to be *N*-[*N*-(1-carboxy-6-hydroxy-3-oxo-heptyl)-L-alanyl]-L-tyrosine (Fig. 7). WF-10129 is a substituted *N*-carboxymethyl dipeptide similar in structure to the potent synthetic ACE inhibitor, enalaprilat (Fig. 8). WF-10129 inhibited ACE in a dose-dependent manner and its IC_{50} was 1.4×10^{-8} M, indicating that it is one of the most potent ACE inhibitors of microbial origin. The IC_{50} for captopril was 1.7×10^{-8} M in a similar experiment. The kinetic study of WF-10129 was carried out and the Dixon plot and Lineweaver-Burk plot for ACE inhibition are shown in Figs. 9 and 10, respectively. WF-10129 was a competitive inhibitor of ACE with a K_i value of 8×10^{-9} M. It was tested intravenously at a dose of 0.3 mg/kg in anesthetized normoten-

Filtrate
|
Dowex 1-X2 (OH⁻)
| eluted with 0.1 M HCl
Dowex 50W-X2 (H⁺)
| eluted with 0.1 M NaCl
Active carbon
| eluted with 80% Me₂CO
DEAE-Sephadex A-25 (PO₄³⁻)
| eluted with 0.03 M NaCl
| pH was adjusted to 2
Diaion HP-20
| eluted with 70% aq. MeOH
CM-Sephadex C-25 (H⁺)
| eluted with H₂O
Sephadex G-15
| eluted with 1% AcOH
HPLC

Isolation of WF-10129 by HPLC

Stationary phase	Cosmosil C_{18} (10 × 250 mm, Nakarai Chemicals Co., Ltd.)
Mobile phase	8% Acetonitrile in 0.05% TFA
Flow rate	5 ml/min
Detector	UV at 254 nm
Retention time	20 min

Fig. 6. Isolation procedure of WF-10129. TFA = trifluoroacetic acid.

Table 4

Physico-chemical properties of WF-10129

Appearance	colorless powder
m.p. (°C)	90–95
Molecular formula	$C_{20}H_{28}N_2O_8$
SI-MS (m/z)	425 (M+H)⁺, 447 (M+Na)⁺
$[\alpha]_D^{23}$ (c 0.375, H₂O)	+ 12.9°
UV: $\lambda_{max}^{H_2O}$ nm (ε)	275 (1060), 280 (930)
$\lambda_{max}^{H_2O+HCl}$ nm	275, 280
$\lambda_{max}^{H_2O+NaOH}$ nm	277, 283, 292
IR: ν_{max}^{KBr} cm⁻¹	3350, 2950, 3000–2300(br), 1720, 1680, 1620, 1540, 1520, 1445, 1380, 1350, 1260, 1230, 1110, 910, 880, 830
TLCᵃ (R_f value)	
BuOH/AcOH/H₂O (4:1:2)	0.4
2-PrOH/H₂O (8:2)	0.6

ᵃStationary phase: silica gel sheet.

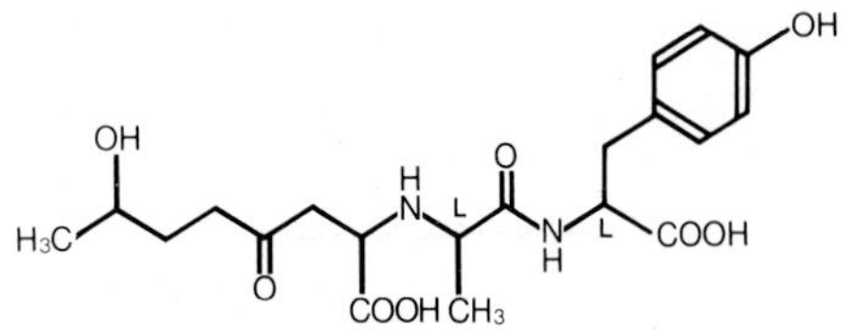

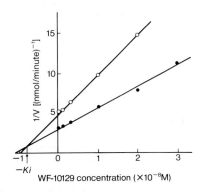

Fig. 7. Structure of WF-10129.

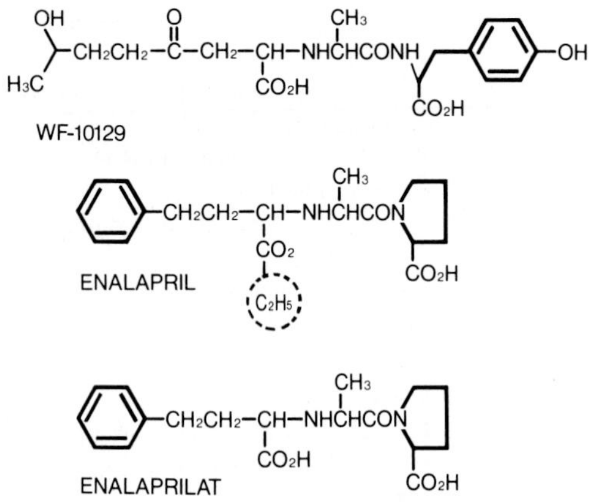

WF-10129

ENALAPRIL

ENALAPRILAT

Fig. 8. Chemical structures of WF-10129, enalapril (MK-421) and enalaprilat (MK-422).

Fig. 9. Dixon plot of inhibition of ACE by WF-10129. Substrate concentration (ABz-Gly-Phe(NO$_2$)-Pro): ●, 0.23 mM; ○, 0.115 mM.

sive rats. As shown in Table 5, WF-10129 inhibited angiotensin I-induced pressor response significantly but had no effect on angiotensin II-induced pressor response.

FR-900452

PAF (1-*O*-alkyl-2-acetyl-*sn*-glycero-3-phospho-

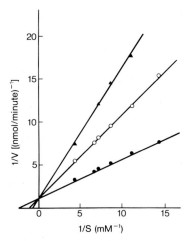

Fig. 10. Lineweaver-Burk plot of inhibition of ACE by WF-10129. WF-10129 concentration: ●, no inhibitor; ○, WF-10129 (1 × 10^{-8} M); ▲, WF-10129 (2 × 10^{-8} M).

Table 5

Inhibition of angiotensin I pressor response by WF-10129 in rats

Dose	Inhibition (%) of angiotensin I[a] response		
	10 min	40 min	50 min
300 μg/kg, i.v.	74.4 ± 5.9	36.9 ± 6.5	25.8 ± 10.3

Results are presented as mean ± S.E. (*n*=4).
[a] 1 μg/kg, i.v.

choline) is a substance secreted by the cells involved in the allergic and inflammatory processes [35], and is an extremely potent inducer of platelet aggregation [9], hypotension [4] and bronchoconstriction [36] (Fig. 11). Recent reports suggest that endogenous PAF is involved in the pathogenesis of endotoxin shock in rats [10]. In our screening program for potential PAF inhibitors [5,25,31], we have tested a wide range of fermented broths for inhibitory effects on PAF-induced rabbit platelet aggregation. As a result, FR-900452 was isolated from the fermentation products of *S. phaeofaciens* (FERM-BP-660) [21]. FR-900452 was purified by extraction with ethyl acetate, column chromatography with silica gel, and finally separated using a pre-packed Lobar silica gel column (E. Merck). It

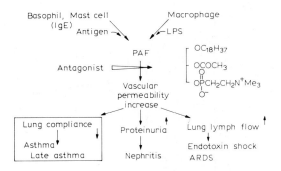

Fig. 11. Strategy for the evaluation of a PAF antagonist in an animal model. LPS = lipopolysaccharide. ARDS = ●—●

was obtained as a pale yellow powder and its molecular formula was $C_{22}H_{25}N_3O_3S$ (Table 6). Its structure was deduced by using chemical modifications, spectroscopic measurements and an X-ray crystal analysis of its dihydro derivative [33] to be (2S,10S,12S,14R)-1-methyl-3-[1-[5-methylthiomethyl-6-oxo-3-(2-oxo-3-cyclopenten-1-ylidene)-2-piperazinyl]ethyl]-2-indolinone (Fig. 12). The oxocyclo-pentenylidene group incorporated as a vinylogous amide in the diketopiperazine skeleton is unique and, as far as we are aware, FR-900452 is the first example of this structural type. It specifically inhibited PAF-induced rabbit platelet aggregation with an IC_{50} of 3.7×10^{-7} M, but was much less active against collagen-, arachidonic acid- or ADP-induced aggregation (IC_{50}: 6.4×10^{-5}, $> 10^{-4}$ or $> 10^{-4}$ M, respectively) (Table 7). As shown in Table 8, FR-900452 at doses of 1 and 10 mg/kg, i.v. given 3 min before PAF injection (1 μg/kg), significantly prevented the PAF-induced hypotension (57% and 96% inhibitions, respectively) [22].

Table 6

Physico-chemical properties of FR-900452

Appearance	pale yellow powder
m.p. (°C)	112–120 (decomp.)
$[\alpha]_D^{23}$ (c 0.5, CHCl$_3$)	+97.0°
UV (MeOH) λ_{max} nm (ε)	246 (13 600), 347 (14 500)
IR (CHCl$_3$) cm^{-1}	3350, 3000, 2900, 1670, 1610, 1595, 1490, 1470, 1445, 1380, 1350, 1340, 1310, 1297, 1220
Molecular formula	$C_{22}H_{25}N_3O_3S$
MS e/z	
obsd.	411.1567
calcd.	411.1618

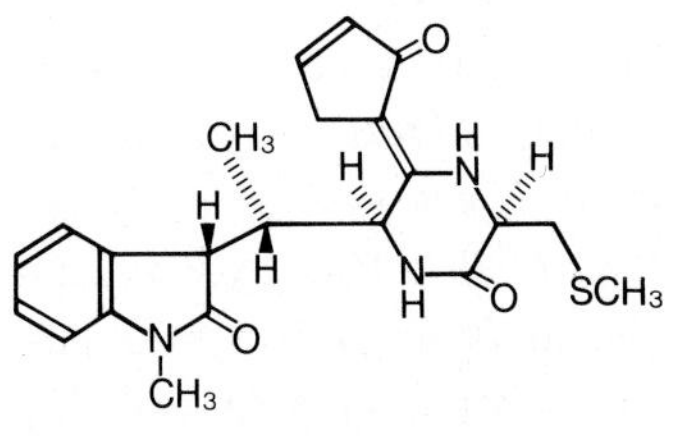

Table 7

Inhibition of rabbit platelet aggregation by FR-900452 and tiaramide

Inducer	IC_{50} value (M)	
	FR-900452	tiaramide
PAF	3.7×10^{-7}	7.9×10^{-5}
Collagen	6.4×10^{-5}	3.3×10^{-6}
Arachidonic acid	$> 10^{-4}$	3.7×10^{-5}
ADP	$> 10^{-4}$	3.3×10^{-5}

Each drug was added 2 min before an aggregating agent, PAF (0.1 μM), collagen (2.5 μg/ml), arachidonic acid (100 μM) or ADP (2.5 μM). Results (n = 4) are presented as the concentration of each drug inhibiting maximal aggregation by 50%.

Table 8

Effects of FR-900452 and tiaramide on PAF-induced hypotension in rats

Drug	Dose (mg/kg)	Time of treatment (min)	n	MABP change (mmHg)	Inhibition (%)
Vehicle	–		8	58.1 ± 3.0	–
FR-900452	0.3	−3	4	53.3 ± 4.4	8
	1	−3	4	$25.0 \pm 7.6^*$	57
	10	−3	4	$2.5 \pm 7.6^*$	96
		−15	5	$11.3 \pm 4.3^*$	82
		−60	5	$33.8 \pm 1.3^*$	42
Tiaramide	10	−3	4	52.5 ± 2.5	10

Sprague-Dawley rats (7 weeks old) were anesthetized with urethane (700 mg/kg, i.p.). Drug and PAF (1 μg/kg) were administered i.v. Each value expresses the mean arterial blood pressure (MABP) change (means ± S.E.).
* Significantly different from the control (P < 0.001).

Fig. 12. Structure of FR-900452.

PAF (1 μg/kg) injected intravenously into anesthetized rabbits resulted in marked loss of circulating platelets and leukocytes, but this loss did not occur when 10 mg/kg of FR-900452 was given i.v. before the PAF injection (Fig. 13). Additionally we assessed the effect of FR-900452, which is a specific PAF inhibitor, on thrombocytopenia and leukopenia induced by bolus i.v. injection of *E. coli* endotoxin (0.03 mg/kg) in rabbits, since PAF is known to contribute to these two signs in endotoxin shock [23]. As shown in Fig. 14, pretreatment with the compound (10 mg/kg, i.v.) significantly reduced the thrombocytopenia at 60 and 180 min after endotoxin injection, but did not reduce the leukopenia. These results indicate that PAF might be involved in the occurrence of thrombocytopenia but not of leukopenia in rabbit endotoxemia. Further chemical variations of this new prototype for optimal PAF inhibitory activity as well as more detailed biological evaluations are in progress [26].

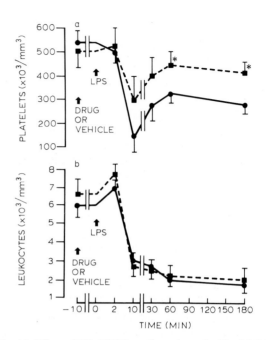

Fig. 14. Effect of FR-900452 on lipopolysaccharide (LPS)-induced thrombocytopenia (a) and leukopenia (b) in rabbits. ■, FR-900452 (10 mg/kg) + LPS (0.03 mg/kg); ●, vehicle + LPS. * Significantly different from vehicle-treated group ($P < 0.05$).

Vinigrol

In the course of our search for antihypertensive compounds with new mechanisms, we discovered the unique antihypertensive and platelet aggregation inhibiting compound vinigrol, by testing culture broths using anesthetized normotensive rats directly [2]. Vinigrol, produced by a fungal strain identified as *Virgaria nigra*, was extracted from the cultured mycelium, purified by extraction with ethyl acetate followed by chromatography on silica gel and then isolated as crystals from heptane and ethyl acetate. Vinigrol was obtained as colorless prisms and its molecular formula was $C_{20}H_{34}O_3$ (Table 9). The structure of vinigrol, a novel diterpenoid with antihypertensive and platelet aggregation inhibiting activities, has been determined by using chemical derivatizations, spectroscopic measurements, and an X-ray crystal analysis to be (1R, 4S,4aS,5S,8R,8aS,9R,12R)-3-hydroxymethyl-12-isopropyl-8,-9-dimethyl-1,4,4a,5,6,7,8,8a-octahydro-1,5-butanonaphthalene-4,8a-diol [32] (Fig. 15). The decahydro-1,5-butanonaphthalene skeleton of

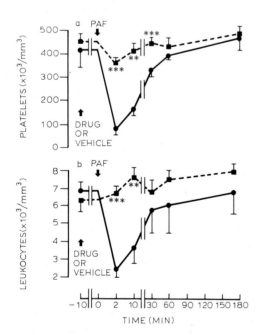

Fig. 13. Effect of FR-900452 on PAF-induced thrombocytopenia (a) and leukopenia (b) in rabbits. ■, FR-900452 (10 mg/kg) + PAF (1 μg/kg); ●, vehicle + PAF. **, *** Significantly different from vehicle-treated group ($P < 0.01$, $P < 0.001$, respectively).

Table 9

Physico-chemical properties of vinigrol

Appearance	colorless prisms
m.p. (°C)	108
$[\alpha]_D^{23}$ (c 1.05, CHCl$_3$)	$-96.2°$
UV (MeOH) λ_{max} nm (ε)	206 (13 000)
IR (CHCl$_3$) cm^{-1}	3450, 2960, 2940, 2870, 1670, 1460, 1380, 1370, 1140, 1100, 1010, 990, 970 (sh), 900
Molecular formula	C$_{20}$H$_{34}$O$_3$
Elemental analysis	
found	C 74.20, H 10.23
calcd. for C$_{20}$H$_{34}$O$_3$	C 74.49, H 10.63
FD-MS m/z	323 (M + H)$^+$

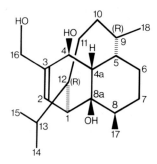

Fig. 15. Structure of vinigrol.

Table 10

Effect of vinigrol on rabbit and human platelet aggregation

Agonist	Rabbit PRP IC$_{50}$ (M)	Human PRP IC$_{50}$ (M)
Epinephrine	1.7×10^{-8}	5.2×10^{-8}
PAF	4.4×10^{-7}	3.3×10^{-8}
ADP	$>1 \times 10^{-6}$	$>1.0 \times 10^{-6}$
Thrombin	$>1 \times 10^{-6}$	n.t.
Collagen	$>1 \times 10^{-6}$	n.t.

Agonist concentration: rabbit – epinephrine 0.4 mM + ADP 0.4 μM, PAF 20 nM, ADP 2.5 μM thrombin 0.5 U/ml, collagen 10 μg/ml; human – epinephrine 5 μM, PAF 1.5 μM, ADP 2.5 μM. Each value is the mean of 3 or 4 determinations.
PRP = platelet-rich plasma; n.t. = not tested.

Table 11

Effect of vasodilators on rat aortic strips contracted with various agonists

Agonist	Antagonist			
	vinigrol (1.5×10^{-7} M)	clonidine (4×10^{-7} M)	phenyl-ephrine (5×10^{-7} M)	KCl (50 mM)
Nilvadipine	1.7×10^{-9}	8.8×10^{-10}	3.9×10^{-7}	9.3×10^{-10}
Prazosin	$>1 \times 10^{-4}$	8.4×10^{-10}	9.7×10^{-10}	$>3 \times 10^{-5}$
Yohimbine	$>3 \times 10^{-5}$	5.6×10^{-7}	4.9×10^{-7}	$>3 \times 10^{-5}$

ED$_{50}$ values (M) are presented, being the means of 3–5 determinations.

vinigrol is unprecedented, and, as far as we are aware, vinigrol is the first example of this structural type. In SHR, vinigrol at a p.o. dose of 2 mg/kg produced a marked and sustained hypotension of about 15% of the control over 6 h [3] (Fig. 16). Vinigrol also specifically inhibited PAF- and epinephrine-induced human platelet aggregation with IC$_{50}$ values of 3.3×10^{-8} M and 5.2×10^{-8} M, respectively (Table 10). It had no inhibitory effects on other aggregation agents such as ADP, thrombin and collagen, but evoked aggregation at higher concentrations ($>3 \times 10^{-6}$ M). The assay results from radio-receptor binding of vinigrol to α-adrenoceptors of rat cerebral membrane clearly showed that vinigrol had no affinity for these receptors [3]. Vinigrol induced contraction of rat aortic smooth muscle preparations at 1.5×10^{-7} M; this contraction was blocked by nilvadipine, a calcium blocker, but was not inhibited by prazosin or yohimbine (Table 11). From these results we suppose that vini-

grol is a partial calcium agonist showing inhibitory effects on calcium movement at low concentrations. More study is required in order to define conclusively the mode of action of vinigrol on calcium channels and also to clarify the mechanism of its antihypertensive activity. Vinigrol had a slight antimicrobial activity against *Bacillus subtilis* and *Staph. aureus* at 10 mg/ml, but no activities against *E. coli* or *C. albicans* at the same concentration. The LD$_{50}$ of vinigrol was 23 mg/kg, i.p. in ddy mice.

42

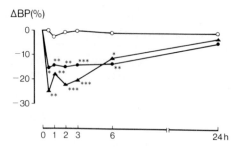

ΔBP(%)

Fig. 16. Effect of orally administered vinigrol on blood pressure in conscious SHR. ○, vehicle control ($n = 8$); ●, vinigrol 2 mg/kg, p.o. ($n = 5$); ▲, vinigrol 20 mg/kg, p.o. ($n = 3$). *, **, *** Significantly different from vehicle-treated group ($P < 0.05$, $P < 0.01$, $P < 0.001$, respectively).

CONCLUSION

The primary goal of any innovative research in the pharmaceutical industry is the identification of new chemical entities. Our intensified and systematic investigation should not only produce useful new pharmacological agents but also, equally important, provide medicinal chemists with new leads for structure-activity relationships. In fact, we have been developing the derivatives of WS-1228B and FR-900452 in late-preclinical studies for angina, endotoxin shock or asthma. If we have the resources to successfully tap the biosynthetic potential of microorganisms and sharpen our analytical tools to test pharmacological targets in a microbiological screening program, we will, in fact, be well prepared to detect many more unexpected compounds from microorganisms.

ACKNOWLEDGEMENT

The authors are indebted to Drs. H. Imanaka, H. Aoki and M. Kohsaka for their encouragement throughout this work.

REFERENCES

1 Ando, T., S. Okada, I. Uchida, K. Hemmi, M. Nishikawa, Y. Tsurumi, A. Fujie, K. Yoshida and M. Okuhara. 1987. WF-10129, a novel angiotensin converting enzyme inhibitor produced by a fungus, Doratomyces putredinis. J. Antibiot. 40: 468–475.

2 Ando, T., Y. Tsurumi, N. Ohata, I. Uchida, K. Yoshida and M. Okuhara. 1988. Vinigrol, a novel antihypertensive and platelet aggregation inhibitory agent produced by a fungus, Virgaria nigra. 1. Taxonomy, fermentation, isolation, physico-chemical and biological properties. J. Antibiot. 41: 25–30.

3 Ando, T., K. Yoshida and M. Okuhara. 1988. Vinigrol, a novel antihypertensive and platelet aggregation inhibitory agent produced by a fungus, Virgaria nigra. 2. Pharmacological characteristics. J. Antibiot. 41: 31–35.

4 Blank, M.L., F. Snyder, L.W. Byers, B. Brooks and E.E. Murirhead. 1979. Antihypertensive activity of an alkyl ether analog of phosphatidylcholine. Biochem. Biophys. Res. Commun. 90: 1194–1200.

5 Buftu, T., N.F. Gamble, T. Doebber, S.B. Hwang, T.Y. Shen, J. Snyder, J.P. Springer and R. Stevenson. 1986. Conformation and activity of tetrahydrofuran lignans and analogues as specific platelet activating factor antagonists. J. Med. Chem. 29: 1917–1921.

6 Bush, K., P.R. Henry and D.S. Slusarchyk. 1984. Muraceins – muramyl peptides produced by Nocardia orientalis as angiotensin converting enzyme inhibitors. 1. Taxonomy, fermentation and biological properties. J. Antibiot. 37: 330–335.

7 Bush, K., P.R. Henry, M. Souser-Woehleke, W.H. Trejo and D.S. Slusarchyk. 1984. Phenacein – angiotensin converting enzyme inhibitor produced by a streptomycete. 1. Taxonomy, fermentation and biological properties. J. Antibiot. 37: 1308–1312.

8 Carmel, A., S. Ehrlich-Rogozinsky and A. Yaron. 1979. A fluorimetric assay for angiotensin-1 converting enzyme in human serum. Clin. Chim. Acta 93: 215–220.

9 Dempoulos, C., R.N. Pinckard and D.J. Hanahan. 1979. Platelet activating factor. J. Biol. Chem. 254: 9355–9358.

10 Doebber, T.W., M.S. Wu, J.C. Robbins, B.M. Choy, M.N. Chang and T.Y. Shen. 1985. Platelet activating factor (PAF) involvement in endotoxin induced hypotension in rats. Studies with PAF-receptor antagonist kadsurenone. Biochem. Biophys. Res. Commun. 127: 799–808.

11 Gaddum, J.H. 1953. The technique of superfusion. Br. J. Pharmacol. 8: 321–326.

12 Hanson, G.J., M.C. Sanquinett, P. Yang, J.G. Campion, O.D. Suleymanov, S.N. Anderson and S.T. McDonald. 1988. Cardiovascular effects of amauromine. Clin. Exp. Hypertension A, in press.

13 Horiai, H., T. Ando, T. Asada, S. Takase, K. Yoshida and F. Shibayama 1989. Hypotensive and calcium antagonistic activities of amauromine, a new fungal alkaloid. Chem. Pharm. Bull. in press.

14 Huang, L., G. Rowin, J. Dunn, R. Sykes, R. Dobna, B.A. Mayles, D.M. Gross and R.W. Burg. 1984. Discovery, purification and characterization of the angiotensin converting enzyme inhibitor, L-681,176, produced by Streptomyces sp. MA 5143a. J. Antibiot. 37: 462–465.

15 Kasai, N., K. Fukuhara, K. Oda and S. Murao. 1983. Inhibition of angiotensin 1 converting enzyme and carboxypepti-

dase A by FMPI, Talopeptin, and their derivatives. Agric. Biol. Chem. 47: 2915–2916.

16 Kido, Y., T. Hamakado, M. Anno, E. Miyagawa, Y. Motoki, T. Wakamiya and T. Shiba. 1984. Isolation and characterization of 15B2, a new phosphorus containing inhibitor of angiotensin 1 converting enzyme produced by *Actinomadura* sp. J. Antibiot. 37: 956–969.

17 Kido, Y., T. Hamakado, T. Yoshida, M. Anno, Y. Motoki, T. Wakamiya and T. Shiba. 1983. Isolation and characterization of ancovenin, a new inhibitor of angiotensin 1 converting enzyme, produced by actinomycetes. J. Antibiot. 36: 1295–1299.

18 Koguchi, T., K. Yamada, R. Okachi, K. Nakayama and H. Kase. 1986. K-4, a novel inhibitor of angiotensin 1 converting enzyme produced by *Actinomadura spiculosospora*. J. Antibiot. 39: 364–371.

19 Mikami, Y. and T. Suzuki. 1983. Novel microbial inhibitors of angiotensin-converting enzyme. Aspergillomarasmines A and B. Agric. Biol. Chem. 47: 2693–2695.

20 O'Connor, S. and P. Somers. 1985. Methods for the detection and quantitation of angiotensin converting enzyme inhibitors in fermentation broths. J. Antibiot. 38: 993–996.

21 Okamoto, M., K. Yoshida, M. Nishikawa, T. Ando, M. Iwami, M. Kohsaka and H. Aoki. 1986. FR-900452, a specific antagonist of platelet activating factor (PAF) produced by *Streptomyces phaeofaciens*. J. Antibiot. 39: 198–204.

22 Okamoto, M., K. Yoshida, M. Nishikawa, K. Hayashi, I. Uchida, M. Kohsaka and H. Aoki. 1986. Studies of platelet activating factor (PAF) antagonist from microbial products. 3. Pharmacological studies of FR-900452 in animal models. Chem. Pharm. Bull. 34: 3005–3010.

23 Okamoto, M., K. Yoshida, M. Nishikawa, M. Kohsaka and H. Aoki. 1986. Platelet activating factor (PAF) involvement in endotoxin induced thrombocytopenia in rabbits: studies with FR-900452, a specific inhibitor of PAF. Thromb. Res. 42: 661–671.

24 Rahwan, R.G. 1983. Mechanism of action of membrane calcium channel blockers and intracellular calcium antagonists. Med. Res. Rev. 3: 21–42.

25 Shen, T.Y., S.B. Hwang, M.N. Chang, T.W. Doebber, M.H. Lam, M.S. Wu, X. Wang, G.Q. Han and R.Z. Li. 1985. Characterization of a platelet activating factor receptor antagonist isolated from haifenteng. Proc. Natl. Acad. Sci. USA 82: 672–676.

26 Shimazaki, N., I. Shima, K. Hemmi and M. Hashimoto. 1987. Diketopiperazines as a new class of platelet activating factor inhibitors. J. Med. Chem. 30: 1706–1709.

27 Takase, S., Y. Itoh, I. Uchida, H. Tanaka and H. Aoki. 1986. Total synthesis of amauromine. Tetrahedron 42: 5887–5894.

28 Takase, S., M. Iwami, T. Ando, M. Okamoto, K. Yoshida, H. Horiai, M. Kohsaka, H. Aoki and H. Imanaka. 1984. Amauromine, a new vasodilator, taxonomy, isolation and characterization. J. Antibiot. 37: 1320–1323.

29 Takase, S., Y. Kawai, I. Uchida, H. Tanaka and H. Aoki. 1984. Structure of amauromine, a new alkaloid with vasodilating activity produced by *Amauroascus* sp. Tetrahedron Lett. 25: 4673–4676.

30 Tanaka, H., K. Yoshida, Y. Itoh and H. Imanaka. 1981. Structure and synthesis of a new vasodilator isolated from *Streptomyces aureofaciens*. Tetrahedron Lett. 22: 3421–3422.

31 Terashita, Z., S. Tsushima, Y. Yoshioka, H. Nomura, Y. Inada and K. Nishikawa. 1983. CV-3988, a specific antagonist of platelet activating factor (PAF). Life Sci. 32: 1975–1982.

32 Uchida, I., T. Ando, N. Fukami, K. Yoshida, M. Hashimoto, T. Tada, S. Koda and Y. Morimoto. 1987. The structure of Vinigrol, a novel diterpenoid with antihypertensive and platelet aggregation inhibitory activities. J. Org. Chem. 52: 5292–5293.

33 Uchida, I., S. Takase, M. Okamoto, K. Yoshida, T. Tada, S. Kohda and M. Hashimoto. 1987. Structure of FR-900452, a novel PAF antagonist from microbial products. J. Org. Chem. 52: 3485–3487.

34 Umezawa, H., T. Aoyagi, K. Ogawa, T. Iinuma, H. Naganawa, M. Hamada and T. Takeuchi. 1985. Foroxymithine, a new inhibitor of angiotensin converting enzyme, produced by actinomycetes. J. Antibiot. 38: 1813–1815.

35 Vargaftig, B.B., M. Chignard, J. Benveniste, J. Lefort and F. Wal. 1981. Background and present status of research on platelet activating factor (PAF-acether). Ann. N.Y. Acad. Sci. 370: 119–137.

36 Vargaftig, B.B., J. Lefort, M. Chignard and J. Benveniste. 1980. Platelet activating factor induces a platelet dependent bronchoconstriction unrelated to the formation of prostaglandin derivatives. Eur. J. Pharmacol. 65: 185–193.

37 Yamato, M., T. Koguchi, R. Okachi, K. Yamada, K. Nakayama and H. Kase. 1986. K-26, a novel inhibitor of angiotensin 1 converting enzyme produced by an actinomycete K-26. J. Antibiot. 39: 44–52.

38 Yoshida, K., M. Okamoto, K. Umehara, M. Iwami, M. Kohsaka, H. Aoki and H. Imanaka. 1982. Studies on new vasodilators, WS-1228A and B. 1. Discovery, taxonomy, isolation and characterization. J. Antibiot. 35: 151–156.

Novel Microbial Products for Medicine and Agriculture
Editors: A.L. Demain, G.A. Somkuti, J.C. Hunter-Cevera and H.W. Rossmoore
© 1989, Society for Industrial Microbiology

CHAPTER 4

Screening of immunomodulating agents

Masayuki Asano, Masanobu Kohsaka, Hatsuo Aoki and Hiroshi Imanaka

Exploratory Research Laboratories, Fujisawa Pharmaceutical Co., Ltd., Ibaragi, Japan

SUMMARY

A system of screening for immunomodulating agents in microbial products was developed in our laboratory. Two active compounds were found, one an immunostimulating agent which has been named FK-156, and the other an immunosuppressive agent named FK-506. FK-156 is an acidic tetrapeptide produced by *Streptomyces olivaceogriseus* sp. nov. Chemical procedures yielded a derivative, FK-565, which is much stronger than FK-156. FK-156 and FK-565 augment many immunological parameters, and are very effective against microbial infections. FK-506 is a macrocyclic lactone produced by *S. tsukubaensis*. It suppresses remarkably the production of interleukin 2 without cytotoxicity, and it is very effective for use in organ transplants.

INTRODUCTION

In searching for new antibiotics, we observed that some microbial metabolites show superior *in vivo* antibacterial activities compared to their *in vitro* minimum inhibitory concentration values. This led us to the hypothesis that microorganisms produce immunostimulating agents which enhance host resistance to bacterial infections. Using this hypothesis, we devised a new screening system and found FK-156 [1, 2]. Chemical procedures yielded a derivative, FK-565 [8].

Success in discovering FK-156 encouraged us to devise a new method for finding immunosuppressive agents from microbial products. We examined various fermentation broths as to whether or not they suppressed immune response, and we found an active compound which has been named FK-506 [5, 6].

MATERIALS AND METHODS

Screening systems

FK-156. Samples were injected subcutaneously into ddy mice, 1, 4, 5, and 6 days before infection. At day 0, mice were challenged intraperitoneally with the minimum lethal dose of *Escherichia coli* No. 22 (10^7 cells/mouse). Forty-eight hours after the infection, the surviving mice were counted.

FK-506. We examined samples by mixed lymphocytes reaction (MLR) assay. BALB/C mice spleen cells were used as responder cells, and mitomycin C-treated C57BL/6 mice spleen cells used as stimulator cells. They were placed on 96-well tissue culture plates containing complete medium. Samples were added to the cultures, which were then incubated at 37°C in 5% CO_2. Seventy-two hours later, [^{3}H]thymidine which had been incorporated into the reaction mixtures was measured [6].

RESULTS

Structures

The structures of FK-156 and FK-565 are shown in Fig. 1 [4, 8].

The structure of FK-506 is shown in Fig. 2 [10].

Biological properties

FK-156 and FK-565. The effects of FK-156 and

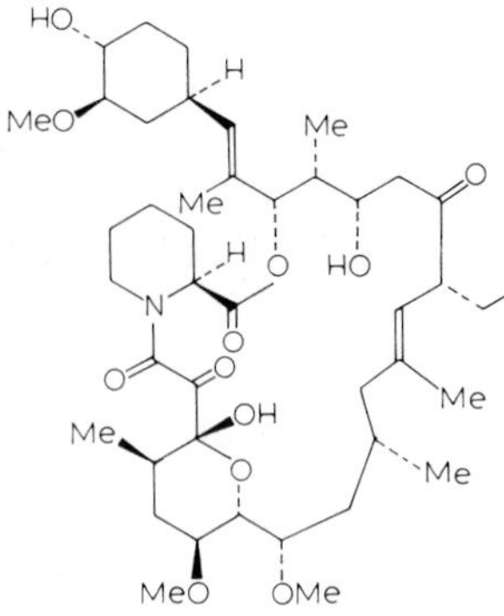

Fig. 2. Structure of FK-506.

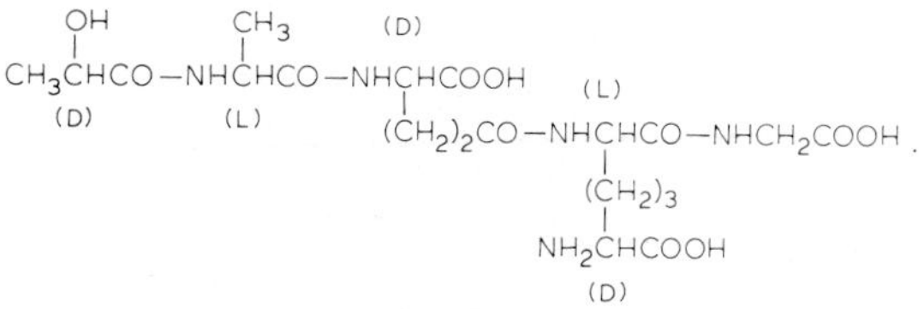

FK-156

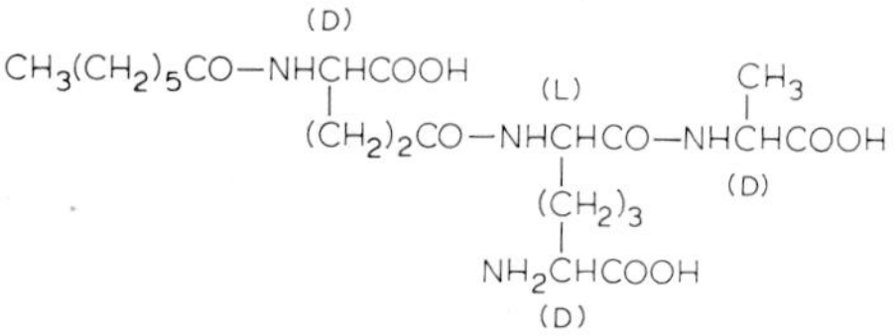

FK-565

Fig. 1. Structure of FK-156 and of FK-565.

FK-565 on the defense of mice against various microbial infections is shown in Table 1. FK-156 prevented various extracellular and intracellular infections to a remarkable extent. FK-565, much more potent than FK-156, was effective via oral administration [8].

FK-156 and FK-565 were also effective in protecting animals against viral infections, for example the herpes simplex virus and the influenza virus (data not shown). Furthermore, FK-565 restored the host defense activity against microbial infections in immunosuppressed animals [11].

The data suggest that FK-565 may be useful in preventing both microbial and viral infections in

Table 1

Defense of mice given FK-156 and FK-565 against various microbial infections

Organism (route)	Survival rate (%)			
	FK-156[a]		FK-565[b]	
	1 mg/kg	control	0.1 mg/kg	control
Escherichia coli No. 22 (i.p.)	90	0	60	10
Klebsiella pneumoniae No. 57 (i.p.)	70	0	40	20
Serratia marcescens No. 32 (i.p.)	80	20	80	20
Pseudomonas aeruginosa No. 97 (i.p.)	100	10	70	10
Candida albicans FP633 (i.v.)	30	0	80	40
Listeria monocytogenes FP566 (i.p.)	40	0	90	0
Salmonella enteritidis FP233 (i.v.)	50	10	80	20
Salmonella enteritidis FP233 (p.o.)	70	40	80	40

[a] FK-156 was given subcutaneously 4 and 1 day before challenge.

[b] FK-565 was given orally 6,5,4 and 1 day before challenge.

patients in an immunosuppressed state, as in cases of cancer or acquired immunodeficiency syndrome (AIDS).

We suspect that in clinical situations FK-565 may be effective against granulocytopenia caused by cancer chemotherapy. It has been shown to very strongly induce colony stimulating factors (CSF) [7]. CSF increased rapidly within 2 h after injection of FK-565 (0.1 μg/kg), reached a peak in 4 h, and then declined to the basal level in 24 h (Fig. 3). Significantly, activity was observed with a dose as low as 0.1 μg/kg.

It has been reported that CSF is able to accelerate recovery of granulopoiesis after the administration of cyclophosphamide [9]. Therefore, we hope that a granulocyte level which has been depressed by cancer chemotherapy may be restored with FK-565, and that a stronger chemotherapy may be administered with no risk.

FK-506. FK-506 first attracted our attention because at 1 nM it inhibited mouse MLR almost completely. This activity is about 100 times stronger than that of cyclosporin A (CsA) (Fig. 4). FK-506 at 1 nM dosage inhibits human MLR as well as mouse MLR, and suppresses the production of interleukin 2. At the 1 nM dose it also inhibits the expression of the interleukin 2 receptor [6].

FK-506 is able to suppress immune response *in vivo.* It suppresses remarkably mouse PFC response (antibody production) and DTH response (cell-mediated immunity) at a dose of 10 mg/kg [6].

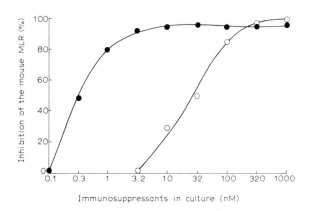

Fig. 4. Inhibition of mouse MLR by FK-506 and CsA. FK-506 and CsA were added throughout the assay. The data are expressed as inhibition based on response in a control diluent. ●, FK-506; ○, CsA.

We examined the effect of FK-506 on organ transplants in animals [3]. Ear skin grafts of complete skin were transplanted onto the backs of recipient rats. FK-506 was administered intramuscularly for 2 weeks. Treatment with FK-506 at a dose of 0.32 mg/kg or higher significantly prolonged the survival time of the skin grafts. CsA was effective at doses of 32 mg/kg or higher (Table 2). FK-506

Table 2

Rat skin allograft survival with various doses of FK-506 and CsA

Agent[a]	Dose (mg/kg/day)	n	MST[b] (range)	P[c]
Placebo		8	6.0 (6–7)	
FK-506	0.032	8	6.5 (6–7)	n.s.
	0.1	8	8.0 (7–10)	<0.01
	0.32	8	12.5 (10–20)	<0.01
	1.0	8	27.0 (26–33)	<0.01
	3.2	8	43.0 (39–47)	<0.01
Placebo		8	6.0 (5–7)	
Cyclosporin A	3.2	8	7.0 (6–7)	<0.05
	10	8	8.0 (7–11)	<0.01
	32	8	22.0 (19–26)	<0.01
	100	8	40.0 (39–46)	<0.01

[a] Recipient WKA rats transplanted with F344 skin allografts were given i.m. FK-506 or CsA 5 days a week for 2 weeks.
[b] MST = median survival time (days).
[c] Significance determined by Mann-Whitney U test.

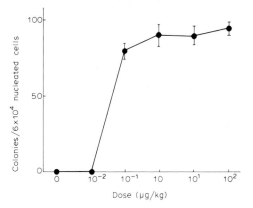

Fig. 3. Effect of FK-565 dosage on CSF. C57BL/6 mice were injected subcutaneously with FK-565, and sera drawn after 4 h. Results are expressed as the mean ± S.E. of triplicate cultures.

is about 100 times as potent as CsA.

Next we tested intermittent administrations. WKA recipients of F344 skin grafts were treated with 3.2 mg/kg FK-506, 5 days a week for 2 weeks, and were given subsequent maintenance doses of 0.32 or 3.2 mg/kg intermittently twice a week for 120 days. As long as the treatment continued all animals retained healthy grafts [3].

FK-506 and CsA are good immunosuppressive drugs. Conventional immunosuppressive drugs, such as azathioprine, prednisolone, and bredinin, have only marginal effectiveness on graft rejection [3]. However, FK-506 and CsA result in graft acceptance as long as their use is continued. FK-506 and CsA show no myelotoxicity, whereas conventional drugs cause a drastic decrease in blood leukocytes.

Recently CsA has been used worldwide in organ transplants. In spite of its good efficacy, very serious side effects include nephrotoxicity, hepatotoxicity, and mild CNS disturbance.

FK-506 can be administered effectively at doses which are only 1% of the effective dose of CsA. Although the exact toxicity of FK-506 is not clear, we expect that FK-506 therapy may be safer than CsA.

CONCLUSION

We obtained novel immunomodulating agents from microbial products. Microorganisms have historically provided many antibiotics useful for clinical therapy. Recently, microorganisms have been demonstrated to have even greater potential pharmacologically, and in the future they will probably provide many new and useful products for medicine.

REFERENCES

1 Gotoh, T., K. Nakahara, M. Iwami, H. Aoki and H. Imanaka. 1982. Studies on a new immunoactive peptide, FK-156. 1. Taxonomy of the producing strains. J. Antibiot. 35:1280–1285.

2 Gotoh, T., K. Nakahara, T. Nishiura, S. Hashimoto, T. Kino, Y. Kuroda, M. Okuhara, M. Kohsaka, H. Aoki and H. Imanaka. 1982. Studies on a new immunoactive peptide, FK-156. 2. Fermentation, extraction and chemical and biological characterization. J. Antibiot. 35:1286–1292.

3 Inamura, N., K. Nakahara, T. Kino, T. Goto, H. Aoki, I. Yamaguchi, M. Kohsaka and T. Ochiai. 1988. Prolongation of skin allograft survival in rats by a novel immunosuppressive agent, FK-506. Transplantation 45:201–206.

4 Kawai, Y., K. Nakahara, T. Gotoh, I. Uchida, H. Tanaka and H. Imanaka. 1982. Studies on a new immunoactive peptide, FK-156. 3. Structure elucidation. J. Antibiot. 35:1293–1299.

5 Kino, T., H. Hatanaka, M. Hashimoto, M. Nishiyama, T. Goto, M. Okuhara, M. Kohsaka, H. Aoki and H. Imanaka. 1987. FK-506, a novel immunosuppressant isolated from a Streptomyces. 1. Fermentation, isolation, and physico-chemical and biological characteristics. J. Antibiot. 40:1249–1255.

6 Kino, T., H. Hatanaka, S. Miyata, N. Inamura, M. Nishiyama, T. Yajima, T. Goto, M. Okuhara, M. Kohsaka, H. Aoki and T. Ochiai. 1987. FK-506, a novel immunosuppressant isolated from a Streptomyces. 2. Immunosuppressive effect of FK-506 in vitro. J. Antibiot. 40:1256–1265.

7 Kozo, N., K. Nakahara and H. Aoki. 1984. Induction of colony-stimulating factor (CSF) by FK-156 and its synthetic derivative, FK-565. Agric. Biol. Chem. 48:2579–2580.

8 Mine, Y., Y. Yokota, Y. Wakai, S. Fukuda, M. Nishida, S. Goto and S. Kuwahara. 1983. Immunoactive peptides, FK-156 & FK-565. 1. Enhancement of host resistance to microbial infection in mice. J. Antibiot. 36:1045–1050.

9 Tamura, M., K. Hattori, H. Nomura, M. Oheda, N. Kubota, I. Imazeki, M. Ono, Y. Ueyama, S. Nagata, N. Shirafuji and S. Asano. 1987. Induction of neutrophilic granulocytosis in mice by administration of purified human native granulocyte colony-stimulating factor. Biochem. Biophys. Res. Commun. 142:454–460.

10 Tanaka, H., A. Kuroda, H. Marusawa, H. Hatanaka, T. Kino, T. Goto and M. Hashimoto. 1987. Structure of FK-506: a novel immunosuppressant isolated from Streptomyces. J. Am. Chem. Soc. 109:5031–5033.

11 Yokota, Y., Y. Mine, Y. Wakai, Y. Watanabe, M. Nishida, S. Goto and S. Kuwahara. 1983. Immunoactive peptides, FK-156 & FK-565. 2. Restoration of host resistance to microbial infection in immunosuppressed mice. J. Antibiot. 36:1051–1058.

Novel Microbial Products for Medicine and Agriculture
Editors: A.L. Demain, G.A. Somkuti, J.C. Hunter-Cevera and H.W. Rossmoore
© 1989, Society for Industrial Microbiology

CHAPTER 5

Enzymic synthesis of immunomodulators[*]

Horst Kleinkauf, Hans von Döhren, Andreas Billich, Alfons Lawen, Hugo Peeters and Reiner Zocher

Institut für Biochemie und Molekulare Biologie, Technische Universität Berlin, Berlin, F.R.G.

INTRODUCTION

Two lines of evidence encourage the researcher to tackle the generally complex enzymology of metabolites, especially peptides, with immunomodulating properties. First, the need of drug development, to fight infections not only conventionally by classical antibiotic treatments, but by stimulating the defense system, to follow up the increasing developments of autoimmune diseases and immunodeficiencies; second, the increasing knowledge of drug–receptor interactions, the sensing of minute structural changes of complex molecules in the elucidation of the selection of wanted and unwanted targets. We thus appreciate that structure-function studies are at least as important as the screening for new effectors. Our deeper understanding of the structural features required for a certain target depend largely on synthesis and modification of the respective compounds and their analogs.

Of considerable help in such studies are enzymatically catalyzed modifications, and of increasing importance, the total enzymic synthesis, in our case of peptides from their constituent amino acids. Such a total synthesis may be accomplished by a stable complex integrating the complete sequence of reactions, as will be described below for cyclosporin and related compounds.

PEPTIDE BIOSYNTHESIS

The principle approaches to peptide biosynthesis found in nature are (a) the ribosomal route, (b) the protein template, and (c) the step-by-step mechanism (Fig. 1).
The principle approaches to peptide biosynthesis found in nature are (1) the ribosomal route, (2) the protein template, and (3) the step-by-step mechanism (Fig. 1).

While the ribosomal route is clearly restricted to its 20 protein components, the stepwise procedure to small products of three to five reactions, the protein template represents a versatile system for a variety of compounds [9]. Starting from an unlimited pool of carboxyl compounds, including amino acids and hydroxy acids, these are activated by ATP consumption, and polymerized in sequence from their thiol ester intermediates. Products include cyclic and branched cyclic peptides, peptidolactones, depsipeptides, and linear peptides with modified termini (Table 1).

The characterization and handling of these systems still depend heavily on empirical trials, but several recent advances are very promising.

IMMUNOMODULATORS AND THEIR PATHWAYS

Muramyl peptides and their derivatives show a variety of effects including activation of B and T cells by stimulation of macrophages. MDP (Fig. 2), a minimal adjuvant active structure, can be derived

[*]Dedicated to Professor Hamao Umezawa.

SYSTEM	PRODUCT

nucleic acid dependent

Type 1
choice of program
assembly line

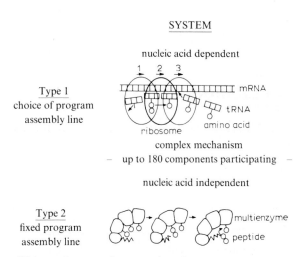

complex mechanism
– up to 180 components participating –

ribosomal
– linear polypeptides of any sequence and length from 20 proteinogenic amino acids
– activation as aminoacyladenylates
– high specificity
– high energy requiring
– proof reading mechanisms
– processing of propeptides

nucleic acid independent

Type 2
fixed program
assembly line

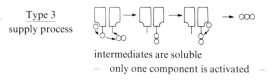

all intermediates remain enzyme-bound
the sequence is determined on the multifunctional enzyme-chain
4′-phosphopantetheine is cofactor
enzymes identified so far only in bacteria or fungi

enzymatic
– linear, branched and cyclic peptides and depsipeptides, e.g. gramicidin S
– activation as aminoacyladenylates
– low specificity
– incorporation of analogs
– non-protein amino acids (D-configuration, ornithine, diaminobutyrate)
– modification, e.g. N-methylation
– length of peptides up to about 30 amino acids

Type 3
supply process

intermediates are soluble
– only one component is activated –

– linear peptides, e.g. glutathione
– activation as phosphates or as aminoacyladenylates
– synthesis of short peptides (approximately 5 amino acids)
– non-protein amino acids are components
– low specificity

Fig. 1. Biosynthetic mechanisms of peptide and protein formation.

by fragmentation of the bacterial cell wall. Biosynthesis of the peptide moiety of peptidoglycan clearly represents a step-by-step mechanism. The amino acid adding enzymes were partially purified in the sixties and early seventies mainly by Strominger's laboratory. Each peptide carboxyl is activated as a phosphate intermediate, and addition of the particular amino group is directed [8]. Due to the many synthetic efforts in this field [1], application of these enzymes has not been exploited. The isolation of the immunostimulant FK-156 (Fig. 2) from strains of *Streptomyces* [7] shows that these types of compounds can even be prepared by fermentation, although still at low levels. This implies some applications of future studies of single-step enzymes in production, expression and protein engineering.

Among others, natural peptides, especially cyclopeptides, have been discovered showing highly selective effects. Structurally homologous peptides containing the unusual Aoe-moiety (2-amino-8-oxo-9,10-epoxydecanoic acid) [9] have been identi-

fied as fungal products (Fig. 3). Chlamydocin has been studied for its cytostatic action, it being degraded rapidly *in vivo*, however, possibly by opening the epoxide function. HC-toxin, a host-specific toxin produced by *Cochliobolus carbonum* parasitizing maize, does not cause immediate cell death. It does not act on replication, transcription or translation, but selectively enhances nitrate uptake [17]. Tentoxin, produced by *Alternaria alternata*, is a nonselective cyclotetrapeptide binding to chloroplast ATPase of toxin-sensitive plants.

The most potent known phytotoxins, the victorins isolated from *C. victoriae* (Fig. 4), invading oat, act through a single specific target, possibly a receptor protein with a high turnover, since translational inhibitors protect the plant. Destruxins, peptidolactones produced by insect pathogenic strains of *Metarhizium anisopliae* (Fig. 3), have also been shown to affect host-specific infection of rape seed by *A. brassicae* [2]. For HC-toxin, tentoxin, victorin, and destruxin some evidence for a multienzymic type of

Table 1

Current enzymology of bioactive peptides

Peptide	Organisms	Structure	State
Linear			
edein	*Bacillus brevis* Vm4	β-Tyr-Ise-Dpr-Dahaa-Gly-spermidine	pp, 3 me
gramicidin	*Bacillus brevis* (ATCC 8185)	f-Val-Gly-Ala-D-Leu-Ala-D-Val-Val-D-Val-Trp-(D-Leu-Trp)$_3$-ethanolamine	pp, 4 me?
alamethicin	*Trichoderma viride*	AcAib-Pro-Aib-Ala-Aib-Ala-Gln-Aib-Val-Aib-Gly-Leu-Aib-Pro-Val-Aib-Aib-Glu-Gln-Pheol	pp, me?
Cyclic			
cyclopeptin	*Penicillium cyclopium*	c(anthranilate-Phe)	pp
enterochelin	*Escherichia coli*	c(Dhb-Ser)	pp, 3 e
ferrichrome	*Aspergillus quadricinctus*	c(Gly$_3$-HyOrn$_3$)	p, me
gramicidin S	*Bacillus brevis* (ATCC 9999)	c(D-Phe-Pro-Orn-Val-Leu)$_2$	p, 2 me
tyrocidin	*Bacillus brevis* (ATCC 8185)	c(D-Phe-Pro-Phe-D-Phe-Asn-Gln-Tyr-Val-Orn-Leu)	p, 3 me
cyclosporin A	*Beauvaria nivea*	c(NMeBmt-Abu-Sar-NMeLeu-Val-NMe-Leu-Ala-D-Ala-NMeLeu-NMeLeu-NMeVal)	p, me
mycobacillin	*Bacillus subtilis*	c(Pro-D-Asp-D-Glu-(γ)-Tyr-Asp-Tyr-Ser-D-Asp-Leu-D-Glu-(γ)-D-Asp-Ala-D-Asp)	p, 3 me
Lactones			
destruxin	*Metarhizium anisopliae*	c(D-Hib-Pro-Ile-NMeVal-NMeAla-β-Ala)	pp, me?
actinomycin	*Streptomyces clavuligerus*	Mha-c(Thr-D-Val-Pro-NMeGly-Val)/$_2$	p, e + 2me
Branched cyclic			
polymyxin	*Bacillus polymyxa*	Oct-Dab-Thr-Dab-c(Dab-Dab-Leu-Leu-Thr-Dab-Dab)	pp, e + me?
bacitracin	*Bacillus licheniformis*	(Ile-Cys)-Leu-D-Glu-Ile-c(Lys-D-Orn-Ile-Phe-Asn-D-Asp-His)	p, 3 me
Depsipeptides			
enniatin B	*Fusarium oxysporum*	c(NMeVal-D-Hiv)$_3$	p, me
beauvericin	*Beauveria bassiana*	c(NMePhe-D-Hiv)$_3$	p, me

Abbrevations

pp-partially purified, p-purified, e-enzyme, me-multienzyme

Aib-aminoisobutyric acid, Dahaa-2,7-dihyroxyazaleic acid, Dhb-dihydroxybenzoic acid, D-Hib – D-hydroxyisobutyric acid, D-Hiv – D-hydroxyisovaleric acid, Dpr-diaminopropionic acid, HyOrn N^6-hydroxy-ornithine, Ise-isoserine, NMeBmt- (4R)-4-((E)-2-butenyl)-4-methyl-L-threonine, Mha-4-methylhydroxyanthranilic acid.

synthesis has been obtained. Partially purified enzyme extracts containing high molecular weight proteins catalyzing the amino acid-dependent formation of ATP from PP$_i$ indicate the presence of acyl- or aminoacyladenylates [Von Döhren and Macko, unpublished data, 16, 18].

Currently most advanced are the studies on the HC-toxins, where genetic data point to a single gene locus being involved. Such a single gene, or multigene coding for a single multienzyme, is strongly supported by the studies on the biosynthesis of enniatin (*Fusarium oxysporum*) and beauvericin (*Beauveria bassiana*), where single multifunctional enzymes catalyze the formation of the cyclohexadepsipeptides (Fig. 5). This has been in accord with the observations that not more than six amino acid residues are added by a single multienzyme species in the bacterial enzyme systems stud-

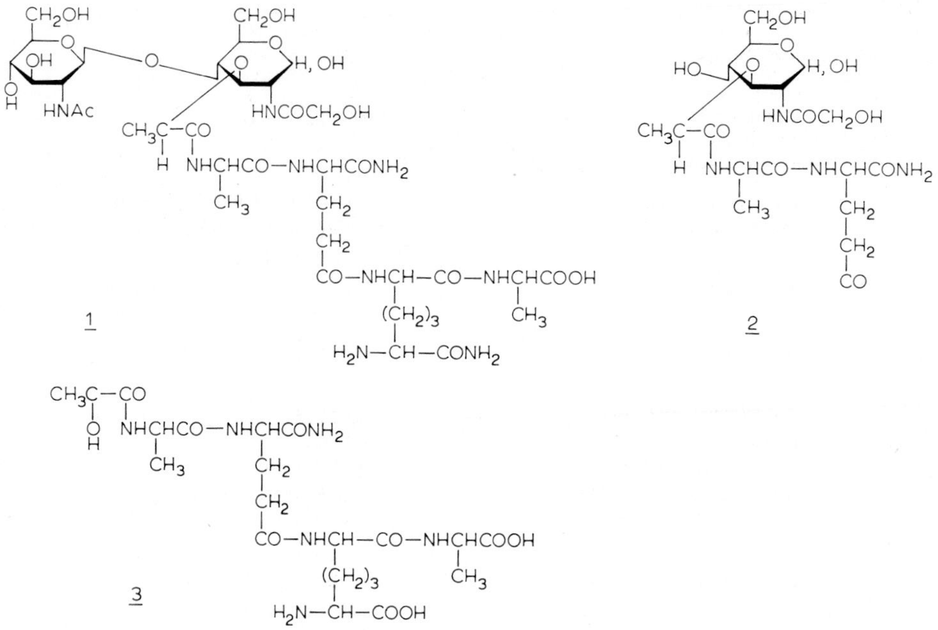

Fig. 2. Immunoactive peptidoglycan-derived structures. 1, monomer of the peptidoglycan of mycobacteria; 2, *N*-acetyl-muramyl-L-alanyl-D-isoglutamine, MDP, the smallest synthetic adjuvant active molecule to replace whole mycobacteria in Freund's adjuvant; 3, FK-156, an immunostimulant produced by *S. olivaceogriseus* and *S. violaceus* [7].

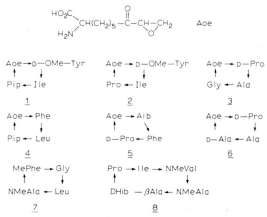

Fig. 3. Bioactive fungal metabolites. 1, Cyl-1 and 2, Cyl-2, both from *Cylindrocladium scoparum*; 3 and 6, HC-toxins from *Helminthosporium carbonum*; 4, WF-3161 from *Petriella guttulata*; 5, chlamydocin from *Diheterospora chlamydosporia*; 7, tentoxin from *A. tenus* or *A. mali*; and 8, destruxin from *Metarhizium anisopliae* or *A. brassicae*. Pip-pipecolic acid. See Refs. 2, 9 and 17.

ied. Peptides containing more than six residues have been found to be formed by a set of several interacting multienzymes, each adding two to six constituents. Structural genes for such enzyme systems are apparently clustered [9].

Recent studies on cyclosporin synthetase produced by *Beauveria nivea* have indicated a more complex type of enzyme, or a stable complex of multienzymes, since synthesis of this cycloundecapeptide (Fig. 6) has been shown to proceed on a single enzyme fraction of very high molecular weight [3]. Thus according to the precursor selection, cyclosporins A, B, C, D or [D-Ser^8]cyclosporin A have been produced enzymatically, yet in trace amounts.

As has been shown before with gramicidin S synthetase from *Bacillus brevis*, and later in more detail with enniatin synthetase [11, 13], a scale-up should present no severe problems. Enniatin synthetase (ESyn) has been immobilized by adsorption or covalent attachment, and synthesis has been conducted according to the overall equation 3 D-Hiv + 3 L-aa + 3 SAM + 6 ATP $\xrightarrow{\text{ESyn}}$ enniatin + 3 SAhC + 6 AMP + 6 PP$_i$ where Hiv is hydroxyisovalerate, aa stands for aliphatic amino acid, SAM for *S*-adenosylmethionine, methylating the activated amino acid via an integrated methyltransferase function prior to peptide bond formation [4], and SAhC is *S*-adenosylhomocysteine.

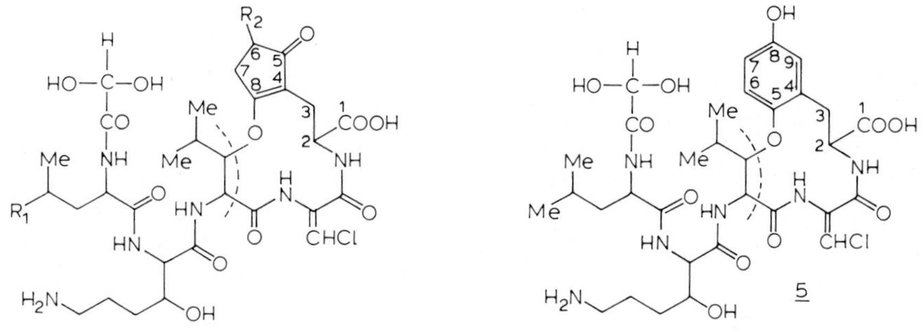

$R_1 = CH_2Cl/CHCl_2/CCl_3$
$R_2 = OH/H$

Fig. 4. Highly specific phytotoxins produced by strains of *C. victoriae* [19].

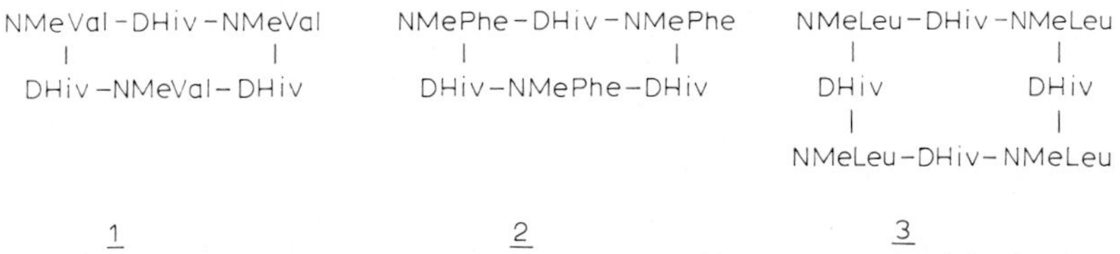

NMeVal – DHiv – NMeVal
| |
DHiv – NMeVal – DHiv

NMePhe – DHiv – NMePhe
| |
DHiv – NMePhe – DHiv

NMeLeu – DHiv – NMeLeu
| |
DHiv   DHiv
| |
NMeLeu – DHiv – NMeLeu

1   2   3

Fig. 5. Enniatin, beauvericin, and bassianolide, cyclodepsipeptides produced by strains of *Fusarium, Beauveria,* and *Verticillium.* Enniatin B (1) is used as a general antibiotic in bacterial and viral therapy; beauvericin (2) and bassianolide (3) are insect toxins, their producers being used in plant protection.

Likewise, the synthesis of various analogs of beauvericin has been conducted, with several analogs of phenylalanine, and in addition some aliphatic amino acids with side chains extending the propyl group [12]. The structural proofs of these have yet to be completed.

The similar attempt to produce cyclosporins will be limited by the requirement for the unusual constituent (4R)-4-((E)-2-butenyl)-4-methyl-L-threonine (Bmt), although several synthetic routes have been worked out. Thus an additional enzyme system for the biosynthesis of this precursor is sought, just as in the case of the toxins mentioned before containing Aoe. Such systems should show some similarity to multienzymic fatty acid synthases.

It is evident from this case that compounds of interest are not limited to certain structural types like peptides. Peptides, however, with their amino acid backbone possess thus an outstanding feature for enzymic modification using amino acid analogs. Quite often peptides may contain constituents of related pathways. Thus the 23-ring lactone virginia-

mycin M, an antibiotic acting on the prokaryotic ribosome, is composed of amino acids and acetate units [10]. Enzymatic studies have not been carried out yet, but the structural homology to another

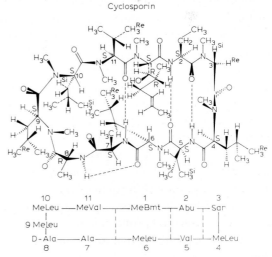

Cyclosporin

10	11	1	2	3
MeLeu	MeVal	MeBmt	Abu	Sar
9 MeLeu				
D-Ala	Ala	MeLeu	Val	MeLeu
8	7	6	5	4

Fig. 6. Structure of cyclosporin in the solid state and structural scheme [19]. Shown is cyclosporin A, while B contains Ala, C Thr, and D Val in position 2, respectively.

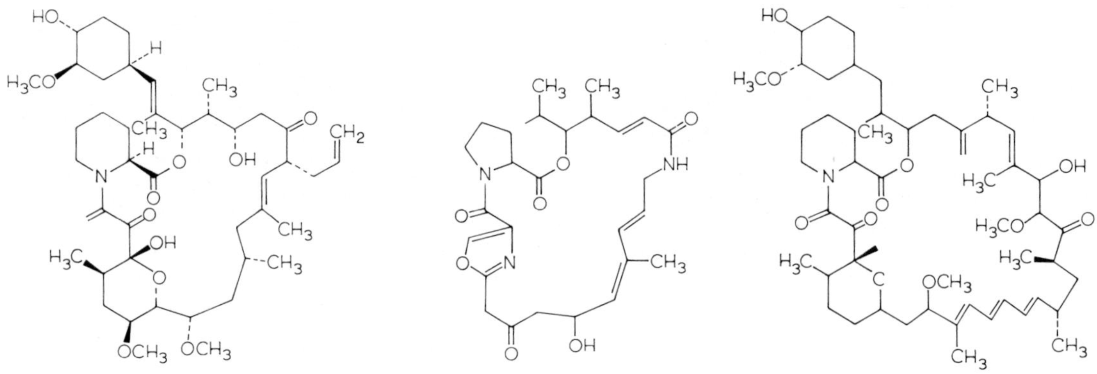

54

Fig. 7. Structures of the immunosuppressor FK-506, recently isolated from *S. tsukubaensis* (1), virginiamycin M, formed by several streptomycetes with a similar 23-ring size (2), and rapamycin, an antifungal macrolide from a *S. hygroscopicus* collected at Easter Island with structural similarities (3).

outstanding immunosuppressor, FK-506, is obvious [14] (Fig. 7).

Enzyme systems, whether fused or single entities, can be expected to share homologies that could prove useful in isolation and characterization. Also a macrolide type of compound, rapamycin (Fig. 7), indicates close biosynthetic relations.

Structural probes for protein structure or genetic information can be of significant use in enzyme identification and analysis. This has recently been shown in the cloning progress of tyrocidine synthetase multienzymes, coding a cyclodecapeptide, with structural probes of the gramicidin S system, and the cloning of isopenicillin *N*-synthase from *Penicillium* and *Aspergillus* with the aid of a *Cephalosporium* gene probe. Likewise, a methyltransferase function integrated into a multienzyme, as in enniatin, beauvericin, destruxin, cyclosporin, or actinomycin systems [5], may be used as a target and perhaps a kind of handle in this sense.

Thus, access to complex enzyme systems can be gained by careful analysis of enzyme production, followed by detailed investigation of enzyme isolation and stability, both processes being enhanced by the use of structural probes and reactions of related systems carrying out multistep synthetic operations.

REFERENCES

1 Adam, M., J.-F. Petit, P. Lefrancier and E. Lederer. 1981. Muramyl peptides. Chemical structure, biological activity and mechanism of action. Mol. Cell. Biochem. 41:27–47.

2 Bains, P.S. and J.P. Tewari. 1987. Purification, chemical characterization and host-specificity of the toxin produced by *Alternaria brassicae*. Physiol. Mol. Plant Pathol. 30:259–271.

3 Billich, A. and R. Zocher. 1987. Enzymic synthesis of cyclosporin A. J. Biol. Chem. 262:17258–17259.

4 Billich, A. and R. Zocher. 1987. *N*-Methyltransferase function of the multifunctional enzyme enniatin synthetase. Biochemistry 26:8417–8423.

5 Billich, A. and R. Zocher. 1987. Unpublished data.

6 Findlay, J. and A. Radics. 1980. On the chemistry and high field nuclear magnetic resonance spectroscopy of rapamycin. Can. J. Chem. 58:579–590.

7 Gotoh, T., K. Nakahara, T. Nishiura, M. Hashimoto, T. Kino, Y. Kuroda, M. Okuhare, M. Kohsake, H. Aoki and H. Imanaka. 1982. Studies on a new immunoactive peptide, FK-156. II. Fermentation, extraction and biological characterization. J. Antibiot. 35:1286–1292.

8 Kleinkauf, H. and H. Koischwitz. 1978. Peptide bond formation in nonribosomal systems. Progr. Mol. Subcell. Biol. 6:59–112.

9 Kleinkauf, H. and H. von Döhren. 1987. Biosynthesis of peptide antibiotics. Ann. Rev. Microbiol. 41:259–289.

10 LeFevre, J.W. and D.G.I. Kingston. 1984. Biosynthesis of the virginiamycin family. 4. Biosynthesis of A2315A. J. Org. Chem. 49:2588–2593.

11 Madry, N., R. Zocher, K. Grodzki and H. Kleinkauf. 1984. Selective synthesis of depsipeptides by the immobilized multienzyme enniatin synthetase. Appl. Microbiol. Biotechnol. 20:83–86.

12 Peeters, H. 1988. Die Biosynthese des Beauvericins. Doctoral thesis, TU Berlin.

13 Siegbahn, N., K. Mosbach, K. Grodzki, R. Zocher, N. Madry and H. Kleinkauf. 1985. Biotechnol. Lett. 7:297–302.

14 Tanaka, H., A. Kuroda, H. Marasuwa, H. Hatanaka, T. Kino, T. Goto and M. Hashimoto. 1987. Structure of FK-506: a novel immunosuppressant isolated from *Streptomyces*. J. Am. Chem. Soc. 109:5031–5033.

15 Von Döhren, H. and V. Macko. 1987. Unpublished data.

16 Walton, J.D. 1987. Two enzymes involved in biosynthesis of the host-selective phytotoxin HC-toxin. Proc. Natl. Acad. Sci. USA 84:8444–8447.

17 Walton, J.D. 1989. Peptide phytotoxins from plant pathogenic fungi. In: Biochemistry of Peptide Antibiotics. (H. Kleinkauf and H.v. Doehren, eds.), De Gruyter, Berlin, New York, in press.

18 Wessel, W.L., K.A. Clare and W.A. Gibbons. 1987. Enzymic biosynthesis of peptide toxins by plant-specific fungi. Biochem. Soc. Trans. 15:917.

19 Wolpert, T.J., V. Macko, W. Acklin, B. Jaun and D. Arigoni. 1986. Structure of minor host-selective toxins from *Cochliobolus victoriae*. Experientia 42:1296–1299.

Novel Microbial Products for Medicine and Agriculture
Editors: A.L. Demain, G.A. Somkuti, J.C. Hunter-Cevera and H.W. Rossmoore
© 1989, Society for Industrial Microbiology

CHAPTER 6

Microbial secondary metabolites inhibiting oncogene functions

Kazuo Umezawa[1], Makoto Hori[2] and Tomio Takeuchi[1]

[1]*Institute of Microbial Chemistry, Tokyo and* [2]*Showa College of Pharmaceutical Sciences, Tokyo, Japan*

SUMMARY

Various oncogenes are considered to act through tyrosine kinase activity. We have isolated erbstatin from *Streptomyces* as an inhibitor of epidermal growth factor (EGF) receptor-associated tyrosine kinase. Erbstatin specifically inhibits tyrosine kinase. Its inhibition is competitive with the peptide substrate and noncompetitive with ATP. It inhibits autophosphorylation of the EGF receptor and the p60^{src} protein in cultured cells, and also inhibits internalization of EGF. Oncogenes such as *ras* and *src* are known to activate phosphatidylinositol turnover. We have isolated psi-tectorigenin from *Nocardiopsis* as an inhibitor of EGF-induced phosphatidylinositol turnover. Herbimycin A, an ansamycin antibiotic, was found to induce reversion of the transformed morphology into the normal morphology in *src*-transformed cells. Oxanosine, a nucleoside analog antibiotic, was found to induce reversion of the transformed phenotypes into the normal phenotypes in *ras*-transformed cells.

INTRODUCTION

Streptomyces and other microorganisms produce not only antibiotics, antitumor agents and enzyme inhibitors but also many compounds that modify the process of carcinogenesis. For example, teleocidin isolated from *Streptomyces* is a typical tumor promoter in mouse skin. Leupeptin, an analog of lecanoric acid and herbimycin, all of microbial origin, are inhibitors of tumor promotion. In the field of carcinogenesis research, oncogene theory has been extensively developed. In the present paper we wish to show that microorganisms produce various inhibitors of oncogene functions.

At least certain types of human neoplasia, such as Burkitt lymphoma, nasopharyngeal carcinoma in the Far East and adult T cell leukemia in Japan, are known to be caused by viruses, and a number of oncogenic viruses have been identified in animals. These oncogenic viruses contain only several genes, which may be either DNA or RNA. The genes of each virus include a viral oncogene or transforming gene which is essential for causing neoplasia in animals or transformation in cell culture. Recently, it was shown that the DNA of some non-virally induced neoplastic cells and tissues contained the oncogenes.

It appears that all oncogenes have a corresponding gene in normal nonneoplastic cells. These cellular counterparts to the viral oncogenes are called cellular oncogenes. These cellular oncogenes are considered to play an important role in normal cell growth. It is now considered that genetic alteration of these normal growth regulatory genes can induce neoplastic transformation.

Over 40 oncogenes have been isolated and characterized. Oncogenes are transcribed and translated into their protein products within the cells. They can be classified into cytoplasmic and nuclear oncogenes by the location of their protein products [31]. The nuclear oncogenes include *myc, fos* and *myb*, however almost nothing is known about the mechanism of their functions. The mechanisms of a few of the cytoplasmic oncogene functions are understood to some extent. The protein product of the *erbB* oncogene is closely related to the receptor for epidermal growth factor (EGF). The *fms* product is similar to the colony stimulating factor receptor. The *neu* product is considered to be similar to the cell surface receptor for an unknown ligand, too. The *src* oncogene group such as *src, yes, ros* and *fgr* are known to possess tyrosine kinase activity. The *sis* product is closely related to platelet-derived growth factor itself. The *ras* product is a guanine nucleotide binding protein. Among the cytoplasmic oncogenes mentioned above, all except *ras* are considered to act through tyrosine kinase activity.

ERBSTATIN, A TYROSINE KINASE INHIBITOR

We screened culture filtrates of microorganisms for an inhibitor of EGF receptor-associated tyrosine kinase and isolated erbstatin [29]. Erbstatin has a simple but novel structure as shown in Fig. 1. It inhibited EGF receptor tyrosine kinase *in vitro* with an IC$_{50}$ of 0.55 μg/ml with EGF receptor and histone as substrates. It did not inhibit protein kinase C or A and weakly inhibited phosphatidylinositol kinase with an IC$_{50}$ of 25 μg/ml.

The synthetic peptide RR-SRC was found to be

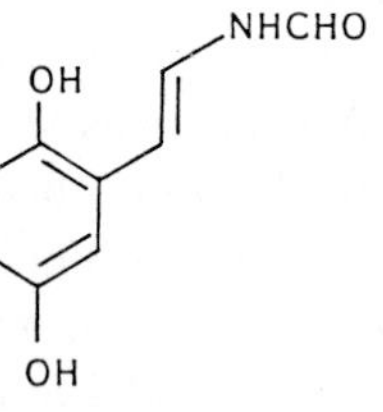

Fig. 1. Erbstatin.

a good substrate for EGF receptor-associated tyrosine kinase [3]. Therefore, using this peptide as a substrate, we were able to study the mechanism of enzyme inhibition by erbstatin. The inhibitory pattern given in the Lineweaver-Burk plot of erbstatin vs. peptide was that of typical competitive inhibition [11]. The inhibitory pattern of erbstatin vs. ATP was noncompetitive. From the Dixon plot analysis the K_i value was found to be about 5.58 μM. On the other hand, inhibition of tyrosine protein kinase by orobol, an isoflavonoid tyrosine kinase inhibitor, was competitive with respect to ATP. The EGF receptor-associated tyrosine kinase was reported to act in the sequential ordered bi bi mechanism, in which the peptide came first and ATP second to the active site of the enzyme [6]. Thus, erbstatin competes with the peptide substrate in the sequential ordered bi bi mechanism, and the mechanism of inhibition is clearly different from that of orobol which competes with ATP. Genistein [21] and amiloride [5], which inhibit tyrosine kinase and H-8 [9], and K-252 compounds [17], which inhibit protein kinase C, are all competitive with ATP.

We have synthesized various erbstatin analogs [14] for the study of structure-activity relationship. The presence of hydroxy groups at 2′ and 5′, 2′ and 4′, or 2′ and 3′ positions appears to be necessary for significant enzyme inhibiting activity. The vinyl structure is essential, but the formamide moiety may not be necessary, because the formamide moiety can be replaced by carboxylic acid without losing the activity. Cytostatic activity of these analogs toward mouse P388 leukemia cells has also been studied. However, the enzyme inhibiting activity does not appear to parallel the cytostatic activity. Thus, the mechanistic relation between them is still unclear.

Erbstatin inhibited tyrosine kinase *in situ* [12]. Addition of erbstatin to A431 cells induced dose-dependent inhibition of EGF-stimulated receptor autophosphorylation. The half-maximal effect was observed at about 15 μg/ml of erbstatin, and 50 μg/ml of the drug inhibited the EGF-stimulated phosphorylation completely. However, the turnover of the EGF receptor as determined by [^{35}S]methionine

incorporation was not influenced either by EGF or by erbstatin at 50 μg/ml. Therefore, *in situ* inhibition of EGF receptor kinase by erbstatin should not be attributed to nonspecific cytotoxicity. Furthermore, phosphorylation of bulk cellular proteins was not inhibited by erbstatin. The *src* gene product, p60^{src}, is known to have tyrosine protein kinase activity [18]. When erbstatin was added to cultured Rous sarcoma virus-infected rat kidney cells, at 25–50 μg/ml it also inhibited autophosphorylation of the p60^{src} protein.

Erbstatin did not inhibit EGF binding to the cell surface receptor up to 100 μg/ml in cultured A431 cells, suggesting direct inhibition of tyrosine protein kinase. On the other hand, erbstatin at a concentration of 25–50 μg/ml clearly inhibited internalization of EGF. The half-maximal effect was observed at about 30 μg/ml. The growth stimulatory effect of EGF is considered to require internalization of the EGF receptor after partial degradation, and this process is suggested to involve EGF receptor tyrosine kinase activation by EGF. Recently, it was reported that inhibition of ATP binding to the EGF receptor suppressed internalization of EGF receptor [4], supporting our observation. Later, it was also reported that microinjection of anti-phosphotyrosine antibodies inhibited EGF receptor internalization [8].

It has been reported that p60^{src} has the capacity *in vitro* to generate polyphosphoinositides [16], suggesting that tyrosine kinase activity is a possible candidate for the signal of phosphatidylinositol turnover. However, we found that erbstatin did not inhibit EGF-induced phosphatidylinositol turnover *in situ* under conditions where it inhibited tyrosine kinase. This result indicates that tyrosine kinase is not signalling the stimulation of phosphatidylinositol turnover in A431 cells.

HERBIMYCIN INHIBITS *src* ONCOGENE EXPRESSION

Herbimycin (Fig. 2) was isolated by Ōmura in 1979 as an ansamycin antibiotic having herbicidal activity [22]. Recently, it was again isolated from *Streptomyces* by Uehara *et al.* as a compound that altered

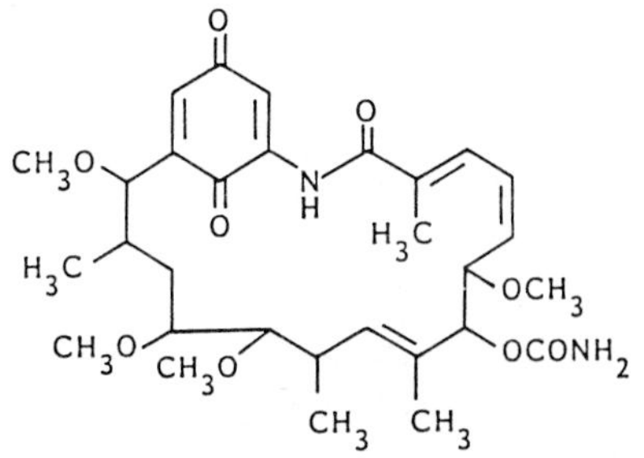

Fig. 2. Herbimycin.

the transformed cell morphology into the normal cell morphology [27].

Temperature-sensitive Rous sarcoma virus-infected rat kidney (RSV^{ts}-NRK) cells show transformed cell morphology at the permissive temperature and normal cell morphology at the nonpermissive temperature. Addition of 0.5 μg/ml of herbimycin at the permissive temperature induced a morphological change of the cells back to their normal morphology within 12–30 h.

One of the transformed phenotypes is the marked decrease in fibronectin expression. We found that the level of fibronectin mRNA was elevated by herbimycin in RSV^{ts}-NRK cells at the permissive temperature [30]. Also herbimycin decreased 2-deoxyglucose transport and induced actin cable formation in Rous sarcoma virus-infected cells. Herbimycin is considered to inhibit *src* oncogene functions by enhancing degradation of the p60^{src} protein [28].

OXANOSINE, AN INHIBITOR OF *ras* ONCOGENE FUNCTIONS

Oxanosine (Fig. 3) was isolated in our institute in 1981 from *Streptomyces* [24]. It is a novel, unusual nucleoside and shows weak antibacterial activity that is antagonized by guanine and guanosine. Oxanosine also has a weak antitumor effect on L1210 mouse leukemia.

Recently, oxanosine was found to alter tumor cell morphology into the normal morphology in temperature-sensitive Kirsten sarcoma virus-infected rat kidney (K-ras^{ts}-NRK) cells [10]. Addition of 2 μg/ml of oxanosine for 2 days at the permissive

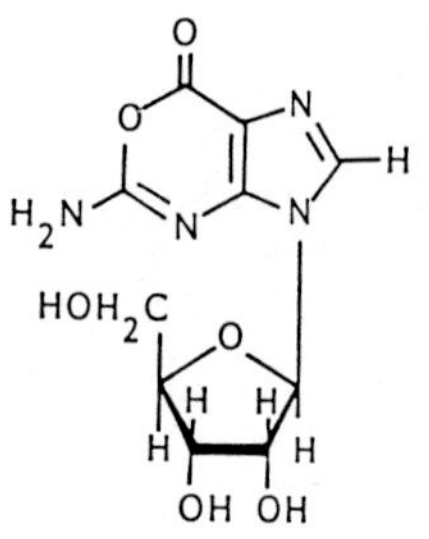

Fig. 3. Oxanosine.

temperature changed the tumor cell morphology into the normal cell morphology.

In Northern blotting analysis, oxanosine increased fibronectin mRNA expression. Using the Western blotting technique we analyzed the cellular levels of fibronectin. Incubation of K-ras[ts]-NRK cells at the permissive temperature with 2 μg/ml of oxanosine for 48 h increased cellular fibronectin content dramatically to the level of normal cells. The fibronectin content in the cells at the nonpermissive temperature did not change in the presence of oxanosine.

For the expression of *ras* oncogene function the p21[ras] protein must bind to guanine nucleotide. Therefore, we have studied whether oxanosine decreases the intracellular level of guanine nucleotides. In the metabolic pathway of GMP synthesis, IMP is converted to XMP by IMP dehydrogenase, and the XMP is converted to GMP by GMP synthetase. Oxanosine itself does not inhibit IMP dehydrogenase, but oxanosine 5'-monophosphate inhibits IMP dehydrogenase almost competitively with the substrate [26]. Therefore, it is likely that oxanosine is phosphorylated in the cells and thereby inhibits IMP dehydrogenase. The intracellular levels of GMP, GDP, or GTP are actually lowered by oxanosine, while the level of ATP is not affected [10].

INHIBITORS OF PHOSPHATIDYLINOSITOL TURNOVER

Various oncogenes such as *ras* [7], *src* [25], *sis* [23], *fms* [15], and *fes* [15] are reported to enhance cellu-

lar phosphatidylinositol turnover. Phosphatidyl breakdown generates two second messengers, diacylglycerol and inositol trisphosphate. Diacylglycerol activates protein kinase C [19], and inositol trisphosphate mobilizes calcium from the endoplasmic reticulum [2]. Therefore, we screened culture filtrates of microorganisms for inhibitors of phosphatidylinositol turnover and thus isolated psi-tectorigenin [13]. A culture broth of a strain of *Nocardiopsis* found in a river near Shanghai showed strong inhibition against phosphatidylinositol turnover. The active principle was purified and its structure was determined to be identical with that of psi-tectorigenin by NMR spectroscopy. As shown in Fig. 4, the structure of psi-tectorigenin is related to that of genistein [20] and of orobol [29], which were isolated from microorganisms as inhibitors of tyrosine protein kinase; however, the IC$_{50}$ of psi-tectorigenin for phosphatidylinositol turnover was several times smaller than those of genistein and orobol. On the other hand, psi-tectorigenin, orobol, and genistein all show similar *in vitro* inhibitory activity against EGF receptor tyrosine kinase, with an IC$_{50}$ of about 0.1 μg/ml.

At 40–100 μg/ml genistein was reported to inhibit both phosphatidylinositol turnover and EGF receptor tyrosine kinase in cultured A431 cells [1]. On the other hand, psi-tectorigenin at 5–50 μg/ml did not inhibit EGF receptor tyrosine kinase in these cells, but only phosphatidylinositol turnover [13]. *In situ* inhibition of tyrosine kinase requires a higher concentration of the inhibitor than *in vitro*, possibly because of slow penetration. Thus, psi-tectorigenin is a more potent and specific inhibitor of phosphatidylinositol turnover than genistein.

Since no potent inhibitors of phosphatidylinosit-

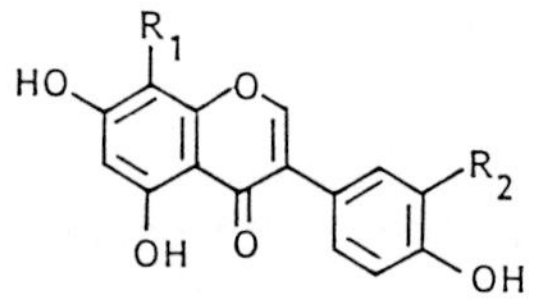

	R$_1$	R$_2$
psi-tectorigenin	OMe	H
orobol	H	OH
genistein	H	H

Fig. 4. Inhibitors of phosphatidylinositol turnover.

ol turnover have previously been reported, psi-tectorigenin may be a useful tool for functional studies on the role of phosphatidylinositol turnover in the mechanism of oncogene functions.

These inhibitors of oncogene functions are all microbial secondary metabolites. They are useful for the mechanistic study of oncogene functions. However, for eventual use in antitumor chemotherapy, we may have to obtain even stronger inhibitors of oncogene functions.

REFERENCES

1 Akiyama, T. and H. Ogawara. 1987. Drugs inhibiting the function of oncogene products, especially tyrosine kinases. Seikagaku 59: 1016–1020.

2 Berridge, M.J. and R.F. Irvine. 1984. Inositol triphosphate, a novel second messenger in cellular signal transduction. Nature 312: 315–321.

3 Casnellie, J.E., M.L. Harrison, L.J. Pike, K.E. Hellstron and E.G. Krebs. 1982. Phosphorylation of synthetic peptides by a tyrosine protein kinase from the particulate fraction of a lymphoma cell line. Proc. Natl. Acad. Sci. USA 79: 282–286.

4 Chen, W.S., C.S. Lazar, M. Poenile, R.Y. Tsien, G.N. Gill and M.G. Rosenfeld. 1987. Requirement for intrinsic protein tyrosine kinase in the immediate and late actions of the EGF receptor. Nature 328: 820–823.

5 Davis, R.J. and M.P. Czech. 1985. Amiloride directly inhibits growth factor receptor tyrosine kinase activity. J. Biol. Chem. 260: 2543–2551.

6 Erneux, C., S. Cohen and D.L. Garbers. 1983. The kinetics of tyrosine phosphorylation by the purified epidermal growth factor receptor kinase of A431 cells. J. Biol. Chem. 258: 4137–4142.

7 Fleischman, L.F., S.B. Chahwala and L. Cantley. 1986. Ras-transformed cells: altered levels of phosphatidylinositol-4,5-bisphosphate and catabolites. Science 231: 407–410.

8 Glenney, J.R., Jr., W.S. Chen, C.S. Lazar, G.M. Walton, L.M. Zokas, M.G. Rosenfeld and G.N. Gill. 1988. Ligand-induced endocytosis of the EGF receptor is blocked by mutational inactivation and by microinjection of anti-phosphotyrosine antibodies. Cell 52: 675–684.

9 Hidaka, H., M. Inagaki, S. Kawamoto and Y. Sasaki. 1984. Isoquinoline sulfonamide, novel and potent inhibitors of cyclic nucleotide dependent protein kinase and protein kinase C. Biochemistry 23: 5036–5041.

10 Itoh, O., S. Kuroiwa, S. Atsumi, K. Umezawa, T. Takeuchi and M. Hori. 1989. Oxanosine, a guanosine analog, alters the transformed phenotypes of rat kidney cells integrating K-ras into the normal phenotypes. Cancer Res. in press.

11 Imoto, M., K. Umezawa, K. Isshiki, S. Kunimoto, T. Sawa,

12 Imoto, M., K. Umezawa, T. Sawa, T. Takeuchi and H. Umezawa. 1987. In situ inhibition of tyrosine protein kinase by erbstatin. Biochem. Int. 15: 989–995.

13 Imoto, M., T. Yamashita, T. Sawa, S. Kurasawa, H. Naganawa, T. Takeuchi, Z. Bao-quan and K. Umezawa. 1988. Inhibition of cellular phosphatidylinositol turnover by psi-tectorigenin. FEBS Lett. 230: 43–46.

14 Isshiki, K., M. Imoto, T. Sawa, K. Umezawa, T. Takeuchi, H. Umezawa, T. Tsuchida, T. Yoshioka and K. Tatsuta. 1987. Inhibition of tyrosine protein kinase by synthetic erbstatin analogs. J. Antibiot. 40: 1209–1210.

15 Jackowski, S., C.W. Rettenmier, C.J. Sherr and C.O. Rock. 1986. A guanine nucleotide-dependent phosphatidylinositol 4,5-diphosphate phospholipase C in cells transformed by the v-fms and v-fes oncogenes. J. Biol. Chem. 261: 4978–4985.

16 Kaplan, D.R., M. Whitman, B. Schaffhausen, L. Raptis, R.L. Garcea, D. Pallas, T.M. Roberts and L. Cantley. 1986. Phosphatidylinositol metabolism and polyoma-mediated transformation. Proc. Natl. Acad. Sci. USA 83: 3624–3628.

17 Kase, H., K. Iwahashi, S. Nakanishi, Y. Matsuda, K. Yamada, M. Takahashi, C. Murakata, A. Sato and M. Kaneko. 1986. K-252 compounds, novel and potent inhibitors of protein kinase C and cyclic nucleotide-dependent protein kinases. Biochem. Biophys. Res. Commun. 135: 397–402.

18 Levinson, A.D., H. Oppermann, L. Levintow, H.E. Varmus and J.M. Bishop. 1978. Evidence that the transforming gene of avian sarcoma virus encodes a protein kinase associated with a phosphoprotein. Cell 15: 561–572.

19 Nishizuka, Y. 1984. The role of protein kinase C in cell surface signal transduction and tumor promotion. Nature 308: 693–698.

20 Ogawara, H., T. Akiyama, J. Ishida, S. Watanabe and K. Suzuki. 1986. A specific inhibitor for tyrosine protein kinase from Pseudomonas. J. Antibiot. 39: 606–608.

21 Ogawara, H., T. Akiyama, J. Ishida, S. Watanabe and K. Suzuki. 1986. A specific inhibitor for tyrosine protein kinase. 14th International Cancer Congress, Abstracts of Lectures, Symposia and Communications, Vol. 3, p. 1139.

22 Ōmura, S., A. Nakagawa and N. Sadakane. 1979. Structure of herbimycin, a new ansamycin antibiotic. Tetrahedron Lett. 1979: 4323–4326.

23 Preiss, J., C.R. Loomis, W.R. Bishop, R. Stein, J.E. Niedel and R.M. Bell. 1986. Quantitative measurement of sn-1,2-diacylglycerols present in platelets, hepatocytes, and ras- and sis-transformed normal rat kidney cells. J. Biol. Chem. 261: 8597–8600.

24 Shimada, N., N. Yagisawa, H. Naganawa, T. Takita, M. Hamada, T. Takeuchi and H. Umezawa. 1981. Oxanosine, a novel nucleoside from actinomycetes. J. Antibiot. 34: 1216–1218.

25 Sugimoto, Y. and R.L. Erikson. 1985. Phosphatidylinositol kinase activities in normal and Rous sarcoma virus-trans-

formed cells. Mol. Cell. Biol. 5: 3194–3198.

26 Uehara, Y., M. Hasegawa, M. Hori and H. Umezawa. 1985. Increased sensitivity to oxanosine, a novel nucleoside antibiotic, of rat kidney cells upon expression of the integrated viral *src* gene. Cancer Res. 45: 5230–5234.

27 Uehara, Y., M. Hori, T. Takeuchi and H. Umezawa. 1985. Screening of agents which convert 'transformed morphology' of Rous sarcoma virus-infected rat kidney cells to 'normal morphology': identification of an active agent as herbimycin and its inhibition of intracellular *src* kinase. Jap. J. Cancer Res. (Gann) 76: 672–675.

28 Uehara, Y., M. Hori, T. Takeuchi and H. Umezawa. 1986. Phenotypic change from transformed to normal induced by benzoquinoid ansamycins accompanies inactivation of p60[src] in rat kidney cells infected with Rous sarcoma virus. Mol. Cell. Biol. 6: 2198–2206.

29 Umezawa, H., M. Imoto, T. Sawa, K. Isshiki, N. Matsuda, T. Uchida, H. Iinuma, M. Hamada and T. Takeuchi. 1986. Studies on a new epidermal growth factor receptor kinase inhibitor, erbstatin, produced by MH435-hF3. J. Antibiot. 39: 170–173.

30 Umezawa, K., S. Atsumi, T. Matsushima and T. Takeuchi. 1987. Enhancement of fibronectin expression by herbimycin A. Experientia 43: 614–616.

31 Weinberg, R.A. 1985. The action of oncogenes in the cytoplasm and nucleus. Science 230: 770–776.

Novel Microbial Products for Medicine and Agriculture
Editors: A.L. Demain, G.A. Somkuti, J.C. Hunter-Cevera and H.W. Rossmoore

CHAPTER 7

Biosynthesis of rebeccamycin, a novel antitumor agent

Kin Sing Lam, Salvatore Forenza, Daniel R. Schroeder, Terrence W. Doyle and Cedric J. Pearce[*]

Bristol-Myers Company, Pharmaceutical Research and Development Division, Wallingford, CT, U.S.A.

SUMMARY

Evidence is presented to demonstrate that the antitumor secondary metabolite rebeccamycin is biosynthesized by *Saccharothrix aerocolonigenes* from one unit of glucose, one of methionine and two of tryptophan, with neither α-amine donating the nitrogen of the phthalimide system.

INTRODUCTION

Rebeccamycin (1) is an antitumor antibiotic isolated from cultures of *Saccharothrix aerocolonigenes*

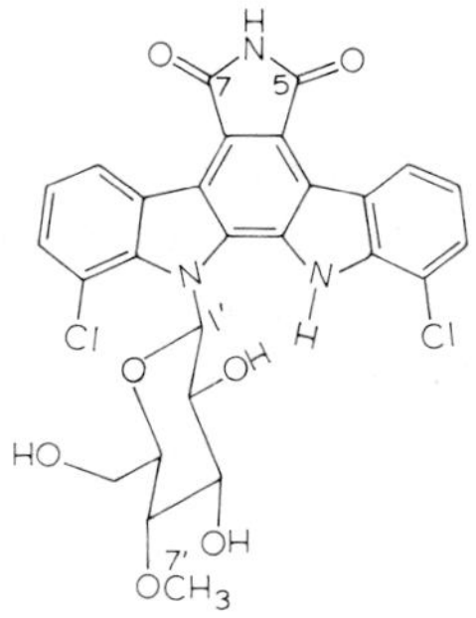

1

[2]. Its structure, consisting of a novel halogenated indolocarbazole chromophore *N*-glycosylated with 4-*O*-methylglucose, was elucidated using a combination of spectroscopic methods [7] and confirmed by X-ray analysis [7] and by total synthesis [6]. This novel chemotype shows good potential to yield a candidate for development toward clinical trials for cancer treatment in humans.

Rebeccamycin, together with staurosporine [4] and the arcyriaflavins [9], represents a unique chemotype which until now has not been investigated biosynthetically. Biogenetic analysis suggests that the indolocarbazole moiety is a tryptophan metabolite with glucose and methionine providing the remainder of the molecule. The chromophore could be derived from two identical tryptophan metabolites with the phthalimide nitrogen originating from a different source, or there could be an intermediate in which the phthalimide nitrogen is derived from one of the tryptophan halves, i.e. the chromophore is not derived from two identical precursors.

MATERIALS AND METHODS

Microorganism

The rebeccamycin-producing culture was identified as a strain of *Saccharothrix aerocolonigenes* [2]. This strain has been deposited with the American Type Culture Collection with the accession number ATCC 39243.

*Visiting Scientist from the School of Pharmacy, University of Connecticut, Storrs, CT, U.S.A.

Media and culture conditions

For this study *S. aerocolonigenes* was grown in a medium containing cerelose 3%, Pharmamedia 1%, Nutrisoy 1% and calcium carbonate 0.3%, at 28°C and 250 rpm on a gyrotary shaker. After 2 days, 3 ml aliquots were transferred to a medium containing soluble starch 1%, ammonium sulfate 0.25%, potassium phosphate 0.2%, magnesium chloride 0.2% and calcium carbonate 0.2%. Labeled precursors were added to the cultures at various times.

Preparation of rebeccamycin

Rebeccamycin was isolated from the cultures following 7 days incubation by extracting the mycelial cake with tetrahydrofuran and the concentrated extract was further purified by HPLC using a C_{18} column (0.1 M ammonium acetate/methanol/acetonitrile, 4:3:3) or using vacuum liquid chromatography [3, 8]. For this latter approach, the crude extract from 500 ml of culture was mixed with 1 g of silica gel H (Merck) and solvent was removed to absorb the material onto the silica gel. The absorbed material was added to the top of a short column prepared using 5 g of silica gel. The column was developed using increasing concentrations of ethyl acetate in hexane and the fraction eluted with 60% ethyl acetate was collected.

Antitumor assay

Test for inhibition of P388 leukemia in mice was performed using a previously described procedure [1, 5].

RESULTS AND DISCUSSION

Physiology of rebeccamycin production

The growth of *S. aerocolonigenes*, the pH of the media and the production of rebeccamycin were followed in a typical culture. The results are given in Table 1 and show a distinct trophophase and idiophase. This was considered promising for efficient utilization of added precursors, a speculation which was later shown to be correct.

Table 1

Production of rebeccamycin in a defined medium

Culture age (h)	% Sediment	pH	Rebeccamycin (μg/ml)
24	5	6.0	0
48	11	6.2	0
72	13	6.6	11.2
96	13	6.7	27.5
120	13	6.6	35.5
144	13	6.6	34.7

Purification and biological activity

Vacuum liquid chromatography was used as the initial purification step for rebeccamycin. Fifteen milligrams of rebeccamycin were recovered from 500 ml of the fermentation broth. This represents an 86.5% yield and rebeccamycin is pure enough for NMR analysis. Rebeccamycin can be further purified by preparative HPLC using a C_{18} column.

Purified rebeccamycin, when tested for activity in a P388 assay, prolonged the survival time of the test mice (Table 2). Thus with a dose of 200 mg/kg the mean survival time was increased by 55%; more than a 25% increase is considered to be significant antitumor activity.

Labeled precursor experiments

Initial experiments using carbon-14-labeled precursors showed that D-glucose, L-methionine and L-tryptophan were incorporated very efficiently into rebeccamycin (Table 3). In addition, these experi-

Table 2

Effect of rebeccamycin on murine P388 leukemia

Dose (mg/kg/injection)	Effectiveness MST % T/C
300	155
200	155
100	145
50	145

Tumor inoculum: 10^6 ascites cells, i.p.; host: CDF_1 mice; evaluation: MST = medium survival time; effectiveness: % T/C = (MST treated/MST control) $\times$ 100; criteria: % T/C $\geq$ 125 considered significant antitumor activity. Treatment schedule: ip, day 1.

Table 3

^{14}C-precursor incorporation into rebeccamycin

Precursor	Time of addition (day)	Incorporation (%)
D-[U-^{14}C]Glucose	0	0.22
	1	0.51
	2	0.29
	3	1.58
L-[3-^{14}C]Tryptophan	0	9.27
	1	9.65
	2	9.77
	3	6.92
L-[methyl-^{14}C]Methionine	0	0.88
	1	1.91
	2	4.48
	3	4.24

ments showed that the best time to add the precursors to obtain maximal incorporation was between 2 and 3 days, which corresponds to the appearance of rebeccamycin.

This feeding approach was repeated but replacing radiolabeled precursors with ^{13}C-enriched glucose, methionine or tryptophan. The labeling pattern in the resulting antibiotic was deduced using ^{13}C-NMR analysis. The enriched carbons are given in Table 4. These results confirm those obtained using radiolabeled precursors and demonstrate incorporation of glucose, methionine and tryptophan without extensive scrambling. To determine the source of the phthalimide nitrogen the following experiment was performed. A defined medium for re-

Table 4

^{13}C-precursor incorporation into rebeccamycin

Precursor	Position enriched	Enrichment factor
D-[1-^{13}C]Glucose	1′	5.2
L-[2-^{13}C]Tryptophan	5	3.4
	7	4.2
L-[methyl-^{13}C]Methionine	7′	4.4

beccamycin production was prepared using nitrogen-15-enriched ammonium sulfate as the sole nitrogen source. After 3 days incubation [2-^{13}C]tryptophan was added to the medium. Following a further 4 days incubation, the antibiotic was extracted, purified and analyzed using proton-decoupled ^{13}C-NMR. The spectrum shows signals for carbons 5 and 7 as both singlets and doublets (Fig. 1). The doublets A and B in Fig. 1 correspond to carbons 5 and 7 respectively, which are enriched 3–4-fold, and result from incorporated ^{13}C label being adjacent to ^{15}N. The minor singlets a and b from carbons 5 and 7 respectively are from ^{13}C which is not coupled to ^{15}N. This pattern is consis-

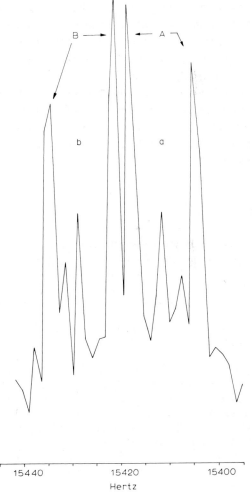

Fig. 1. ^{13}C-NMR spectrum of the phthalimide system of rebeccamycin showing ^{13}C-^{15}N and ^{13}C-^{14}N signals.

tent with ^{13}C and ^{15}N enrichment in the same molecule; thus the majority of molecules which are ^{13}C-enriched at position 5 also contain ^{15}N at position 6, the phthalimide system, and similarly for carbon 7. Since the only source of ^{13}C-enrichment is tryptophan and the only source of ^{15}N is the ammonium sulfate, this excludes the possibility that either of the α-amines of tryptophan are incorporated into rebeccamycin.

CONCLUSION

Rebeccamycin is derived from two molecules of tryptophan, one of glucose and one of methionine. Glucose and methionine are probably incorporated via UDP-glucose and *S*-adenosylmethionine respectively. That tryptophan is possibly incorporated following deamination to yield indolepyruvic acid is supported by the following observation. In competition experiments we have been able to demonstrate decreased incorporation of labeled tryptophan into rebeccamycin to one third of control values by adding indolepyruvic acid together with the tryptophan.

REFERENCES

1 Bradner, W.T. 1980. Transplanted animal tumors. In: Cancer and Chemotherapy, Vol. 1 (Crooke, S.T. and A.W. Prestayko, eds.) pp. 221–227, Academic Press, New York.

2 Bush, J.A., B.H. Long, J.J. Catino, W.T. Bradner and K. Tomita. 1987. Production and biological activity of rebeccamycin, a novel antitumor agent. J. Antibiot. 40: 668–678.

3 Coll, J.C. and B.F. Bowden. 1986. The application of vacuum liquid chromatography to the separation of terpene mixtures. J. Nat. Prod. 49: 934.

4 Furusaki, A., N. Hashiba, T. Matsumoto, A. Hirano, Y. Iwai and S. Ōmura. 1978. X-ray structure of staurosporine: a new alkaloid from a *Streptomyces* strain. J. Chem. Soc. Chem. Commun. 1978: 800–801.

5 Geran, R.I., N.H. Greenberg, M.M. MacDonald, A.M. Schumacher and B.J. Abbot. 1972. Protocols for screening chemical agents and natural products against tumors and other biological systems (3rd Edn.). Cancer Chemother. Rep. Part 3, 3: 1–103.

6 Kaneko, T., H. Wong, K.T. Okamoto and J. Clardy. 1985. Two synthetic approaches to rebeccamycin. Tetrahedron Lett. 26: 4015–4016.

7 Nettleton, D.E., T.W. Doyle, B. Krishnan, G.H. Matsumoto and J. Clardy. 1985. Isolation and structure of rebeccamycin: a new antitumor antibiotic from *Nocardia aerocolonigenes*. Tetrahedron Lett. 25: 4011–4014.

8 Pelletier, S.W., H.P. Choksie and H.K. Desai. 1986. Separation of diterpenoid alkaloid mixtures using vacuum liquid chromatography. J. Nat. Prod. 49: 892–900.

9 Steglich, W., B. Steffan, L. Kopanski and G. Eckhardt. 1980. Indole pigments from the fruiting bodies of the slime mold *Arcyria denudata*. Angew. Chem. Int. Ed. Engl. 19: 459–461.

Novel Microbial Products for Medicine and Agriculture
Editors: A.L. Demain, G.A. Somkuti, J.C. Hunter-Cevera and H.W. Rossmoore

CHAPTER 8

New adenosine deaminase inhibitors, adechlorin and adecypenol

Haruo Tanaka and Satoshi Ōmura

School of Pharmaceutical Sciences, Kitasato University, and The Kitasato Institute, Tokyo, Japan

SUMMARY

Adenosine deaminase inhibitors such as coformycin and deoxycoformycin have been of interest in the chemotherapy of viral diseases and cancer. During our screening work for new inhibitors of the enzyme from microorganisms, two new inhibitors, adechlorin and adecypenol, were isolated from the culture broths of *Actinomadura* sp. OMR-37 and *Streptomyces* sp. OM-3223, respectively. The aglycones of the inhibitors were identical to those of coformycin and deoxycoformycin. The K_i values for adechlorin and adecypenol against calf intestinal adenosine deaminase were determined to be 5.3×10^{-10} and 4.7×10^{-9} M, respectively. Adechlorin is an inhibitor of the tight-binding type like coformycin and deoxycoformycin, and enhanced the antiviral activity of Ara-A when HeLa S3 cells infected with HSV-1 were incubated with Ara-A in the presence of adechlorin (2.5 μM). Adecypenol is a semitight-binding inhibitor of adenosine deaminase. The double-reciprocal plot yielded patterns consistent with classical competitive inhibition. It was also found that adecypenol highly enhanced the cytotoxicity of Ara-A against HeLa S3 cells and that adecypenol greatly potentiated the antitumor activity of Ara-A against mouse leukemia L-1210 *in vivo*.

INTRODUCTION

The enzyme adenosine deaminase (ADA) (adenosine aminohydrolase, EC 3.5.4.4), which is widespread in mammalian tissue, is involved in the regulation of the intracellular levels of adenosine and deoxyadenosine, which control a number of important physiological functions and serve as precursors of nucleic acid biosynthesis. A congenital defect of ADA in lymphocytes and erythrocytes results in severe combined immunodeficiency, suggesting that the presence of ADA is essential for lymphocytic functions. Many adenosine analogs, which are important in cancer chemotherapy, immunology and virology, are substrates for ADA and are often inactivated by the enzyme. Thus, ADA inhibitors are responsible for alterations in adenosine and deoxyadenosine levels, lymphocytic growth and functions, and also enhance the chemotherapeutic effects of adenosine [1].

Two antibiotics, coformycin and 2'-deoxycoformycin (pentostatin), are known to be very potent inhibitors of ADA. Coformycin was discovered as a byproduct of formycin fermentations of *Nocardia interforma* and *Streptomyces kaniharaensis* [11, 15, 16]. In the studies of antitumor and antimicrobial activities of formycin, it was found that the purified material has much less activity than the crude material, and a minor component preventing the inactivation (deamination) of formycin was isolated from the crude material and named coformycin.

Deoxycoformycin was isolated from the fermentation broth of a strain of *S. antibioticus* in the course of screening work for ADA inhibitors [19]. It is known that the antibiotic possesses a chemotherapeutic effect on hairy cell [7] and adult T-cell leukemia [5, 10, 20].

Recently, we found two new ADA inhibitors, adechlorin (2′-chloropentostatin) [12] and adecypenol [13, 14], during the screening work for new ADA inhibitors from soil actinomycetes. In this paper, we describe their isolation, structures and biological activities including potentiation of *in vitro* cytotoxicity of Ara-A (vidarabine) and of the *in vivo* antitumor activity against L-1210 leukemia.

R
OH : Coformycin (**1**)
H : Deoxycoformycin (**2**)
Cl : Adechlorin (**3**)

Adecypenol (**4**)

SCREENING

Screening work for new ADA inhibitors was performed as follows. The reaction mixture containing adenosine and ADA preparation (Sigma, calf intestinal mucosa, type VI) was incubated at 20°C for 20 min in the presence of a culture filtrate of a soil isolate, and then applied to cellulose TLC with 5% Na_2HPO_4 saturated with isoamyl alcohol. The spots corresponding to adenosine and inosine were determined with a UV scanner.

Among about 8000 strains of soil actinomycetes, new ADA inhibitors, adechlorin (OMR-37 and an additional three strains) and adecypenol (OMR-3227) were discovered, and coformycin and deoxycoformycin producers (20 strains) were also selected. Based on their taxonomic properties, the adechlorin producer OMR-37, which also produced 2′-deoxycoformycin, was classified into the genus *Actinomadura*, and the adecypenol producer OM-3223, which coproduced coformycin, was determined to belong to the genus *Streptomyces* [12, 13].

ISOLATION AND STRUCTURE OF ADECHLORIN

The cultured broth of *Actinomadura* sp. OMR-37 was obtained by incubation in a medium (20 liters) consisting of glucose 0.1%, soluble starch 2.4%, meat extract 0.3%, Bacto-Tryptone 0.5%, yeast extract 0.5%, and $CaCO_3$ 0.2%, pH 7.2, at 30°C for 42 h using a 30-liter jar fermentor. The culture supernatant (55 liters) was subjected to column chromatography on activated carbon, Diaion HP-20 and silica gel to give two active fractions A and B. The fractions A and B provided pure materials of adechlorin (127 mg) and 2′-deoxycoformycin (173 mg), respectively, after gel filtration through a Toyopearl HW-40 column. Adechlorin was obtained as colorless crystals: m.p. 125–131°C, $[\alpha]_D^{20}$ (c 1.0, H_2O) + 21°, UV λ_{max}^{MeOH} nm (ε): 283 (12 080). The molecular formula was established to be $C_{11}H_{15}N_4O_4Cl$ from the results of the elemental analysis and the high-resolution mass spectrum of the tetraacetate. The structure (3) was elucidated by comparison of the ^1H- and ^{13}C-NMR and mass spectra with those of coformycin and 2′-deoxycoformycin and by the NMR analysis of the acetate and its hydrolysate [12]. Independently, Schaumberg *et al.* [17] reported the same compound, which was found by using *Enterococcus faecium* PD 05045 as test organism.

ADA-INHIBITING AND BIOLOGICAL ACTIVITIES OF ADECHLORIN

Kinetics of the ADA inhibition by adechlorin was examined as described by Agarwal et al. [2]. They classified ADA inhibitors into three types of readily-reversible, semitight-binding and tight-binding inhibitors. Adechlorin exhibited complete inhibition against ADA at 100 nM without preincubation. As shown in Fig. 1, when 1.0 nM adechlorin was preincubated in the reaction mixture for 15 min, it exhibited potent inhibitory activity and the inhibition continued for a long time, while almost no inhibition was observed at the same concentration of adechlorin without preincubation. This indicates that adechlorin is an inhibitor of the tight-

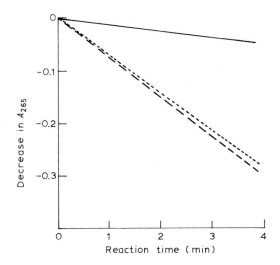

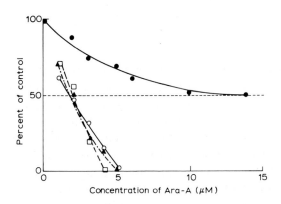

Fig. 2. Enhancement of antiviral activity of Ara-A by adechlorin. ●, Ara-A (ED$_{50}$ = 14 μM); □--□, Ara-A + 2′-deoxycoformycin (2.5 μM); ▲-··-▲, Ara-A + coformycin (2.5 μM); ○—○ Ara-A + adechlorin (2.5 μM).

Fig. 1. Effect of preincubation on ADA inhibition by adechlorin. ⎼⎼, no adechlorin; ⎼⎼⎼⎼, 1.0 nM adechlorin without preincubation; ⎯, 1.0 nM adechlorin with 15 min preincubation.

binding type like coformycin and 2′-deoxycoformycin [1, 3].

The K_i values of adechlorin, coformycin and 2′-deoxycoformycin were determined to be 5.3 × 10^{-10}, 2.1 × 10^{-10} and 7.6 × 10^{-11}M, respectively, as described by Cha *et al.* [3].

Adechlorin did not exhibit antimicrobial activity against various bacteria and fungi at the concentration of 1.0 mg/ml. When adechlorin was administered intravenously to mice at the dose of 100 mg/kg, no acute toxicity was observed although some weight loss was noted.

Because ADA inhibitors are known to enhance the antiviral activity of Ara-A [1], the effect of adechlorin on the antiviral activity of Ara-A was examined by the plaque reduction method [4] using HeLa S3 cells infected with herpes simplex virus type I. As shown in Fig. 2, the enhancing effect of adechlorin was equivalent to those of coformycin and 2′-deoxycoformycin.

Recently, Jackson *et al.* [8] reported that adechlorin (2′-chloropentostatin) potentiates to a considerable extent the cytotoxicity and *in vivo* antitumor activity of Ara-A against L-1210 leukemia.

ISOLATION AND STRUCTURE OF ADECYPENOL

Fermentative production of adecypenol by *Streptomyces* sp. OM-3223 was carried out in a 30-liter jar fermentor containing 20 liters of a medium consisting of glucose 2.0%, peptone 0.5%, meat extract 0.5%, yeast extract 0.1%, NaCl 0.5%, and CaCO$_3$ 0.3%, pH 8.0, at 30°C for 40 h. The broth supernatant (18 liters) was subjected to column chromatography on activated carbon, Amberlite IRC-50 and silica gel-RP-18 to give two active components, which corresponded to adecypenol (19 mg) and coformycin (20 mg). Adecypenol was obtained as colorless needles: m.p. 240–245°C (decomp.), $[\alpha]_D^{24}$ (*c 1.0, H$_2$O*) −31.6°, UV λ_{max}^{MeOH} nm (ε) 279 (7960). The molecular formula was established to be C$_{12}$H$_{16}$N$_4$O$_4$ by high-resolution mass spectroscopy and elemental analysis. The data from ^{1}H- and ^{13}C-NMR and EI-MS confirmed that the chromophore was identical to those of adechlorin, coformycin and 2′-deoxycoformycin. The structure of the other moiety was estimated by ^{1}H-NMR decoupling experiments at 400 MHz to be identical to the cyclopentene system of neplanocin A. Thus, the structure of adecypenol was elucidated to be $\underline{4}$ [14].

70

ADA-INHIBITING AND BIOLOGICAL ACTIVITIES OF
ADECYPENOL

Kinetics of the ADA inhibition by adecypenol was investigated as described by Agarwal *et al.* [2]. As shown in Fig. 3, the inhibitory effect of adecypenol was enhanced by preincubation with the enzyme for 15 min. However, the inhibition was not complete and the enzyme reaction proceeded gradually. Thus, adecypenol was classified as being of the semitight-binding type, like a chemically synthesized inhibitor, *erythro*-9-(2-hydroxyl-3-nonyl)adenosine [1]. The K_i value of adecypenol was calculated according to the Lineweaver - Burk method. The velocity was determined after the attainment of a steady state in the binding between adecypenol and ADA (after about 3 min). The double-reciprocal plots yielded patterns consistent with classical competitive inhibition. The replot of the slope vs. adecypenol concentration was linear and yielded a K_i value of 4.7×10^{-9} M.

Adecypenol did not exhibit antimicrobial activity against various bacteria and fungi tested at 1.0 mg/ml by the paper disc method. When adecypenol was administered intravenously to mice at the dose of 100 mg/kg, no acute toxicity was observed.

Adecypenol was not cytotoxic to cultured cells even at 20 μg/ml (Fig. 5); however, it potentiated the cytotoxicity of adenine nucleosides. Fig. 4 shows the results obtained with HeLa S3 cells. The cells were grown in a medium supplemented with 10% calf serum. Deoxyadenosine at 20 μg/ml gave 28% inhibition of growth; on the other hand, 20 μg/ml of deoxyadenosine plus 5 μg/ml of adecypenol gave 90% inhibition. Fig. 5 shows that the mixture

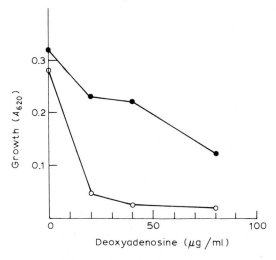

Fig. 4. Potentiation of the cytotoxicity of deoxyadenosine by adecypenol. ●, no adecypenol; ○, 5 μg/ml adecypenol.

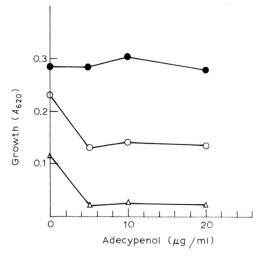

Fig. 5. Reversal of the cytotoxicity in the presence of deoxyadenosine and adecypenol by other deoxyribonucleosides. Deoxyribonucleosides consisted of deoxyadenosine, deoxyguanosine, deoxycytidine and deoxythymidine. ●, no addition; ○, 80 μg/ml of each deoxyribonucleoside; △, 80 μg/ml deoxyadenosine.

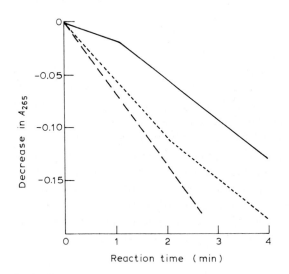

Fig. 3. Effect of preincubation on ADA inhibition by adecypenol. --, no adecypenol; -----, 25 nM adecypenol without preincubation; ——, 25 nM adecypenol with 15 min preincubation.

of deoxynucleosides (deoxyadenosine, deoxyguanosine, deoxycytidine and deoxythymidine, each 80 μg/ml) reversed about a half of the inhibition by deoxyadenosine alone or deoxyadenosine plus adecypenol. These results coincide with the report that dATP, formed from deoxyadenosine and accumulated in the cells, serves as a feedback inhibitor of ribonucleotide reductase and causes a depletion of other deoxyribonucleosides, and as a result DNA synthesis decreases [9]. Thus, it is considered that the mixture of deoxyribonucleosides restores DNA synthesis. The IC_{50} value of Ara-A against HeLa S3 cells was > 100 μM; however, it was decreased to 16.1 and 14.5 μM in the presence of 1.0 μM adecypenol and 0.1 μM 2′-deoxycoformycin, respectively.

The antitumor activity of adecypenol and its ability to potentiate the antitumor effect of Ara-A were studied in L-1210 leukemia. CDF_1 mice were injected intraperitoneally with 1×10^5 L-1210 cells on day 0 and given drugs intraperitoneally twice (9 a.m. and 6 p.m.) a day for 7 days. On this schedule, Ara-A (100 mg/kg/day) or adecypenol (5 mg/kg/day) alone did not show antitumor activity. However, the combination of the drugs gave a greater extension of lifespan as shown in Table 1; for exam-

ple, the optimal combination gave a 94% increase in lifespan.

DISCUSSION

Besides the known ADA inhibitors, coformycin and deoxycoformycin, additional new inhibitors adechlorin and adecypenol were discovered in our screening work for new ADA inhibitors from microorganisms. Consequently, all of the ADA inhibitors which have been discovered from microorganisms have the same chromophore. Although coformycin, 2′-deoxycoformycin and adechlorin have a sugar moiety (ribose, deoxyribose or 2′-chloro-2′-deoxyribose, respectively) and are tight-binding inhibitors of ADA, adecypenol has a cyclopentene moiety instead of a sugar and is a semitight-binding inhibitor.

The cyclopentene moiety is also a structural moiety of neplanocin A, a cyclopentenyl analog of adenosine, which is a specific inhibitor of RNA methylation but is not an RNA synthesis inhibitor and not utilized for transcription [6]. Siaw and Coleman [18] reported that deoxycoformycin is phosphorylated to give mono-, di- and triphosphate derivatives, and that the triphosphate derivative is incorporated into cellular DNA. It is considered that this may result in the unusual organ toxicities which have been associated with the use of high levels of this drug [18]. Recently, 2′-deoxycoformycin therapy at low doses in hairy cell leukemia [7] and adult T-cell leukemia [5, 10, 20] has been reported to give good results.

We have found that the semitight-binding ADA inhibitor adecypenol is also effective in potentiating *in vivo* antitumor activity of Ara-A. Further *in vitro* and *in vivo* studies using adecypenol are of interest because it is expected that the compound is not phosphorylated and has low toxicity *in vivo*.

Table 1

Combination effect of adecypenol and Ara-A on L1210 leukemia in mice

Drug	Dose (mg/kg/day)	Increase in lifespan (%)	Body weight (g)
Adecypenol	5	0	19.2
Ara-A	100	17	18.2
Adecypenol/			
Ara-A	5/100	toxic	
	2/100	94	14.4
	0.4/100	53	17.2
	5/25	44	17.9
	2/25	42	19.4
	0.4/25	28	19.3

Mean survival time and weight at day 6 of control mice (5 mice in a group) was 7.2 ± 0.4 days and 20.6 ± 0.8 g. Mice were administered drugs intraperitoneally twice a day (9 a.m. and 6 p.m.) on days 1–3 and 5–8.

REFERENCES

1 Agarwal, R.P. 1982. Inhibitors of adenosine deaminase. Pharmacol. Ther. 17: 399–429.

72

2 Agarwal, R.P., T. Spector and R.E. Parks, Jr. 1977. Tight-binding inhibitors. IV. Inhibition of adenosine deaminase by various inhibitors. Biochem. Pharmacol. 26: 359–367.

3 Cha, S., R.P. Agarwal and R.E. Parks, Jr. 1975. Tight-binding inhibitors. II. Non-steady state nature of inhibition of milk xanthine oxidase by allopurinol and alloxanthine and of human erythrocytic adenosine deaminase by coformycin. Biochem. Pharmacol. 24: 2187–2197.

4 Conner, J.D., K. Sweetman, S. Carey, M.A. Stuckey and R. Bachaman. 1974. Effect of adenosine deaminase upon the antiviral activity *in vitro* of adenine arabinoside for vaccinia virus. Antimicrob. Agents Chemother. 6: 630–636.

5 Daenen, S., R.A. Rojer, J.W. Smit, M.R. Halle and H.O. Nieweg. 1984. Successful chemotherapy with deoxycoformycin in adult T-cell lymphoma-leukaemia. Br. J. Haematol. 58: 723–727.

6 Glazer, R.I. and M.C. Knode. 1984. Neplanocin A, a cyclopentenyl analog of adenosine with specificity for inhibiting RNA methylation. J. Biol. Chem. 259: 12 964–12 969.

7 Golomb, H.M. and M.J. Ratain. 1987. Recent advances in the treatment of hairy-cell leukemia. New Engl. J. Med. 316: 870–872.

8 Jackson, R.C., W.R. Leopold and D.A. Ross. 1986. The biochemical pharmacology of (2′-R)chloropentostatin, a novel inhibitor of adenosine deaminase. Adv. Enzyme Regul. 25: 125–139.

9 Korte, D., W.A. Haverkort, E.F. Leeuwen, D. Roos and A.H. Gennip. 1987. Biochemical consequences of 2′-deoxycoformycin treatment in a patient with T-cell lymphoma. Some unusual findings. Cancer 60: 750–755.

10 Lofters, W., M. Campbell, W.N. Gibbs and B.D. Cheson. 1987. 2′-Deoxycoformycin therapy in adult T-cell leukemia/lymphoma. Cancer 60: 2605–2608.

11 Niida, T., T. Niwa, T. Tsuruoka, N. Ezaki, T. Shomura and H. Umezawa. 1967. Isolation and characteristics of coformycin. Presented at the 153rd Scientific Meeting of the Japanese Antibiotic Research Association, Jan. 27, 1967.

12 Ōmura, S., N. Imamura, H. Kuga, H. Ishikawa, Y. Yamazaki, K. Okano, K. Kumura, Y. Takahashi and H. Tanaka. 1985. Adechlorin, a new adenosine deaminase inhibitor containing chlorine. Production, isolation and properties. J. Antibiot. 38: 1008–1015.

13 Ōmura, S., H. Ishikawa, H. Kuga, N. Imamura, S. Taga, Y. Takahashi and H. Tanaka. 1986. Adecypenol, a unique adenosine deaminase inhibitor containing homopurine and cyclopentene rings. Taxonomy, production and enzyme inhibition. J. Antibiot. 39: 1219–1224.

14 Ōmura, S., H. Tanaka, H. Kuga and N. Imamura. 1986. Adecypenol, a unique adenosine deaminase inhibitor containing homopurine and cyclopentene rings. J. Antibiot. 39: 309–310.

15 Sawa, T., Y. Fukagawa, I. Homma, T. Takeuchi and H. Umezawa. 1967. Mode of inhibition of coformycin on adenosine deaminase. J. Antibiot. Ser. A 20: 227–231.

16 Sawa, T., Y. Fukagawa, I. Homma, T. Takeuchi and H. Umezawa. 1967. Formycin-deaminating activity of microorganisms. J. Antibiot. Ser. A 20: 317–321.

17 Schaumberg, J.P., G.C. Hokanson, J.C. French, E. Smal and D.C. Baker. 1985. 2′-Chloropentostatin, a new inhibitor of adenosine deaminase. J. Org. Chem. 50: 1651–1656.

18 Siaw, M.F.E. and M.S. Coleman. 1984. *In vitro* metabolism of deoxycoformycin in human T lymphoblastoid cells. Phosphorylation of deoxycoformycin and incorporation into cellular DNA. J. Biol. Chem. 259: 9426–9433.

19 Woo, P.W.K., H.W. Dion, S.M. Lange, L.F. Dahl and L.J. Durham. 1974. A novel adenosine and Ara-A deaminase inhibitor. (*R*)-3-(2-deoxy-β-D-*erythro*-pentofuranosyl)-3,6,7,8-tetrahydroimidazo[4,5-*d*][1,3]diazepin-8-ol. J. Heterocyclic Chem. 11: 641–643.

20 Yamaguchi, K., L.S. Yul, T. Oda, Y. Maeda, M. Ishii, K. Fujita, S. Kagiyama, K. Nagai, H. Suzuki and K. Takatsuki. 1986. Clinical consequences of 2′-deoxycoformycin treatment in patients with refractory adult T-cell leukemia. Leukemia Res. 10: 989–993.

Novel Microbial Products for Medicine and Agriculture
Editors: A.L. Demain, G.A. Somkuti, J.C. Hunter-Cevera and H.W. Rossmoore

CHAPTER 9

Trichostatin and leptomycin: specific inhibitors of the G1 and G2 phases of the eukaryotic cell cycle

Teruhiko Beppu and Minoru Yoshida

Department of Agricultural Chemistry, The University of Tokyo, Tokyo, Japan

SUMMARY

Trichostatins A and C, isolated as potent inducers of erythroid differentiation in murine Friend leukemia cells, caused reversible arrest of rat 3Y1 fibroblast proliferation in phases G1 and G2 without any inhibitory effect on macromolecular synthesis. Leptomycins A and B, isolated as agents to induce morphological abnormalities in fungi and yeast cells, also caused the arrest of the cell cycle in phases G1 and G2 in *Schizosaccharomyces pombe* and 3Y1 cells. Both of the agents showed a selective killing effect on the SV40-transformed fibroblasts, and antitumor activity against transplantable murine tumors was detected with leptomycin B *in vivo*. The possibility of using these specific G1 and G2 phase inhibitors as selective antitumor agents is discussed.

INTRODUCTION

Extensive screening of antitumor agents from microbial sources has provided a variety of chemicals, most being potent inhibitors of cellular DNA synthesis which inevitably have a nonselective toxic effect on the normal proliferative tissues. In order to break through the limitations of the present chemotherapy, development of agents with selective inhibitory effects on proliferation of tumor cells is needed.

The major events in the eukaryotic cell cycle, DNA synthesis in S phase and mitotic cell division in M phase, are completely separated by two gap phases, G1 and G2. In addition, normal proliferating cells can be reversibly introduced into quiescence (G0) by serum deprivation. Several growth factors such as platelet-derived and epidermal growth factors are required for initiation or pro-

gression of G1 phase [10]. Reversible arrest of the cell cycle in G2 phase has also been suggested [3]. There are many indications that regulatory mechanisms in phases G1 and G2 might play an essential role in controlling cellular proliferation, differentiation and carcinogenesis. Thus it seems probable that some events in the gap phases will be potential targets for developing selective antitumor agents.

Trichostatins and leptomycins were the products of *Streptomyces* isolated as potent inducers of erythroleukemia cell differentiation and morphological abnormalities in the lower eukaryotic microorganisms, respectively. Both of these agents were found to possess new activities causing the reversible arrest of the eukaryotic cell cycle in both G1 and G2 phase in normal cells, while they caused irreversible killing of virus-transformed cells. Their characteristic modes of action are dealt with in this paper.

TRICHOSTATINS

The murine erythroleukemia cell line established by Friend *et al.* [1] consists of transformed cells in which erythroid differentiation is blocked by infection with Friend leukemia virus. Differentiation is reinitiated effectively by various polar compounds such as dimethyl sulfoxide (DMSO) [2] and hexamethylene bisacetamide [11]. Relatively weak differentiation is also induced by a variety of agents affecting DNA metabolism such as UV irradiation and mitomycin C. The cell line has been used as a model system of eukaryotic cell differentiation as well as an assay system for screening new agents with differentiation-inducing activities.

As a result of such screening with microbial metabolites, we detected the potent activity in broth of a strain which was identified to be *Streptomyces platensis.* The active agents were found to be trichostatin A (TSA) and trichostatin C (TSC) (Fig. 1) [14, 15], which had been reported to be antifungal antibiotics. TSA and TSC induced efficient differentiation of Friend cells with the maximum induction of about 80% benzidine-positive cells at 1.5×10^{-8} M and 5×10^{-7} M, respectively. Erythroid differentiation by TS was cooperatively enhanced by UV irradiation but not by treatment with DMSO. No inhibitory effect of TS was observed on synthesis of DNA and other macromolecules in Friend cells [15]. These results indicate some similarity of the mode of action of TS to that of DMSO, but the striking feature of TS is their extremely low dosage required for induction of differentiation.

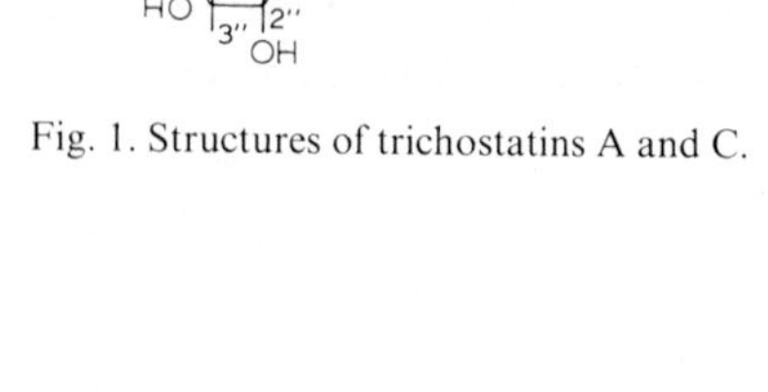

Fig. 1. Structures of trichostatins A and C.

During the course of these studies, we observed that TSA caused inhibition of cell growth without any inhibitory effect on macromolecular synthesis. Detailed analysis of the inhibitory effect was performed with proliferating rat 3Y1 fibroblast cells [13]. Addition of 0.1 μg/ml of TSA caused growth inhibition along with a gradual decrease of the mitotic index of the cell population. DNA synthesis was not inhibited at all during the first 4 h after the drug challenge and was then gradually suppressed to zero after 24 h incubation. These results suggest that TSA caused arrest of the cells at some points in the cell cycle but not in the S and M phases.

When the cells arrested in G0 phase by serum starvation were transferred to fresh minimum essential medium containing 12% fetal calf serum, proliferation of the cells started synchronously from G0 and proceeded through G1 to S phase. Addition of TSA to the synchronous culture within 6 h after the serum stimulation caused complete inhibition of the cells to enter S phase, indicating that arrest occurred with TSA in early G1 phase.

On the other hand, TSA was found to cause arrest in G2 phase in the synchronous culture starting from early S phase. Proliferating 3Y1 cells were accumulated in early S phase by incubation with 1 mM hydroxyurea. Then the cells were released from the hydroxyurea-arrest and challenged with TSA. Distribution of DNA contents in nuclei in the cell population was analyzed during the following cultivation by flow cytometry. As shown in Fig. 2, TSA did not inhibit DNA synthesis in S phase as suggested by transition of the 2C peak toward 4C, but completely blocked the following process to reproduce the 2C peak in the control culture. Thus it is evident that TSA causes arrest of the cell cycle in both the G1 and G2 phases, suggesting involvement of a common molecular mechanism in both gap phases.

Another striking effect of TSA was found when the cells arrested in G2 phase by TSA were released from the inhibition. In such a culture, almost all the cells with 4C DNA skipped M phase and entered S phase after an 18-h lag, resulting in the formation of proliferative tetraploid cells. This characteristic mode of action of TSA on the cell cycle can be illus-

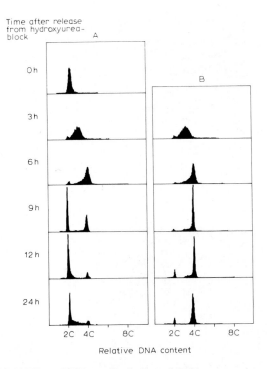

Time after release from hydroxyurea-block

0h

3h

6h

9h

12h

24h

2C 4C   8C   2C 4C   8C

Relative DNA content

Fig. 2. Effect of TSA on distribution of DNA contents in cultures released from hydroxyurea-block. 3Y1 cells were released from hydroxyurea-block in the control (A). TSA (0.1 μg/ml) was added simultaneously with release from the hydroxyurea-block at time 0 (B).

trated as in Fig. 3. TSA seems to be at least a useful tool for analyzing the regulatory mechanisms in the eukaryotic cell cycle.

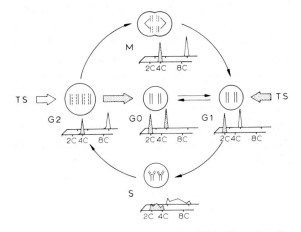

Fig. 3. Points in the cell cycle arrested by TSA. Typical profiles of DNA contents in nuclei at G0, G1, S, G2 and M phases are illustrated. TSA-block in G2 phase causes introduction of 4C cells into G0.

Although this characteristic arrest of the cell cycle with TSA was completely reversible in normal 3Y1 fibroblasts, the same concentration of TSA caused irreversible killing of the SV40 virus-transformed fibroblasts along with a different profile of DNA contents in nuclei. These results suggest an essential difference in the G1 and G2 phases in the transformed cells from those in the normal cells, and also suggest the possibility that the G1- and/or G2-specific inhibitors might be selective antitumor agents.

LEPTOMYCINS

In order to find a new type of antifungal antibiotic, we had conducted a screening project to detect activity to induce morphological abnormalities in various fungi and yeast cells [4]. Leptomycins A and B (LMA, LMB) (Fig. 4) were obtained from the broth of a *Streptomyces* strain as the agents inducing hyphal curling of *Trichophyton mentagrophytes* and cell elongation of fission yeast, *Schizosaccharomyces pombe* (Fig. 5) [5–7].

LMB caused growth inhibition of *S. pombe* following elongation of cells at 2×10^{-8} M, while only slight inhibition of DNA and RNA synthesis was observed at this concentration. Addition of LMB to a synchronous culture in G2 phase blocked subsequent events in the cell cycle. Analysis of the effect of LMB on *cdc2* (nuclear division blocked) and *cdc7* (early cell plate formation blocked) mutants also supported the G2-arrest by LMB in *S. pombe* [8]. In addition, recent results also revealed that LMB caused arrest of the cell cycle not only in G2 phase but also in G1 phase in both *S. pombe* and 3Y1 fibroblast cells. Although the apparent mode of action of LMB closely resembles that of TSA,

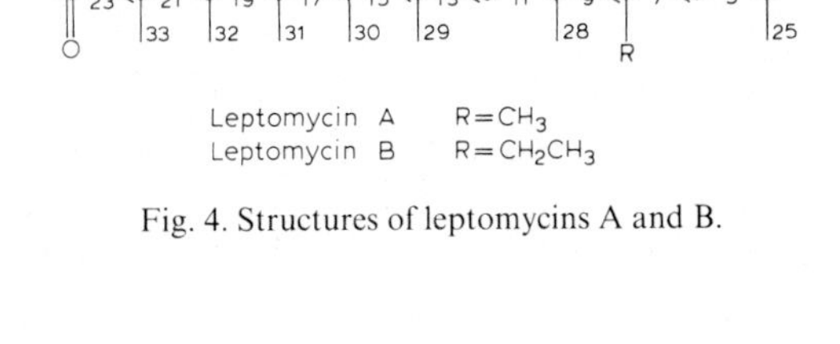

Leptomycin A   R=CH$_3$
Leptomycin B   R=CH$_2$CH$_3$

Fig. 4. Structures of leptomycins A and B.

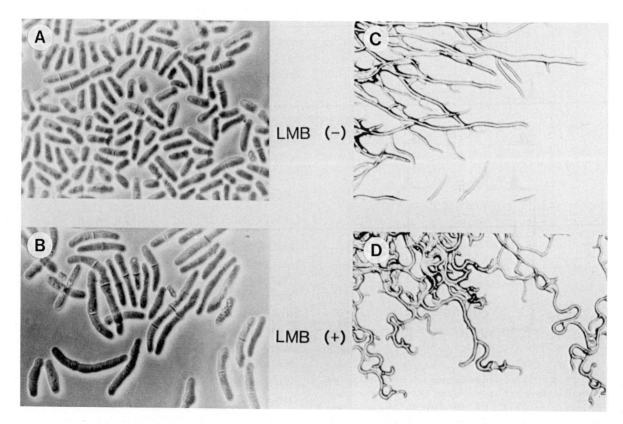

Fig. 5. Cell elongation of *S. pombe* and hyphal curling of *T. mentagrophytes* by LMB. (A) *S. pombe* (control). (B) Elongated cells of *S. pombe*. (C) *T. mentagrophytes* (control). (D) Hyphal curling of *T. mentagrophytes*.

several results indicated that their targets are different. LMB showed a selective killing effect on the SV40-transformed fibroblasts and also showed distinct antitumor activity against several transplantable murine tumors *in vivo* (Table 1) [9].

DISCUSSION

TSA and LMB were found to block the cell cycle progression in both G1 and G2 phases without any extensive killing or inhibition of macromolecular synthesis in normal cells. Both agents showed a marked selective killing effect on the virus-transformed cells. This type of agent has not previously been discovered, except for a high concentration (5 mM) of sodium butyrate [12]. It seems probable that the type of past screening project to find potent killing agents for tumor cells has facilitated the detection of DNA-attacking agents but missed another type of cell cycle inhibitors. Complicated regulatory machineries operating in G1 and G2 phases might be targets of a variety of new agents, whose possibilities in tumor chemotherapy must be explored in the future.

Table 1

Antitumor activity of LMB on murine tumors

Treatment schedule	Total dose (mg/kg)	Increase in life span (%)			
		P388	Lewis lung	B16 melanoma	Ehrlich
Saline	—	0	0	0	0
Day 1	1.25		−31	0	36
	0.625	19	−3	0	23
	0.313	14	21	6	63
	0.156	13			39(1)
	0.078				14
Days 1, 5, 9	1.25	23	−13	6	114(1)
	0.625	23	34	11	49(1)
	0.313	19	13	24	60
	0.156	11	30	15	55(1)
	0.078	14			72
	0.039				24
Days 1–5	0.625	−45			−4
	0.313	4	−42	−18	97(2)
	0.156	47	102	14	125(1)
	0.078	40	48	32	53(1)
	0.039	19	52	43	30

Tumor: P388 leukemia, 1×10^5 cells/CDF; Lewis lung carcinoma, 1×10^6 cells/C57BL; B16 melanoma, 1×10^6 cells/C57BL; and Ehrlich carcinoma, 2.5×10^6 cells/ddY. Mean survival days (range) of controls were as follows: P388 leukemia, 10.6 (10–11); Lewis lung carcinoma, 12.2 (11–14); B16 melanoma, 22.8 (19–28); and Ehrlich carcinoma 21.1 (15–29). Numbers in parentheses indicate the number of cured mice/five treated mice. Cured mice were excluded from the calculation of the increase in life span.

REFERENCES

1 Friend, C., M.C. Patuleia and E. de Harven. 1966. Erythrocytic maturation *in vitro* of murine (Friend) virus-induced leukemia cells. Natl. Cancer Inst. Monogr. 228: 505–520.

2 Friend, C., W. Scher, J.G. Holland and T. Sato. 1971. Hemoglobin synthesis in murine virus-induced leukemic cells *in vitro*: stimulation of erythroid differentiation by dimethyl sulfoxide. Proc. Natl. Acad. Sci. USA 68: 378–382.

3 Gelfant, S. 1977. A new concept of tissue and tumor cell proliferation. Cancer Res. 37: 3845–3862.

4 Gunji, S., K. Arima and T. Beppu. 1983. Screening of antifungal antibiotics according to activities inducing morphological abnormalities. Agric. Biol. Chem. 47: 2061–2069.

5 Hamamoto, T., S. Gunji, H. Tsuji and T. Beppu. 1983. Leptomycins A and B, new antifungal antibiotics. I. Taxonomy of the producing strain and their fermentation, purification and characterization. J. Antibiot. 36: 639–645.

6 Hamamoto, T., H. Seto and T. Beppu. 1983. Leptomycins A and B, new antifungal antibiotics. II. Structure elucidation. J. Antibiot. 36: 646–650.

7 Hamamoto, T., T. Uozumi and T. Beppu. 1985. Biosynthetic studies of leptomycins. J. Antibiot. 38: 533–535.

8 Hamamoto, T., T. Uozumi and T. Beppu. 1985. Leptomycins A and B, new antifungal antibiotics. III. Mode of action of leptomycin B on *Schizosaccharomyces pombe*. J. Antibiot. 38: 1573–1580.

9 Komiyama, K., K. Okada, S. Tomisaka, I. Umezawa, T. Hamamoto and T. Beppu. 1985. Antitumor activity of leptomycin B. J. Antibiot. 38: 427–429.

10 Pardee, A.B., R. Dubrow, J.L. Hamlin and R.F. Kletzien. 1978. Animal cell cycle. Annu. Rev. Biochem. 47: 715–750.

11 Reuben, R.C., R.L. Wife, R. Breslow, R.A. Rifkind and P.A. Marks. 1976. A new group of potent inducers of differentiation in murine erythroleukemia cells. Proc. Natl. Acad. Sci. USA 73: 862–866.

12 Yamada, K. and G. Kimura. 1985. Formation of proliferative tetraploid cells after treatment of diploid cells with sodium butyrate in rat 3Y1 fibroblasts. J. Cell Physiol. 122: 59–63.

13 Yoshida, M. and T. Beppu. 1988. Reversible arrest of proliferation of rat 3Y1 fibroblasts in both the G1 and G2 phases by trichostatin A. Exp. Cell Res. 177: 122–131.

78

14 Yoshida, M., Y. Iwamoto, T. Uozumi and T. Beppu. 1985. Trichostatin C, a new inducer of differentiation of Friend leukemic cells. Agric. Biol. Chem. 49: 563–565.

15 Yoshida, M., S. Nomura and T. Beppu. 1987. Effects of trichostatins on differentiation of murine erythroleukemia cells. Cancer Res. 47: 3688–3691.

Novel Microbial Products for Medicine and Agriculture
Editors: A.L. Demain, G.A. Somkuti, J.C. Hunter-Cevera and H.W. Rossmoore
© 1989, Society for Industrial Microbiology

CHAPTER 10

Rhizoxin, an inhibitor of tubulin assembly

Shigeo Iwasaki

Institute of Applied Microbiology, The University of Tokyo, Tokyo, Japan

SUMMARY

Rhizoxin is a novel 16-membered antifungal and antitumor macrolide isolated from *Rhizopus chinensis*, the pathogen of the rice seedling blight. Rhizoxin inhibited mitosis of tumor cells in a manner similar to that of vincristine, an antitubulin agent, and showed chemotherapeutic effects similar to those of vincristine. Rhizoxin at a concentration of 1×10^{-5} M completely inhibited *in vitro* polymerization of microtubule proteins purified from porcine brain. The activity of rhizoxin against tubulin polymerization, and its binding site on tubulin, were compared with those of other anti-tubulin drugs such as colchicine, vinblastine, and a maytansinoid compound, ansamitocin P-3. Rhizoxin binds to the maytansine binding site. The binding site of rhizoxin is not the same as those of colchicine and vinblastine. The effect of rhizoxin on fungal tubulin was also studied using wild and mutant strains of *Aspergillus nidulans*, whose tubulin genes were identified.

INTRODUCTION

Rhizoxin (RZX, 1a) (Fig. 1a) is a novel 16-member macrolide isolated from the Rh-2 strain of *Rhizopus chinensis*, a rice seedling blight pathogen. The skeletal structure of RZX has been determined by spectroscopy [4], and the absolute structure was assigned based on the chemical interrelation of the compound with compound 4, whose structure has been determined by X-ray crystallography [6]. The fungus produced a variety of homologous compounds (Fig. 1). The structures of compounds 1b–3b, regarded as the biosynthetic precursors of 1a, were elucidated by comparison of their physico-chemical characteristics (Table 1) and NMR data (Table 2) with those of 1a [5]. The structures of 5, a homolog, and the derivatives 6, 7 and 8 (Fig. 1) were elucidated from spectroscopic data.

MATERIALS AND METHODS, RESULTS

Effects of RZX and its homologs (1a–3b) on rice seedling roots

The characteristic early symptom of rice seedling blight is an abnormal swelling of the seedling roots [10]. When the symptoms were induced by RZX at a concentration of less than 10 ng/ml, the malformed shape suggested that the compound interferes with the formation of the cell skeleton (Fig. 2). Compounds 1b, 2a, 2b, 3a and 3b, at the same concentration, caused the same symptoms.

Antifungal activity of RZX

The potent activity of RZX against a variety of phytopathogenic fungi was determined by assaying mycelium growth inhibitory activity (Table 3) [4]. Mycelium inhibitory concentrations against 10 tested fungi was less than 1 μg/ml, except for *R*.

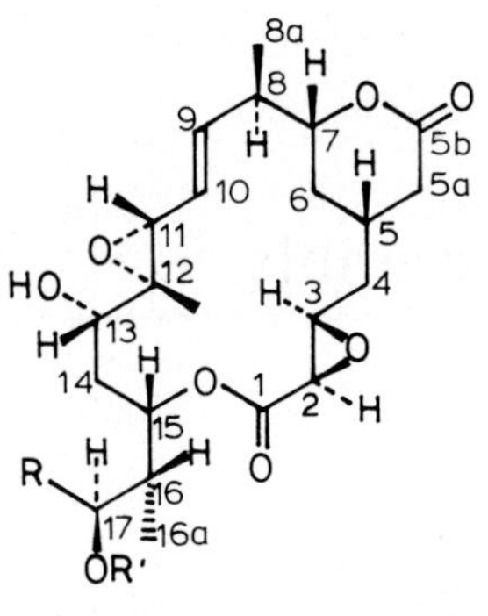

Fig. 1. Structures of RZX homologs and derivatives.

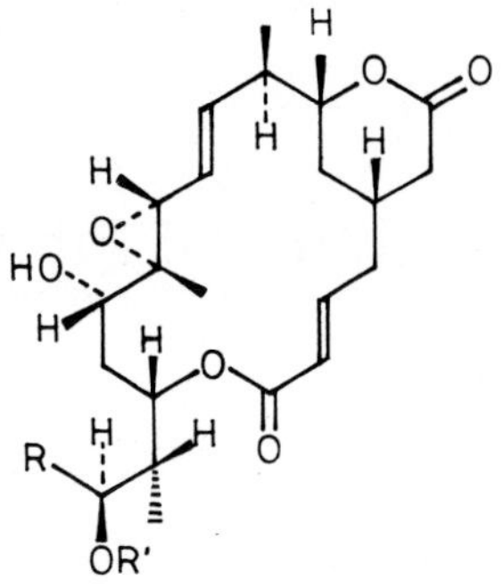

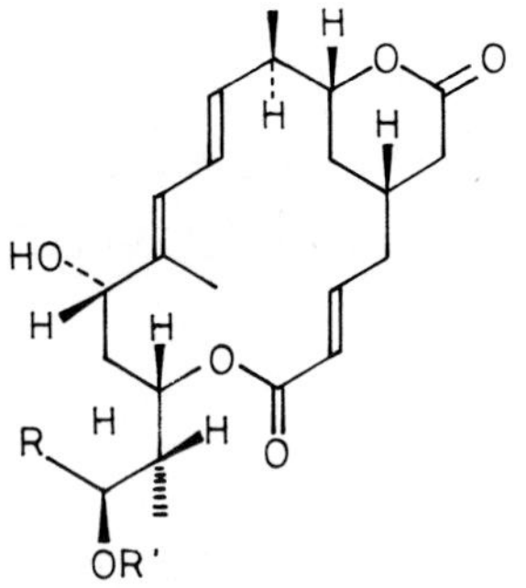

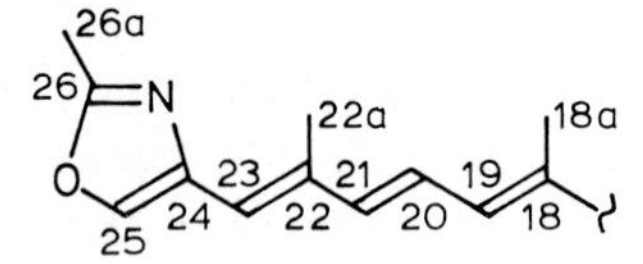

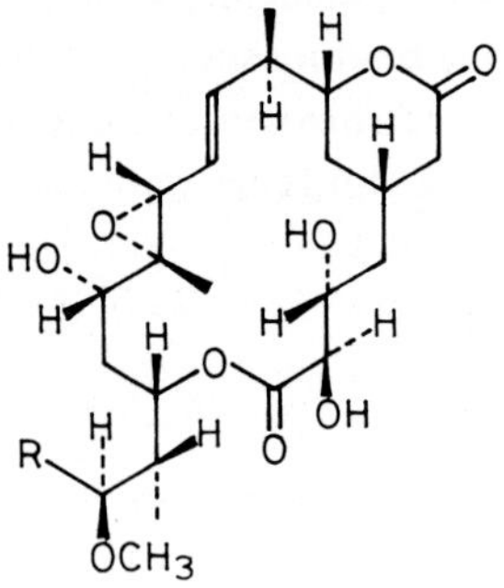

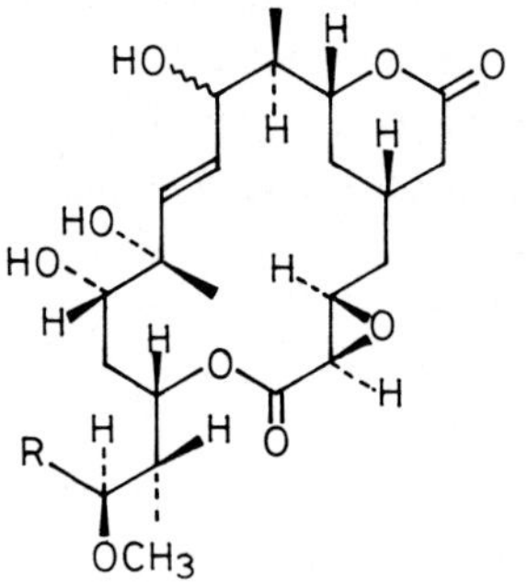

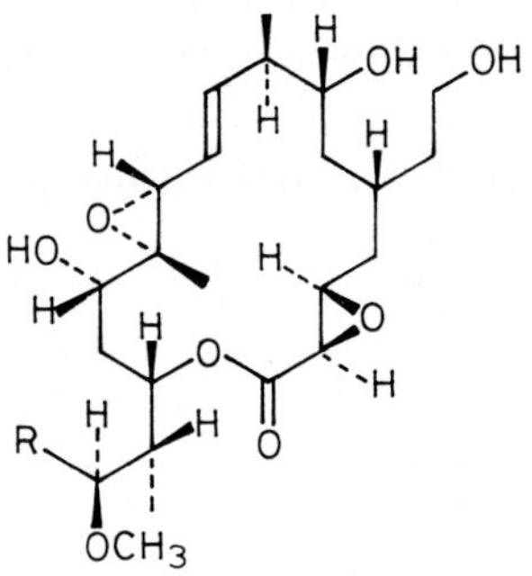

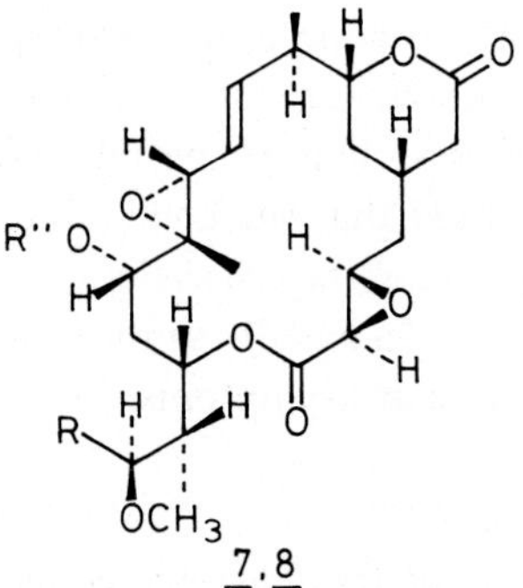

Table 1

Physico-chemical characteristics of 1a – 3b

Compd.	Molecular formula	HREIMS[a] (calcd. value)	α_D^{24} (MeOH)	UV (MeOH)	λ_{max} nm (ε)
1a	$C_{35}H_{47}O_9N$	M^+ 625.3233 (625.3250)	$+155.5°(c = 0.80)$	295 (42 300),	308 (54 000), 325 (39 000)
1b	$C_{34}H_{45}O_9N$	M^+-1 610.3009 (610.3012)	$+116.3°(c = 0.11)$	297 (32 300),	309 (41 000), 323 (30 100)
2a	$C_{35}H_{47}O_8N$	M^+ 609.3300 (609.3299)	$+136.8°(c = 0.71)$	297 (46 000),	308 (64 400), 323 (46 300)
2b	$C_{34}H_{45}O_8N$	M^+ 595.3135 (595.3142)	$+\ 99.3°(c = 0.61)$	297 (39 100),	308 (50 300), 323 (36 600)
3a	$C_{35}H_{47}O_7N$	M^+ 593.3382 (593.3414)	$+287.1°(c = 0.48)$	216 (25 900), 238 (24 500), 309 (49 900),	235 (24 700), 297 (38 700), 323 (36 500)
3b	$C_{34}H_{45}O_7N$	M^+ 597.3165 (597.3137)	$+246.0°(c = 0.66)$	215 (28 400), 238 (25 700), 308 (55 100),	232 (26 200), 297 (42 500), 323 (40 300)

HREIMS = high-resolution electron impact mass spectrometry.

Table 2

Chemical shifts of ^{1}H-signals of 1a – 3b (δ value)

Protons	1a	1b	2a	2b	3a	3b
H-2 (d)	2.96	2.98	5.61	5.72	5.61	5.63
H-3 (ddd)	3.27	3.29	6.82	6.85	6.77	6.79
H-11 (d)	3.20	3.23	3.24	3.27	5.81	5.79
H-12a (s)	1.45	1.43	1.42	1.44	1.79	1.81
H-17 (d)	3.23	3.89	3.25	3.91	3.26	3.89
17-OCH$_3$(s)	3.15	–	3.15	–	3.17	–

Table 3

Antifungal activity[a] of RZX

Phytopathogenic fungi	RZX (μg/nl)		
	10	1	0.1
Alternaria kikuchiana	+	+	–
Colletotrichum lindemuthianum	+	+	+
Fusarium nivale	+	+	+
Fusarium oxysporum f. *lycopersici*	–	–	–
Helminthosporium oryzae	+	+	+
Pyricularia oryzae	+	+	–
Pythium aphanidermatum	+	+	+
Rhizoctonia solani	+	+	–
Rhizopus chinensis	–	–	–
Sclerotinia trifoliorum	+	+	+

[a] Mycelium growth inhibitory activity: +, inhibition; –, no inhibition.

chinensis (a RZX-producing fungus) and *Fusarium oxysporum*. Growth of some of the tested fungi was inhibited even at 0.1 μg/ml. Potent activities of the RZX homologs 1b–3b were also observed against *Pyricularia oryzae*. Little activity was observed against bacteria.

Antitumor activity of RZX and its homologs

RZX strongly inhibits the mitosis of a variety of tumor cells [15]. The cytotoxicity of RZX against drug-resistant tumor cells led to interest in the development of a new antitumor agent. The cytotoxi-city of RZX against vincristine (VCR)- and adriamycin (ADM)-resistant tumor cells was examined by comparison of RZX cytotoxicity with that of VCR cytotoxicity. P388/VCR, P388/ADM and K562/VCR tumor cells showed 15.4-, 25.7- and 21-

82

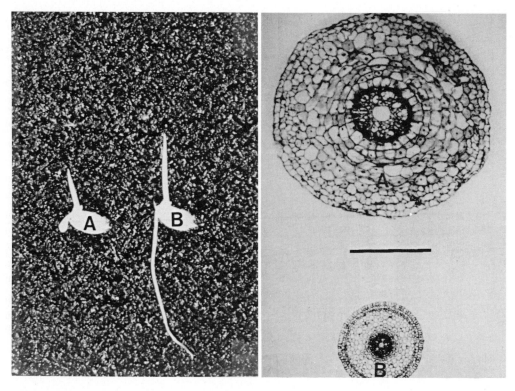

Fig. 2. Typical symptoms of rice seedlings treated with RZX (A), compared with a healthy root (B). Bar represents 0.5 mm.

fold resistance, respectively, to VCR, when the IC_{50} values of the tumor cells and the parent cells were determined. The tumor cells showed only 4.2-, 4.5- and 2.1-fold resistance to RZX (Table 4). These results clearly show that RZX is more effective than VCR against tumor cells, especially VCR- and ADM-resistant tumor cells.

To compare the *in vivo* effects of RZX and VCR, different doses of the drugs were administered to L1210-bearing CD2F mice (Table 5). RZX given on 4 successive days after tumor inoculation increased the life span of the L1210 bearing mice by 81%, 67% and 43% at doses of 1.6, 0.8 and 0.4 μmol/kg, respectively. VCR was slightly less effective. Similar chemotherapeutic effects of RZX were observed against B16 melanoma which had been in-

Table 4

Cytotoxicity of RZX and VCR in mouse and human tumor cell lines sensitive and resistant to VCR and ADM

Compound	IC_{50} (nM)				
	P388	P388/VCR	P388/ADM	K562	K562/VCR
RZX	0.91 ± 0.01	3.84 ± 0.39 (4.2)[a]	4.13 ± 0.49 (4.5)	0.51 ± 0.04	1.28 ± 0.05 (2.5)
VCR	2.10 ± 0.10	32.4 ± 2.3 (15.4)	54.0 ± 2.3 (25.7)	2.68 ± 0.25	56.3 ± 1.3 (21.0)

[a] Degree (*x*-fold) of resistance as compared to parent cells.

Table 5

Comparison of antitumor activity of RZX and VCR against L1210 leukemia

Compound	Dose (μmol/kg)	Body weight change[a] (g)	Mean survival time (day) experiment 1	experiment 2	ILS (%)
Control		+2.3	8.4 ± 1.1	9.0 ± 1.0	
RZX	0.4 (0.25)[b]	+0.4	12.0 ± 1.0		43
	0.8 (0.5)	−0.7	14.0 ± 1.7		67
	1.6 (1.0)	−2.9	15.2 ± 2.2		81
	3.2 (2.0)	−3.6		9.0 ± 5.0	0
VCR	0.54 (0.5)	−1.9		13.0 ± 2.1	44
	1.08 (1.0)	−6.4	14.0 ± 2.5		67
	2.17 (2.0)		5.2 ± 0.8		toxic

L1210 cells (10^5/mouse) were implanted i.p. into CD2F$_1$ mice (5 mice/group) on day 0, and drug was administered i.p. daily from day 1 to day 4.

[a] Difference in body weight (g) between days 7 and 1.

[b] The dose in mg/kg is given in parentheses.

oculated. RZX given at 0.8 μmol/kg resulted in an increased life span (ILS) of 91%. Even at doses as low as 0.4 μmol/kg, 24% ILS was observed.

The chemotherapeutic effect of RZX against VCR-resistant tumor-bearing mice was also tested by comparison with VCR. VCR at doses ranging from 0.11 to 1.1 μmol/kg, 1, 5 and 9 days after tumor inoculation, showed no chemotherapeutic effects in mice bearing P388 leukemia resistant to VCR. RZX given at the same schedule resulted in 30% ILS at 0.32 μmol/kg, with a maximum ILS of about 60% at doses of 2.4–3.2 μmol/kg. These results demonstrate that RZX is effective against VCR-resistant tumor cells *in vivo*.

Cytotoxicity of RZX homologs 1b–3b was tested against HeLa cells. All of the compounds show about the same growth inhibitory activity, as compared to RZX.

Morphological changes and cell cycle analysis of tumor cells

Light microscopic examination of L1210 cells taken from the peritoneal cavity of CD2F mice given 2 mg/kg RZX 6 h prior to the experiment showed the cells to be elongated. Many metaphase-arrested L1210 cells were observed [15]. Similar morphological changes have been observed for VCR-treated cells [15].

Cell cycle analysis by flow cytometry indicated that RZX inhibits mitosis in tumor cells in a manner similar to that of VCR. L1210 cells recovered from mice 24 h after RZX treatment were blocked in the G2–M phase (Table 6). More than 50% of the cells were distributed in the G2–M phase. These results clearly indicate that VCR and RZX both have the same mode of action, the inhibition of mitosis.

Table 6

Cell cycle phase distribution of L1210 cells treated with RZX or VCR

Treatment	Cell cycle distribution (%) G_0–G_1	S	G_2–M
Control	44.0 ± 1.0	42.4 ± 2.7	13.5 ± 2.0
RZX	17.2 ± 1.7	29.3 ± 1.6	53.5 ± 1.7
VCR	15.5 ± 3.1	23.7 ± 2.5	60.7 ± 5.6

CD2F$_1$ mice were inoculated with 10^5 L1210 cells. After 6 days, RZX or VCR was given at 2 mg/kg. L1210 cells were recovered from the peritoneal cavity 24 h after drug administration and examined by flow cytometry.

Effect of RZX on cleavage of fertilized sea urchin eggs

RZX was added to sea urchin embryo suspension 5 min after fertilization. At a concentration of 0.8×10^{-8} M RZX, fertilized eggs did not cleave and remained at the 1-cell stage. At 0.16×10^{-8} M concentration, development of some of the embryos progressed normally or slowly, and the development of others did not progress. When sperm was added to the egg suspension after the addition of RZX, fertilized membrane formed and subsequent development was the same as above [14].

In sea urchin eggs treated with 1.6×10^{-8} M RZX, fusion of the male and female pronuclei did not occur during the 140-min observation time, during which control embryos reached the 4-cell stage. This action of RZX was approximately 3000-, 300- and 4-fold more effective in inhibiting mitosis, compared with the reported activities of colchicine (CLC), vinblastine (VLB) and maytansine, respectively. The structures of CLC, VLB, maytansine, and ansamitocin P-3 (P-3) are shown in Fig. 4.

Effects of RZX on the polymerization of tubulin and on polymerized microtubule proteins [14]

Microtubule protein was prepared from porcine brains using the polymerization/depolymerization method of Shelanski [12], repeating the procedure twice. The protein concentration of the solution was determined by the method of Lowry *et al.* [8]. The microtubule protein thus prepared consisted of approximately 75% tubulin and 25% microtubule-associated proteins (MAP 1, MAP 2, tau). Immediately before use, the protein was further purified from the stock solution by a repeated cycle of polymerization/depolymerization. Turbidity was then measured at 37°C, in a buffer solution.

The polymerization reaction of 2 mg of porcine microtubule protein in 1 ml buffer and the inhibitory effects of RZX at various concentrations are shown in Fig. 3A. Polymerization of tubulin occurred rapidly, with the curve flattening at approximately 30 min incubation. By adding RZX at various concentrations, polymerization of the tubulin was inhibited in a concentration-dependent manner. At 5×10^{-6} M and 1×10^{-5} M, 50% and almost 100% inhibition was observed, respectively. Under the electron microscope, no polymerized microtubule was observed when 1×10^{-5} M of the drug was added.

The time dependence of depolymerization of polymerized microtubules by the addition of various concentrations of RZX is shown in Fig. 3B. The

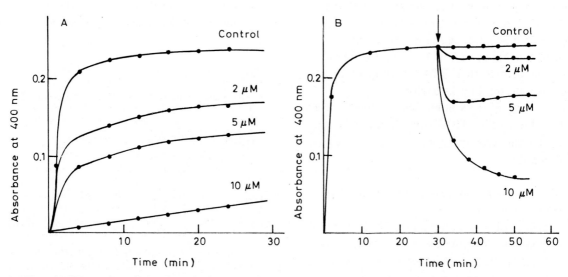

Fig. 3. Effect of RZX on microtubule polymerization. (A) Microtubule protein (2 mg/ml) was mixed with RZX at 0°C and incubated at 37°C. (B) Microtubule proteins were incubated at 37°C. RZX solutions were added 30 min later.

85

drug was added after 30 min incubation of the microtubule protein. Following addition of 5×10^{-6} M and 1×10^{-5} M of the drug, approximately 30% and 70% depolymerization occurred, respectively.

Comparison of the effects of RZX, VLB, P-3 and CLC on tubulin polymerization

RZX inhibits pronuclear fusion and cleavage in sea urchin eggs, prevents the polymerization of tubulin, depolymerizes microtubules, and causes morphological changes in rice and tumor cells. These activities are, in general, similar to those of spindle poisons such as CLC, podophyllotoxin, steganacin, *Vinca* alkaloids and maytansinoids (Fig. 4) [14].

Anti-tubulin activities of RZX (1a), VLB and P-3 were compared by adding various concentrations of the drugs to the brain microtubule protein solution (Fig. 5). RZX and P-3 inhibited polymerization of brain tubulin in a similar manner. The activity of VLB is about twice as strong as that of RZX and P-3, and the activity of CLC is weaker than that of RZX. IC$_{50}$ values of RZX, P-3, VLB and CLC were determined to be 5×10^{-6}, 5×10^{-6}, 2×10^{-6} and 1×10^{-5} M, respectively, under the same assay conditions.

Fig. 5. Comparison of the effects of three antimitotic drugs on microtubule assembly. Microtubule protein (2 mg/ml) was mixed with various concentrations of the drugs RZX (●), P-3 (ASM P-3, ○), and VLB (■) and was incubated at 37°C. Relative absorbance after 20 min is plotted vs. drug concentration.

Aggregation, observed as an increase in relative absorption, occurred with VLB at a concentration of 1×10^{-5} M or greater. No aggregation was observed with RZX or P-3, even at concentrations as high as 1×10^{-4} M (Fig. 5).

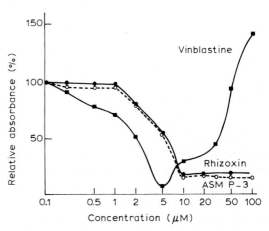

Maytansine : R = COCH(CH₃)N(CH₃)COCH₃
Ansamitocin P-3 : R = COCH(CH₃)₂

Colchicine

Vinblastine

Fig. 4. Structures of antimitotic drugs: maytansine, P-3 (ASM P-3), CLC, and VLB.

Effect of RZX homologs and derivatives on the polymerization of tubulin [14]

Different concentrations of RZX homologs (1b–3b, 4, 5) and RZX derivatives (6–8) were added to microtubule protein, and their ability to inhibit tubulin polymerization was measured. IC$_{50}$ values obtained are shown in Table 7.

The homologs 1b–3b showed high activities as compared to that of RZX. Compounds 4 and 5 showed lower activities, whereas compound 6 had notably high activity. Derivatives 7 and 8 were inactive at the tested concentrations. Higher concentrations of 7 could not be examined because of the insolubility of the compound. These results show that two epoxy groups present on the RZX molecule are not essential for the activity. This may indicate that the fixation of molecular geometry either by epoxy groups or by olefinic linkages is important for interaction with the protein. Inactivity of compounds 7 and 8 against microtubule polymerization would suggest a significant role of the hydroxy group at C-13 in RZX binding to tubulin.

Determination of RZX binding to tubulin [13]

In vitro binding of RZX to tubulin was examined using [^{14}C]RZX, prepared biosynthetically by feeding [*methyl*-^{14}C]methionine [7]. The binding was evaluated by the ultrafiltration method using a YMT-membrane, Amicon centrifree MPS-3. Porcine brain tubulin (5 μM) was incubated in the microtubule assembly buffer with various concentrations of drugs for appropriate periods of time at 37°C. The samples (0.5 ml) were added to a reservoir of MPS-3 and centrifuged at 1000 × *g*. Ninety

percent of the unbound drugs were filtered off through the membrane into filtrate caps, and 10% of the free ligand was adsorbed by the membrane. Unbound drug concentrations were corrected.

RZX binds to tubulin rapidly, and the binding is reversible. Unlabeled RZX rapidly displaced labeled RZX bound to tubulin (Fig. 6). The stoichiometry of RZX binding on tubulin and the dissociation constant (K_d) were determined by Scatchard plots (Fig. 7), and shown to be 0.87 and 1.7 × 10^{-7} M, respectively. Under the same experimental conditions, those values for VLB were determined to be 0.89 and 1.5 × 10^{-7} M, respectively, in good agreement with values reported in the literature [1].

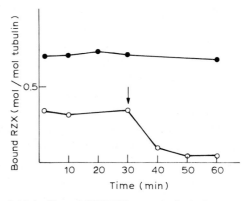

Fig. 6. Mol of bound [^{14}C]RZX per mol of tubulin. ●, 7.8 μM of [^{14}C]RZX was added to 5 μM of tubulin and incubated at 37°C. ○, 1.5 μM of [^{14}C]RZX was added to 5 μM of tubulin. After 30 min of incubation 20 μM of unlabeled RZX was added (arrow).

Table 7

Inhibitory activity of RZX and its homologs against porcine microtubule polymerization

	1a	1b	2a	2b	3a	3b	4	5	6	7	8
IC$_{50}$ (μM)	5	7	5	7	7	7	50	> 100	20	> 20	> 100

Microtubule protein (2 mg/ml) was mixed with various concentrations of the compounds and incubated for 30 min at 37°C. IC$_{50}$ values were determined by measuring turbidity at 400 nm.

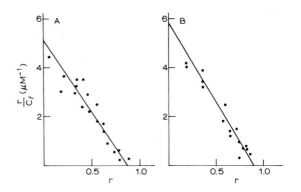

Fig. 7. Scatchard plots of RZX (A) and VLB (B) binding to porcine brain tubulin. r: mol of bound drug per mol of tubulin. Cf: molar concentration of unbound RZX.

Determination of the RZX binding site on tubulin [13]

To determine the RZX binding site on tubulin, we examined inhibition of RZX binding by CLC, VLB and P-3. The inhibitory effects of each of these three drugs on RZX binding was different (Table 8). Unlabeled P-3 caused strong inhibition of labeled RZX binding. Inhibition by unlabeled VLB was much weaker, with 25-fold more being required for 46% inhibition, despite almost the same K_d for the two drugs. CLC had no effect on RZX binding.

Double-reciprocal plots for RZX binding by P-3 and VLB (Fig. 8) show the P-3 inhibition constant (K_i, 1.3×10^{-7} M). The K_i of P-3 was estimated to be almost equal to the P-3 K_d, because of inhibitory

Table 8

Inhibition of RZX binding to porcine brain tubulin by CLC, VLB, and P-3

Drug concentration (μM)	Bound RZX (μM)	Inhibition of RZX binding (%)
RZX (1.8)	1.7	–
+ CLC (50)	1.6	6
+ VLB (20)	1.3	24
+ VLB (50)	0.91	46
+ P-3 (5)	1.0	41
+ P-3 (20)	0.3	82

1.8 μM of [^{14}C]RZX and various concentrations of the drugs were added to 5 μM of tubulin. Bound RZX was determined after 20 min incubation at 37°C.

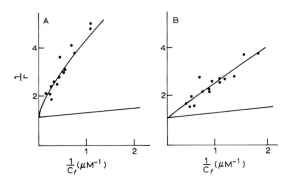

Fig. 8. Double-reciprocal plots for the inhibition of RZX binding by 5 μM of P-3 (A) and 20 μM of VLB (B). r: mol of bound RZX per mol of tubulin. Cf: molar concentration of unbound RZX. Control: line obtained from double-reciprocal plots for RZX binding.

activity against tubulin assembly similar to those of RZX and VLB [12]. The K_i value of VLB (2.9×10^{-6} M) was 20-times larger than the K_d of VLB. Data shown in Table 8, and the K_i values of P-3 and VLB, indicate that RZX and P-3, and accordingly maytansine, share the same binding site on tubulin, and that the VLB binding site is not identical to that of RZX. The CLC binding site is different from the RZX binding site.

It was also observed that RZX and VLB affect each other's binding. This may be explained by one or both of the following mechanisms: (a) conformational changes of the protein induced by binding of each ligand; (b) binding of the two ligands close to each other in the same binding region (overlapping binding sites resulting in partially competitive binding).

Although RZX and maytansine were shown to bind to tubulin at the same site, RZX was effective against human and murine tumor cells resistant to VCR and ADM, both *in vitro* and *in vivo* [15]. In addition, RZX exhibits potent antifungal activity. Therefore, RZX appears to be worthy of further evaluation of its utility as a clinical drug and a biochemical tool.

Differential effect of RZX and benomyl on mutant strains of Aspergillus nidulans

Several benzimidazole compounds have been widely used as fungicides. These compounds, which interfere with fungal microtubule assembly, are known to be antimitotic agents [2].

The tubulins of *A. nidulans* have been characterized in a wild type strain, and benomyl-resistant *ben*A, -B, and -C mutant strains electrophoretically and by copolymerization with porcine brain tubulin [11]. Evidence obtained from experiments using these mutants suggests that the benomyl binding site is on β-tubulin, and that *ben*A is a structural gene for β-tubulin in *A. nidulans*, although *ben*B and -C have not been identified.

Growth inhibitory activities of RZX, P-3, benomyl (methyl 1-(butylcarbamoyl)benzimidazole-2-carbamate) and thiabendazole (2-thiazol-4-ylbenzimidazole) were examined against a wild-type strain of *A. nidulans*. The IC$_{50}$ value of RZX (0.5 μM) was less than that of benomyl (approximately 1.2 μM) and thiabendazole (approximately 20 μM) and its action was shown to be fungistatic. P-3 was active against the fungus in a manner similar to RZX, but with a much weaker IC_{50} (50 μM).

The activities of these drugs were examined against a wild-type strain (FGSC No. 188), and against *benA* (FGSC No. 524), *benB* (FGSC No. 565), and *benC* (FGSC No. 529) mutant strains of *A. nidulans*. The results indicate that the *benA, -B* and *-C* mutants are as sensitive as the wild strain to RZX and P-3 (Table 9). The fact that the *benA* benomyl-resistant mutant, a β-tubulin gene mutant, did not show cross-resistance against RZX indicates the difference in tubulin binding sites between RZX and benomyl. Since benzimidazole compounds have been reported to bind to mammalian brain tubulin at the CLC binding site [3], the above is in agreement with our results using porcine brain tubulin [13]. In addition, it was observed that an α-tubulin mutant of *A. nidulans* (L014) [9] supersensitive to benomyl was also as sensitive to RZX. The sensitivity was as great as that of the wild strains.

We have isolated RZX-resistant mutants of *A. nidulans* which are sensitive to benomyl. Genetic analysis of these strains and study of RZX binding to their tubulins are under way.

DISCUSSION

RZX, a novel 16-member macrolide, has been shown to inhibit mitosis in fungi, plant, and mammalian cells, both *in vitro* and *in vivo*. It has also been established that the drug interferes with the formation of microtubules and causes microtubule depolymerization. In summary, we conclude that RZX binds to tubulin at a different site than CLC, and that RZX and maytansine share the same binding site. The RZX and maytansine binding site is not in the same location as the VLB binding site, but they may overlap.

Since RZX has potent antifungal activity, it was possible to compare its activity with that of other anti-tubulin agents against various mutant strains of *A. nidulans* whose genotypes have been characterized. In *A. nidulans*, benomyl-resistant tubulin mutants have been isolated, and it should be possible to isolate tubulin mutants resistant to other drugs, such as RZX. By determining the tubulin structure of sensitive and resistant mutants, valuable information about the relationship between the tubulin structure and the binding of antimitotic drugs should be obtained.

ACKNOWLEDGEMENTS

I would like to acknowledge all of my coworkers, and also colleagues included in the references. I would also like to thank the Takeda Chemical Industry Central Research Institute for supplying ansamitocin P-3. The tubulin mutant of *A. nidulans* was provided by Professor N.R. Morris of Rutgers University Medical School, and is gratefully acknowledged.

Table 9

Activity of RZX, P-3, and benomyl against wild-type, *benA*, *benB* and *benC* mutant strains of *A. nidulans*

Strain	ED$_{50}$ (μM)		
	RZX	P-3	benomyl
wild type	0.2	16	1.4
benA	0.25	18	28[a]
benB	0.25	15	7.6[a]
benC	0.2	10	2

[a]From Ref. 16.

REFERENCES

1 Bhattacharyya, B. and J. Wolff. 1976. Tubulin aggregation and disaggregation: mediation by two distinct vinblastine-binding sites. Proc. Natl. Acad. Sci. USA 73: 2375–2378.
2 Davidse, L.C. and W. Flach. 1977. Differential binding of methyl benzimidazole-2-yl carbamate to fungal tubulin as a mechanism of resistance to this antimitotic agent in mutant strains of *Aspergillus nidulans*. J. Cell Biol. 72: 174–193.
3 Hoebeke, J., G. van Nijen and M. DeBrabander. 1976. Interaction of oncodazole (R17934), a new antifungal drug, with rat brain tubulin. Biochem. Biophys. Res. Commun. 69: 319.

4 Iwasaki, S., H. Kobayashi, J. Furukawa, M. Namikoshi, S. Okuda, Z. Sato, I. Matsuda and T. Noda. 1984. Studies on macrocyclic lactone antibiotics VII. Structure of a phytotoxin 'rhizoxin' produced by *Rhizopus chinensis*. J. Antibiot. 37: 354–362.

5 Iwasaki, S., M. Namikoshi, H. Kobayashi, J. Furukawa and S. Okuda. 1986. Studies on macrocyclic lactone antibiotics IX. Novel macrolides from the fungus *Rhizopus chinensis*: precursors of rhizoxin. Chem. Pharm. Bull. 34: 1384–1390.

6 Iwasaki, S., M. Namikoshi, H. Kobayashi, J. Furukawa, S. Okuda, A. Itai, A. Kasuya, Y. Iitaka and Z. Sato. 1986. Studies on macrocyclic lactone antibiotics VIII. Absolute structure of rhizoxin and a related compound. J. Antibiot. 39: 424–429.

7 Kobayashi, H., S. Iwasaki, E. Yamada and S. Okuda. 1986. Biosynthesis of the antimitotic antitumour antibiotic, rhizoxin, by *Rhizopus chinensis*; origin of the carbon atoms. J. Chem. Soc. Chem. Commun. 1701–1702.

8 Lowry, O.H., N.J. Rosebrough, A.L. Farr and R.J. Randall. 1951. Protein measurement with the folin phenol reagent. J. Biol. Chem. 193: 265–275.

9 Morris, N.R., M.H. Lai and C.E. Oakley. 1979. Identification of a gene for β-tubulin in *Aspergillus nidulans*. Cell 16: 437–442.

10 Noda, T., T. Hashiba and Z. Sato. 1980. The structure changes in young swollen roots of rice seedlings infected with *Rhizopus chinensis* Saito. Ann. Phytopathol. Soc. Japan 46: 40–45.

11 Sheir-Neiss, G., M.H. Lai and N.R. Morris. 1978. Identification of a gene for β-tubulin in *Aspergillus nidulans*. Cell 15: 639–647.

12 Shelanski, M.L. 1973. Microtubule assembly in the absence of added nucleotides. Proc. Natl. Acad. Sci. USA 70: 765–768.

13 Takahashi, M., S. Iwasaki, H. Kobayashi, S. Okuda, T. Murai and Y. Sato. 1987. Rhizoxin binding to tubulin at the maytansine-binding site. Biochim. Biophys. Acta 926: 215–223.

14 Takahashi, M., S. Iwasaki, H. Kobayashi, S. Okuda, T. Murai, Y. Sato, T. Haraguchi-Hiraoka and H. Nagano. 1987. Studies on macrocyclic lactone antibiotics XI. Anti-mitotic and anti-tubulin activity of new antitumor antibiotics, rhizoxin and its homologues. J. Antibiot. 40: 66–72.

15 Tsuruo, T., T. Oh-hara, H. Iida, S. Tsukagoshi, Z. Sato, I. Matsuda, S. Iwasaki, S. Okuda, F. Shimizu, K. Sasagawa, M. Fukami, K. Fukuda and M. Arakawa. 1986. Rhizoxin, a macrocyclic lactone antibiotic, as a new antitumor agent against human and murine tumor cells and their vincristine-resistant sublines. Cancer Res. 46: 381–385.

16 Van Tuyl, J.M. 1975. Genetic aspects of acquired resistance to benomyl and thiabendazole in a number of fungi. Med. Fac. Landbouww. Rijksuniv. Gent. 40: 691–697.

Novel Microbial Products for Medicine and Agriculture
Editors: A.L. Demain, G.A. Somkuti, J.C. Hunter-Cevera and H.W. Rossmoore
© 1989, Society for Industrial Microbiology

CHAPTER 11

Reverse transcriptase inhibitors

Shoshiro Nakamura and Yoshio Inouye

Institute of Pharmaceutical Sciences, Hiroshima University School of Medicine, Hiroshima, Japan

SUMMARY

More than 400 microbial metabolites, antibiotics and synthetic quinones have been screened for their inhibitory activity against reverse transcriptase of avian myeloblastosis virus. Glysperins, luzopeptins, streptonigrin and its derivatives, thielavins and synthetic quinones were all potent inhibitors. Among them, only those of low cytotoxicity, evaluated using murine lymphoblastoma L5178Y cells, were tested in the *in vitro* human immunodeficiency virus/T_4 cell antiviral test system. Adriamycin, luzopeptin C and sakyomicin A were found to suppress viral replication at concentrations which hardly affected cell viability. Chromostin, a novel enzyme inhibitor obtained in our laboratory, and streptonigrin inhibited the *in vitro* replication of the Friend strain murine leukemia virus.

INTRODUCTION

Reverse transcriptase, namely RNA-directed DNA polymerase, is considered to play a crucial role in the life cycle of retroviruses. Specific inhibitors of the enzyme might be promising candidates for the chemotherapy of retroviral diseases. Cultural broths of more than 200 microbial strains, *ca.* 150 antibiotics and various kinds of synthetic compounds have been tested for their inhibitory activity against reverse transcriptase of avian myeloblastosis virus (AMV-RTase). The potent inhibitors with low cytotoxicity toward murine lymphoblastoma L5178Y cells have been further examined for their effects on the *in vitro* replication of human immunodeficiency virus (HIV) and the *in vivo* splenomegaly induced by the Friend murine leukemia virus strain (FLV). The sensitivities of HIV-RTase and AMV-RTase to various compounds were also studied comparatively.

MATERIALS AND METHODS

Assay methods for enzyme activities

Reverse transcriptase [11]. The assay solution was composed of 100 mM Tris-HC1 buffer (pH 8.0), 5 mM $MgCl_2$, 5 mM dithiothreitol, 60 mM NaC1, 0.2 mM [^{3}H]TTP (12.5 μCi/ml), 20 μg/ml poly(rA), 0.02 U/ml oligo(dT)$_{12-18}$ and 3.0 U/ml AMV-RTase. A test sample was dissolved in dimethyl sulfoxide (DMSO) at 5 mg/ml and diluted with distilled water to make a test solution. A mixture of the assay solution (50 μl) and the reaction mixture (50 μl) was incubated at 37°C for 60 min with shaking. The reaction was terminated by cooling in an ice bath and the reaction mixture (50 μl) was soaked onto a 2.4-cm round piece of DEAE-filter paper. The filter paper was washed three times with 5% $Na_2HPO_4 \cdot 12H_2O$ within 30 min, once with water and finally with ethanol. The radioactivity of the fraction remaining on the filter paper was measured in a toluene-based scintillation cocktail.

DNA-directed DNA polymerase I and alpha [1]. The assay solution was composed of 80 mM glycine-NaOH buffer (pH 9.2), 10.0 mM $MgCl_2$, 1.4 mM dithiothreitol, 50 μg/ml activated calf thymus DNA, 40 μM each of dATP, dCTP, dGTP and [^{3}H]TTP (6.0 μCi/ml for DNA polymerase I or 14.0 μCi/ml for alpha, respectively) and DNA polymerase I (*Escherichia coli*, 12.5 U/ml) or alpha (calf thymus, 30.0 U/ml). A mixture of the assay solution (50 μl) and the test solution prepared as described above (50 μl) was incubated at 37°C for 60 min.

DNA-directed RNA polymerase [1]. The assay solution was composed of 80 mM Tris-HCl buffer (pH 8.0), 20 mM $MgCl_2$, 300 mM KCl, 0.2 mM EDTA, 0.2 mM dithiothreitol, 0.8 mM Na_2HPO_4, 0.3 mM each of ATP, GTP, CTP and [^{3}H]UTP (20 μCi/ml), 0.3 mg/ml calf thymus DNA and 12 U/ml RNA polymerase of *E. coli*. The following procedures were the same as those for AMV-RTase and DNA polymerases.

Determination of cytotoxicity toward L5178Y cells [4]

A test sample was dissolved in DMSO at 2.5 mg/ml and diluted with serum-free Fischer's medium. A mixture of the test solution (0.2 ml) and the cell suspension ($5.0-6.0 \times 10^4$ cells/1.8 ml) in Fischer's medium supplemented with 10% horse serum (Grand Island Biological Co.) was incubated at 37°C for 72 h. The cell numbers were counted in a Coulter counter.

The in vitro replication of HIV [2]

One of the strains of HIV was obtained from the culture supernatant of Molt-4/HTLV-III. MT-4 cells, an HTLV-I-carrying T_4 cell line, were maintained in RPMI 1640 medium supplemented with 10% fetal calf serum (FCS), 100 IU/ml benzylpenicillin and 100 μg/ml streptomycin at 37°C in a CO_2

incubator. MT-4 cells were exposed to the viral preparation at a multiplicity of infection (MOI) of 0.002 for 1 h. After infection, the cells were washed and resuspended in fresh medium at 3×10^5 cells/ml. The cells were cultured in the absence or presence of various concentrations of a test sample for 3–6 days. Half of the culture medium was changed on day 3. The expression of HIV-specific antigens was visualized by indirect immunofluorescence (IF) assay and the cell viability was measured by the trypan blue dye exclusion method.

The in vivo replication of FLV [3]

Either ddY or DBA/2 mice were sacrificed 12 days after FLV infection and a 10% homogenate of the enlarged spleens was used as a viral source. Female DDD mice, 6 weeks old and weighing about 25 g, or male ddY mice, 5 weeks old and weighing about 23 g, were injected with the viral inoculum on day 0. In group I, daily i.p. inoculation of a test sample at different concentrations was started on day 0 and continued for 5 days. In group II, the treatment was started on day 5 and lasted for 5 days. Twelve days after the viral infection, all mice were killed and the spleen weights were measured.

RESULTS AND DISCUSSION

Screening for AMV-RTase inhibitors

Cultured broths of more than 200 strains of freshly isolated Streptomycetaceae were screened for inhibitory activity against AMV-RTase. The broth filtrate was heated at 80°C for 3 min to inactivate proteinases, DNases, RNases, etc., and 100-fold diluted to make the test solution. Fourteen out of 200 strains showed more than 30% inhibition.

Retrostatin [10]. Isolate H 1058-MY2, named *Streptomyces retrostaticus* sp. nov., was shown to produce two RTase inhibitors of acidic and lipophilic nature. Both were extracted from the broth filtrate with ethyl acetate at acidic pH. The main component was found to be identical with streptonigrin (ID_{50}, 3 μg/ml) and the minor one was proven to be a novel compound and named retrostatin

(RTS). RTS was isolated as a red amorphous powder and the existence of a hydrogen-bonded quinone group was supported by IR (KBr):$\nu_{C=O}$ 1595 cm^{-1}. The ID$_{50}$ values of RTS and adriamycin (ADM) were 50 μg/ml and 25 μg/ml, respectively. DNA polymerase I and RNA polymerase of *E. coli* were inhibited by ADM but not RTS. RTS was labile, losing most of its biological activity when standing in air at room temperature for 2 weeks.

Chromostin [3]. The active principle produced by isolate H 1196-MY6, an unidentified actinomycete of cell wall type IIIC, was precipitated from the broth filtrate with ammonium sulfate. The precipitate was further purified by DEAE-cellulose column chromatography followed by gel filtration on Sephadex G-75. The principle proved to be new and was named chromostin (CHS) because of its chromogenic protein nature (MW 20 000–30 000; UV λ_{max} H$_2$O nm ($\varepsilon_{1 cm}^{1\%}$). 325 (64)). CHS did not show any antimicrobial activity at a concentration of 1600 μg/ml and was not toxic to mice by i.p. injection of 500 mg/kg. CHS preferentially inhibited AMV-RTase (ID$_{50}$ 12 μg/ml), showing no significant inhibition of *E. coli* DNA and RNA polymerases at concentrations as high as 400 μg/ml.

Limocrocin [1]. The precipitate from the broth filtrate of isolate H 1180-MY8 at acidic pH showed strong inhibition of AMV-RTase. The active principle was purified as red needles and identified as limocrocin, a pigment produced by *Streptomyces limosus*, with an ID$_{50}$ against AMV-RTase of 50 μg/ml. The inhibitory activity against AMV-RTase was not affected by changing the concentration of template-primer, substrate or carrier protein. Enhancement of the inhibition of AMV-RTase was observed when the concentration of the enzyme was increased.

Sakyomicin A [14] inhibitor obtained from the culture filtrate of *Nocardia* sp. as red prisms was identified as sakyomicin A (SKM), with an ID$_{50}$ against AMV-RTase of 33 μg/ml.

Inhibition of AMV-RTase by known antibiotics

Besides broth filtrates, more than 150 antibiotics were employed in our screening for inhibitors of AMV-RTase. Individual antibiotics were tested at final concentrations of 40 and 10 μg/ml and the results are shown in Table 1. Significant inhibition of AMV-RTase was observed with colistin, enduracidin A, janiemycin, luzopeptins, aminocidin, ADM, streptonigrin (STN), bleomycins, glysperins, julimycin and thielavins.

Cytotoxicity of AMV-RTase inhibitors

Cytotoxicities of the antibiotics showing strong inhibition of AMV-RTase were measured using L5178Y cells. Luzopeptins A and B, aclacinomycin A, baumycin, figaroic acid, bleomycins and STN were too toxic to be applied to the HIV/MT-4 cell system (Table 2).

Effect on the in vitro replication of HIV

Among the peptide antibiotics, luzopeptins A, B and C showed the most potent inhibition of both AMV- and HIV-RTases. However, luzopeptins A and B, bis- and mono-acetates of luzopeptin C, respectively, could not be applied to the HIV/MT-4 system. In one experiment, specific viral antigens were induced in 6, 9 and 10% of MT-4 cells treated with 2.5, 1.25 and 0.625 μg/ml luzopeptin C, while 40% of the untreated cells gave a positive IF reaction [6]. Both colistin and janiemycin were specific for AMV-RTase and the replication of HIV was not affected by these antibiotics at concentrations up to 8 μg/ml [6].

As for the anthracyclines, ADM was the sole candidate as an anti-HIV substance in terms of the inhibition of RTase and cytotoxicity [9]. Although ADM was not inhibitory against HIV-RTase, the replication of HIV in MT-4 cells was susceptible to ADM, probably due to its interference in the transcriptional step.

Quinone antibiotics were another source of inhibitors of AMV-RTase [11, 14]. STN was comparable to luzopeptins as an inhibitor of AMV-RTase. Further, HIV-RTase was inhibited by STN as in the case of luzopeptins. However, inhibition of the *in vitro* replication of HIV by STN was secondary to its cytotoxic effect. The glycine derivative (STN-Gly) was as potent as STN as an inhibitor of RTases with negligible cytotoxicity [11]. Probably due to a lack of membrane transport [5], STN-Gly

Table 1

Inhibitory activity (%) of antibiotics against AMV-RTase

Antibiotics	µg/ml		Antibiotics	µg/ml	
	40	10		40	10
Peptides			polyoxin C	3	2
actinomycin D	6	0	tubercidin	8	0
amidinomycin	5	4	Anthracyclines		
bacitracin A	0	0	aclacinomycin A	19	9
capreomycin	16	0	ADM	70	30
colistin	89	49	baumycin	36	15
echinomycin	11	0	daunomycin	54	5
enduracidin A	67	50	figaroic acid	51	18
ilamycin B1	40	18	marcellomycin	68	40
janiemycin	80	59	Ansamycins		
luzopeptin A	100	89	ansamitocin	5	0
luzopeptin B	96	97	geldanamycin	2	0
luzopeptin C	100	100	rifampicin	17	12
pyridomycin	10	0	Macrolides		
siomycin	29	0	cirramycin	3	0
triostin A	33	10	erythromycin	3	4
BU-2470 A	52	60	leucomycin	18	13
Aminoglycosides			Bleomycins		
aminosidin	70	26	bleomycin A2	51	38
butirosin	0	9	bleomycin A5	52	46
glebomycin	13	1	bleomycin B2	23	12
inosamycin A	22	14	pepleomycin	59	13
inosamycin D	11	10	platomycin A	77	70
neomycin B	46	19	tallysomycin A	63	31
paromomycin	0	11	tallysomycin B	50	39
sorbistin A1	0	0	Pluramycins		
xylostatin	27	0	neopluramycin	24	0
Bu-1975	8	5	pluramycin	72	43
Nucleosides			Polyethers		
amicetin	8	0	dianemycin	18	0
Ara-C	3	0	leuseramycin	0	0
blasticidin S	6	1	lonomycin	0	0
bredinin	3	1	moyukamycin	10	5
cadeguomycin	0	0	Miscellaneous		
ezomycin A1	2	0	aureomycin	16	13
ezomycin A2	5	4	azomycin	14	11
formycin A	1	6	chartreucin	12	0
herbicidin A	5	0	chloramphenicol	15	2
minimycin	11	15	chromomycin	0	0
neplanomycin A	4	6	cumermycin A1	44	9
neplanomycin B	0	0	cycloserine	0	1
neplanomycin D	10	14	danomycin	2	0
nucleocidin	0	0	elsamycin	38	4
oxamicetin	0	0	glysperin A	74	60
polyoxin A	6	1	glysperin B	53	25

Table 1 (cont'd.)

Inhibitory activity (%) of antibiotics against AMV-RTase

Antibiotics	μg/ml		Antibiotics	μg/ml	
	40	10		40	10
Miscellaneous			SKM	63	26
glysperin C	5	10	streptolydigin	10	10
histidinomycin	25	14	STN	93	84
julimycin	62	30	STN-Gly	93	91
lyncomycin	28	0	STN-OCH$_3$	12	0
miharamycin A	8	0	thielavin A	89	56
mitomycin A	40	16	thielavin B	80	56
mitomycin C	0	0	tomaymycin	4	0
mycoplanecin	11	11	trichomycin	25	0
neothramycin	8	0	vancomycin	3	5
novomycin	17	4			
pholipomycin	78	8	Control		
pyrrolnitrin	2	0	suramin	96	81

Table 2

ID$_{50}$ (μg/ml) of antibiotics against AMV-RTase and lymphosarcoma L5178Y cells

Antibiotics	AMV-RTase	L5178Y
Colistin	36	>4.0
Enduracidin A	36	>4.0
Luzopeptin A	1	0.0003
Luzopeptin B	1	0.016
Luzopeptin C	2	0.8
BU-2470	7	>4.0
Aclacinomycin A	>80	0.004
ADM	22	0.49
Baumycin	>80	<0.001
Daunomycin	35	0.04
Figaroic acid	35	<0.001
Marcellomycin	29	0.012
Bleomycin A2	15	0.006
Bleomycin B2	>40	0.005
Pepleomycin	35	0.119
Pluramycin	15	0.000063
Glysperin	8	>4.0
SKM	33	0.49
STN	3	0.0043
STN-Gly	2	>4.0
STN-OCH$_3$	>40	0.017
Thielavin A	7	>4.0
Thielavin B	6	>4.0
Suramine	6	>16

was found to be inactive against the *in vitro* replication of HIV [6]. Though SKM was a much less active inhibitor of AMV-RTase than STN, the former seemed to be superior to the latter as an inhibitor of HIV replication.

Effect on the in vitro replication of FLV

CHS [3]. CHS inhibited splenomegaly dose-dependently when administered on days 5–9 (group II), while no distinctive protection of mice in group I was observed. Similar results were obtained by Numata *et al.* using revistin, another inhibitor of RTase of acidic protein nature, as a therapeutic agent (Table 3).

STN. In contrast to CHS, suppression of the replication of FLV was observed in mice in groups I and II at sublethal concentrations (Table 4).

ADM. No protection against FLV infection was observed when ADM was administered on days 0–4 (data not shown).

Biological properties of STN derivatives

The amide and ester derivatives on C-2' of STN were newly synthesized [8]. In general, the inhibition of AMV-RTase by the individual amide derivatives was favorably comparable to that of STN

Table 3

Therapeutic effect of CHS on FLV-infected mice

	FLV, 0.1 ml, i.p. ↓												Splenomegaly ↑
Day	0	1	2	3	4	5	6	7	8	9	10	11	12
Group I	↑	↑	↑	↑	↑								CHS
Group II						↑	↑	↑	↑	↑			or saline

Dose of CHS (mg/mouse/day)		Weight of spleen (mg), mean ± S.D.		
		V^+C^+	V^-C^+ (control)	% Inhibition[a]
Group I	1.0	432 ± 69	130 ± 23	4.4
	0.5	396 ± 98	142 ± 23	19.6
	0.25	454 ± 107	132 ± 15	−1.9
Group II	1.0	290 ± 106	150 ± 40	55.7
	0.5	386 ± 80	180 ± 45	34.8
	0.25	410 ± 95	148 ± 22	17.1
Control	$V^+ C^-$	426 ± 73		
	$V^- C^-$	110 ± 20		

[a] $\% \text{ Inhibition} = (1 - \dfrac{V^+C^+ - V^-C^+}{V^+C^- - V^-C^-}) \times 100$

V^+ = infected with FLV; V^- = not infected with virus; C^+ = CHS administered; C^- = CHS not administered.

Table 4

Therapeutic effect of STN on FLV-infected mice

	FLV, 0.2 ml, i.p. ↓												Splenomegaly ↑
Day	0	1	2	3	4	5	6	7	8	9	10	11	12
Group I	↑	↑	↑	↑	↑								STN
Group II						↑	↑	↑	↑	↑			or saline

Dose of STN (mg/kg/day)		Weight of spleen (mg), mean ± S.D.		
		$V^+ S^+$	$V^- S^+$ (control)	% Inhibition[a]
Group I	0.8	no survivor	no survivor	toxic
	0.2	219.7 ± 129.7	139.4 ± 45.9	93.5
	0.05	303.2 ± 181.0	212.9 ± 41.5	92.7
	0.0125	951.0 ± 447.3	164.4 ± 1.4	36.7
Group II	0.8	28.8 ± 6.3	70.8	103.4
	0.2	365.4 ± 297.2	139.3 ± 29.0	81.8
	0.05	1283.1 ± 347.4	158.9 ± 7.7	9.6
	0.0125	752.0 ± 173.5	217.9 ± 35.0	
Control	$V^+ S^-$	1363.2 ± 517.2		
	$V^- S^-$	119.8 ± 6.2		

[a] $\% \text{ Inhibition} = (1 - \dfrac{V^+S^+ - V^-S^+}{V^+S^- - V^-S^-}) \times 100$

V^+ = infected with FLV; V^- = not infected with virus; S^+ = STN administered; S^- = STN not administered.

[11]. Furthermore, they showed specificity for AMV-RTase as in the case of STN. The minimal cytotoxicity of the amide derivatives was partially reversed provided that the N,N'-dimethylamino group existed in the amine moiety. The lack of inhibitory activity against AMV-RTase in the ester derivatives was fully reversed by the existence of the N,N'-dimethylamino group in the substituent.

Inhibition of AMV-RTase by the quinones

By using various synthetic quinones, the naphthoquinone and quinoline quinone moieties were

Table 5

Biological activities (ID_{50}: $\mu g/ml$) of STN derivatives

Compound	L5178Y/S	L5178Y/ ADM^R	AMV-RTase	DdDP[a]	DdDP[b]	DdRP[c]	MIC[d]
1. STN-OH	0.0043	0.00026	3	>160	>160	100	<0.05
2. STN-OCH$_3$	0.017	0.0013	>40	>160	>160	>160	25
3. STN-NH$_2$	1.3	0.55	5	>160	160	33	>25
4. STN-NH(CH$_2$)$_2$OH	1.4	0.62	2	>160	>160	NT	>25
5. STN-NH(CH$_2$)$_3$-N(CH$_3$)$_2$	0.33	0.058	3	37	43	NT	25
6. STN-NHCH$_2$COOH	>4.0	2.5	2	160	>160	NT	>25
7. STN-NHOH	0.12	0.33	5	140	>160	20	3.12
8. STN-NHNH$_2$	0.014	0.00098	6	80	>160	27	3.12
9. STN-NHNHCONH$_2$	0.17	0.038	2	>160	>160	NT	>25
10. STN-NH(CH$_2$)$_3$NH-(CH$_2$)$_4$NH-STN	0.57	0.41	7	86	150	NT	25
11. ADM	0.12	1.5	22	4	7	24	NT

[a] DNA-directed DNA polymerase (*E. coli*).
[b] DNA-directed DNA polymerase (calf thymus).
[c] DNA-directed RNA polymerase (*E. coli*).
[d] MIC ($\mu g/ml$) against *Bacillus subtilis*.

Table 6

Biological activities of STN derivatives

Compound	ID_{50} ($\mu g/ml$)		Inhibition (%) against HIV-RTase	
	AMV-RTase	L5178Y/S	50 $\mu g/ml$	10 $\mu g/ml$
1. STN-OH	3	0.00025	87	81
2. STN-NHCH$_2$COOH	2	>4.0		
3. STN-L-Ala (U)	3	>8.0	84	79
4. STN-L-Ala (L)	2	>8.0	87	81
5. STN-D-Ala (U)	2	0.04	88	83
6. STN-D-Ala (L)	2	0.13	87	78
7. STN-NH(CH$_2$)$_4$COOH	5	>4.0	88	86
8. STN-NH(CH$_2$)$_7$COOH	8	>4.0	90	70
9. STN-NH(CH$_2$)$_2$N(CH$_3$)$_2$	7	0.2	90	88
10. STN-NH(CH$_2$)$_3$N(CH$_3$)$_2$	3	0.5	90	89
11. STN-O-(CH$_2$)$_2$CH$_3$	>40	0.004	66	24
12. STN-O-(CH$_2$)$_3$CH$_3$	>40	0.004	67	0
13. STN-O- (CH$_2$)$_2$N(CH$_3$)$_2$	5	0.003	93	83
14. STN-O-(CH$_2$)$_3$N(CH$_3$)$_2$	4	0.004	83	84

shown to be minimum requisites for the inhibitory activities of STN and SKM against AMV-RTase [7, 13]. Interestingly, isoquinoline quinones were as potent as quinoline quinones. Furthermore, AMV-RTase was inhibited by o- and p-quinoline (or isoquinoline) quinones to the same extent as STN, with ID_{50} values ranging between 1 and 5 μg/ml. The cytotoxicities of the quinones were much lower than that of STN; the ID_{50} values were higher than 0.15 μg/ml. In particular, the ID_{50} value of 8-methoxy-7-methyl-5,6-dihydroquinoline-5,6-dione was as high as 16 μg/ml, while 50% inhibition of cell growth was seen in the presence of 0.0025 μg/ml STN [12]. This favors its use as an antiviral substance, although its solubilization remains a problem.

Table 7

ID_{50} (μg/ml) of various quinones against AMV-RTase

		R_1	R_2	R_3	ID_{50} (μg/ml)
	1	—H	—H		2.0
	2	—OCH_3	—H		2.3
	3	—OCH_3	—CH_3		7.2
	4	—H	—OCH_3		<1.25
	5	—CH_3	—OCH_3		8.0
	6	—H	—H		3.1
	7	—H	—CN		<1.2
	8	—CH_3	—H		5.1
	9	—CH_3	—H		2.0
	10	—CH_3	—CH_3		18.0
	11	—H			2.0
	12	—CH_3			2.0
	13	—H			4.0
	14	—CH_3			2.0
	15	—H	—H	—H	10.0
	16	—H	—H	—OH	2.0
	17	—CH_3	—H	—H	17.0
	18	—CL	—CL	—H	17.0
	19	—OH	—H	—H	>40.0
	20	—OH	—$(CH_2)_2COOH$	—H	>40.0
	21	—OH	—$(CH_2)_2COOC_2H_5$	—H	>40.0
	STN				3.0
	SKM				26.5

REFERENCES

1 Hanajima, S., K. Ishimaru, K. Sakano, S.K. Roy, Y. Inouye and S. Nakamura. 1985. Inhibition of reverse transcriptase by limocrocin. J. Antibiot. 38: 803–805.

2 Harada, S., Y. Koyanagi and N. Yamamoto. 1985. Infection of human T-lymphotropic virus type-I (HTLV-I)-bearing MT-4 cells with HTLV-III (AIDS virus): chronological studies of early events. Virology 14: 272–281.

3 Inouye, Y., N. Manabe, H. Mukai, S. Nakamura, T. Matsugi, H. Amanuma and Y. Ikawa. 1985. Chromostin, a novel specific inhibitor against reverse transcriptase. J. Antibiot. 38: 519–521.

4 Inouye, Y., H. Okada, S.K. Roy, T. Miyasaka, S. Hibino, N. Tanaka and S. Nakamura. 1985. Biological properties of streptonigrin derivatives. I. Antimicrobial and cytocidal activities. J. Antibiot. 38: 1429–1432.

5 Inouye, Y., H. Okada, J. Uno, T. Arai and S. Nakamura. 1986. Effects of streptonigrin derivatives and sakyomicin A on the respiration of isolated rat liver mitochondria. J. Antibiot. 39: 550–556.

6 Inouye, Y., Y. Take, S. Nakamura, H. Nakashima, N. Yamamoto and H. Kawaguchi. 1987. Screening for inhibitors of avian myeloblastosis virus reverse transcriptase and effect on the replication of AIDS-virus. J. Antibiot. 40: 100–104.

7 Inouye, Y., Y. Take, K. Oogose, A. Kubo and S. Nakamura. 1987. The quinoline quinone as the minimum entity for reverse transcriptase inhibitory activity of streptonigin. J. Antibiot. 40: 105–107.

8 Miyasaka, T., S. Hibino, Y. Inouye and S. Nakamura. 1986. Synthesis of novel streptonigrin-2-amide derivatives with 3,3'-(phenylphosphoryl)-bis(1,3-thiazolidine-2-thione). J. Chem. Soc. Perkin Trans. I 1986: 479–482.

9 Nakashima, H., N. Yamamoto, Y. Inouye and S. Nakamura. 1987. Inhibition by doxorubicin of human immunodeficiency virus (HIV) infection and replication in vitro. J. Antibiot. 40: 396–399.

10 Nishio, M., A. Kuroda, M. Suzuki, K. Ishimaru, S. Nakamura and R. Nomi. 1983. Retrostatin, a new specific enzyme inhibitor against avian myeloblastosis virus reverse transcriptase. J. Antibiot. 36: 761–769.

11 Okada, H., H. Mukai, Y. Inouye and S. Nakamura. 1986. Biological properties of streptonigrin derivatives. II. Inhibition of reverse transcriptase activity. J. Antibiot. 39: 306–308.

12 Take, Y., K. Oogose, T. Kubo, Y. Inouye, S. Nakamura, Y. Kitahara and A. Kubo. 1987. Comparative study on biological activities of heterocyclic quinones and streptonigrin. J. Antibiot. 40: 679–684.

13 Take, Y., M. Sawada, H. Kunai, Y. Inouye and S. Nakamura. 1986. Role of the naphthoquinone moiety in the biological activities of sakyomicin A. J. Antibiot. 39: 557–563.

14 Tanaka, N., T. Okabe, N. Tanaka, Y. Take, Y. Inouye, S. Nakamura, H. Nakashima and N. Yamamoto. 1986. Inhibition by sakyomicin A of avian myeloblastosis virus reverse transcriptase and proliferation of AIDS-associated virus (HTLV-III/LAV). Jpn. J. Cancer Res. (Gann) 77: 324–326.

Novel Microbial Products for Medicine and Agriculture
Editors: A.L. Demain, G.A. Somkuti, J.C. Hunter-Cevera and H.W. Rossmoore

CHAPTER 12

Low molecular weight enzyme inhibitors produced by microorganisms

Takaaki Aoyagi and Tomio Takeuchi

Institute of Microbial Chemistry, Tokyo, Japan

SUMMARY

A large number of enzymes work in complicated pathways for the expression of various biological functions in organisms. Enzyme inhibitors are likely to become useful tools for the analysis of these functions, as well as for the study of reaction mechanisms and the three-dimensional structures of enzymes. Already of great value in elucidating disease processes, enzyme inhibitors even seem to be useful in the treatment of various diseases. In searching for enzyme inhibitors in culture filtrates of microbes we discovered many substances which specifically inhibit various enzymes, such as serine-, cysteine-, aspartic- and metalloproteinases, aminopeptidases, dipeptidyl aminopeptidases, carboxypeptidases, dipeptidyl carboxypeptidases, etc. These inhibitors have low molecular weights and unique structures. We found significant activity of numerous exopeptidase enzymes on the surface membranes of various mammalian cells, e.g., aminopeptidases, carboxypeptidases, alkaline phosphatase, esterase, etc. Searching for specific inhibitors against these cell surface enzymes, we discovered inhibitors such as amastatin, bestatin, arphamenines A and B, actinonin, probestin, prostatin, formestin, diprotins A and B, histargin, foroxymithine, forphenicine, ebelactones A and B, esterastin, etc. These inhibitors bind to the cell surface, modifying the functions of cells involved in immune responses. Studies on these enzyme inhibitors may provide important keys to understanding various aspects of biological phenomena and many diseases, including inflammation, immune response, complement reaction, carcinogenesis, metastasis, viral infection, autoimmune diseases, muscular dystrophy, demyelination diseases, etc. Because of their interesting pharmacological activities, some of the inhibitors are currently under evaluation for use as medical drugs. Enzyme inhibitors seem to be a promising new field of study.

INTRODUCTION

It is more than 20 years since we began the study of low molecular weight (LMW) enzyme inhibitors, in collaboration with the late Professor Hamao Umezawa. When we discovered leupeptin in 1969, the first inhibitor to be found, we did not foresee the great growth that would occur in this field of research.

Initially screening for inhibitors against plasmin, trypsin, and/or kallikrein, we found leupeptin. Encouraged by this success, we continued to search for inhibitors of various endopeptidases, finding antipain, chymostatin, pepstatin, etc. This directed our interest to other enzymes, such as cell surface enzymes, including exopeptidases, alkaline phosphatase, esterase, etc., as well as glycosidases. Assisted by many coworkers, we eventually succeeded in obtaining more than 60 LMW inhibitors possessing novel structures.

DISCUSSION

Endopeptidase inhibitors

For many years we have searched for inhibitors of various proteinases, including cell surface enzymes, and have found more than 60 kinds of small molecular size enzyme inhibitors from culture filtrates of microbes [1, 2, 13, 24, 25, 27]. These inhibitors, in contrast to those discovered in animals and plants, are characterized by their LMW and novel structures. The structures were completely unforeseen, stimulating work on the mechanism of inhibition and the structure-activity relationship of the inhibitors.

Searching for inhibitors in culture filtrates of microbes, we discovered many substances which specifically inhibit various enzymes, such as serine-, cysteine-, aspartic-, and metalloproteinases.

Screening culture filtrates of microbes for inhibitory activities against trypsin, plasmin, papain, chymotrypsin, and elastase led to the discovery of the inhibitors leupeptin, antipain, chymostatin, and elastatinal (Fig. 1).

Leupeptin, which contains L-argininal, inhibits trypsin, plasmin, papain, cathepsin B, etc. Antipain, which also contains L-argininal, inhibits papain, trypsin, cathepsin B, etc. Chymostatin, which contains L-phenylalaninal, inhibits chymotrypsins. Elastatinal, which contains L-alaninal, inhibits pancreas elastase [11, 21, 29, 35]. Leupeptin, antipain, chymostatin, and elastatinal contain C-terminal aldehyde groups. When these aldehyde groups are oxidized or reduced to give an acid or an alcohol, the compounds lose their activities.

Pepstatin, pepstanone, and hydroxypepstatin were found by screening for inhibitors of pepsin (Fig. 1) [16, 30, 39]. They inhibit pepsin, cathepsin D, chymosin, renin, etc. Pepstatin, widely used in biochemical studies, contains the isovaleryl group. Pepstatins, pepstanones, and hydroxypepstatins were found to show almost equal activity against pepsin and cathepsin D [4, 5]. However, pepstatins are more effective against renin than either pepstanone or hydroxypepstatin, and the activity of pepstatin increases with increasing number of carbon atoms in the fatty acid moiety.

As inhibitors of metalloproteinases, we obtained phosphoramidon as a thermolysin inhibitor and steffimycins as collagenase inhibitors (Fig. 1) [22].

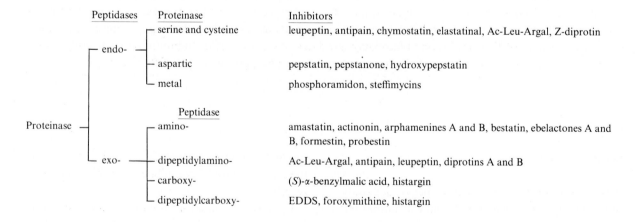

Peptidases	Proteinase	Inhibitors
	serine and cysteine	leupeptin, antipain, chymostatin, elastatinal, Ac-Leu-Argal, Z-diprotin
endo-	aspartic	pepstatin, pepstanone, hydroxypepstatin
	metal	phosphoramidon, steffimycins
	Peptidase	
	amino-	amastatin, actinonin, arphamenines A and B, bestatin, ebelactones A and B, formestin, probestin
exo-	dipeptidylamino-	Ac-Leu-Argal, antipain, leupeptin, diprotins A and B
	carboxy-	(S)-α-benzylmalic acid, histargin
	dipeptidylcarboxy-	EDDS, foroxymithine, histargin

Proteinase

Fig. 1. Proteinases and their LMW inhibitors. EDDS = (S,S)-N,N'-ethylenediaminedisuccinic acid.

Inhibitors of cell surface enzymes

Inhibitors of exopeptidases. During the early stages of infection with the influenza virus, we observed the rearrangement of sialic acid-containing glycoconjugates, a constituent of the plasma membrane of host cells. At the same time, the fluidity of the plasma membrane is decreased when a virion is adsorbed on the cell membrane, causing a drastic change in the activities of enzymes located on the cell membrane [3, 7, 10].

We observed aminopeptidase, alkaline phosphatase, and esterase activity on the surface of lymphocytes, macrophages, normal or virus-transformed cells, tumor cells, etc. [6, 9, 14]. Considering the biological role of these cell membrane enzymes, we undertook a search for inhibitors of cell surface enzymes. Inhibitors of these enzymes form an enzyme-inhibitor complex on the cellular membrane. Studies of the effect of this complex on cellular function will form a new approach to elucidating the relationship between the membrane phenomena and the corresponding cellular function.

Amastatin, bestatin, arphamenines A and B, α-aminoacylarginine, actinonin, probestin, prostatin, formestin A and B, ebelactones A and B, leupeptin, Ac-Leu-Argal, diprotins A and B, benzylmalic acid, histargin, chymostatin, foroxymithine, etc., were found to be inhibitors of enzymes, including aminopeptidases, dipeptidylaminopeptidases, carboxypeptidases, and dipeptidylcarboxypeptidases. They specifically inhibit the corresponding enzymes. Exopeptidase inhibitors were discovered, as well as inhibitors against plasma membrane enzymes.

Amastatin strongly inhibits aminopeptidase A (AP-A), Leu-AP, Tyr-AP, and tripeptidyl and tetrapeptidyl aminopeptidases [12]. Amastatin has five asymmetric carbon atoms in its molecular structure.

Bestatin strongly inhibits AP-B, Leu-AP, Ala-AP, and tripeptidyl and tetrapeptidyl aminopeptidases [36]. Bestatin has three asymmetric centers, and eight stereoisomers have been synthesized. The *S*-configuration of the C-2 of the (2*S*, 3*R*)-3-amino-2-hydroxy-4-phenylbutanol moiety is the stereochemical form important for activity. All four ste-reoisomers of bestatin with the 2*S*-configuration display inhibitory activity against AP-B and Leu-AP, whereas the four stereoisomers of 2*R*-configuration show no activity or slight activity [18].

Three main effects of bestatin have been elucidated to date: immunological effects, antitumor effects, and what we call other effects. Immunological effects include increases in E-rosette-forming T-cells, OKT4 cells and the OKT4/8 ratio, and enhanced lymphocyte blastogenesis to phytohemagglutinin (PHA), skin reaction to purified protein derivative (PPD) and PHA, and cytolytic action of NK cells against tumor cells. Antitumor effects include inhibition of growth of cultured tumor cells *in vitro*, *N*-methyl-*N'*-nitro-*N*-nitrosoguanidine-induced gastric cancer in rats, lymphocyte metastasis of P388 leukemia, and prolongation of the remission period of acute nonlymphocytic leukemia in adult human patients. Other effects include suppression of the onset of hypertension in spontaneously hypertensive rats, and the onset of muscular dystrophy in man [26].

We further screened for inhibitors of AP-B and discovered another group of inhibitors which we named arphamenines A and B [34]. These inhibitors have a methylene ketone (-CO-CH₂-) in place of the scissile peptide bond (-CO-NH-) of L-arginyl-L-phenylalanine, the substrate of AP-B. Formation of the methylene ketone moiety represents a new biosynthetic pathway [19]. Furthermore, we also found L-isoleucyl-L-arginine, L-leucyl-L-arginine, and L-valyl-L-arginine by screening for AP-B [40].

It is known that aminopeptidase-M (AP-M) is located in mammals in the microsomal fraction of the brush border of renal tubules. We discovered actinonin as a specific inhibitor of AP-M [37]. Actinonin had previously been known as an antibiotic and its structure has been reported [20].

We searched for inhibitors of *N*-formylmethionine aminopeptidase (fMet-AP), which is also located on the cell surface and has been reported to play an important role in chemotaxis. We were successful in obtaining inhibitors, which we named formestins A and B [8]. In addition, ebelactones A and B, found by screening for inhibitors of esterase, inhibited not only esterase but also fMet-AP (Fig. 1) [38].

We screened for inhibitors of dipeptidylamino-peptidase (DAP). Ac-Leu-Argal and leupeptin, specific inhibitors of DAP-III, and diprotins A and B, specific inhibitors of DAP-IV, were discovered [17, 32].

An inhibitor of carboxypeptidase A (CP-A) was identified as (S)-α-benzylmalic acid [23]. A specific inhibitor of CP-A, it also weakly inhibits CP-B. A specific inhibitor of CP-B was found and named histargin [31]. It inhibits dipeptidylcarboxypeptidases, including angiotensin converting enzyme (ACE) (Fig. 1).

The type of inhibition of these inhibitors against exopeptidases is shown in Tables 1 and 2. All of the

inhibitors we discovered are listed in relation to the classification of the peptidases in Fig. 1.

Inhibitors of other enzymes. Our previous studies demonstrated the activities of exopeptidases, carboxypeptidases, alkaline phosphatase, esterase, etc., on the surface of lymphocytes, macrophages, normal or virus-transformed cells and tumor cells. Searching for specific inhibitors of exopeptidases, we discovered various kinds of inhibitors, described above. We also discovered inhibitors of alkaline phosphatase, esterase, and phospholipase, such as forphenicine, esterastin, ebelactones A and B, and plipastatins A1, A2, B1, and B2. All these inhibitors enhance immune responses, except for esterastin,

Table 1

Kinetic constants of aminopeptidase inhibitors

Inhibitor	Enzyme	Substrate	K_m ($\times 10^{-4}$ M)	K_i ($\times 10^{-7}$ M)	Type of inhibition
Amastatin	AP-A	Glu·NA	8.0	2.5	competitive
Amastatin	Leu-AP	Leu·NA	37.0	16.0	competitive
Bestatin	AP-B	Arg·NA	1.0	0.6	competitive
Bestatin	Leu-AP	Leu·NA	5.8	0.2	competitive
Arphamenine A	AP-B	Arg·NA	1.0	0.025	competitive
Arphamenine B	AP-B	Arg·NA	1.0	0.008	competitive
Ile-Arg	AP-B	Arg·NA	1.0	5.0	competitive
Val-Arg	AP-B	Arg·NA	1.0	21.0	competitive
Actinonin	AP-M	Leu·NA	0.8	1.7	competitive
Formestin A	fMet-AP	fMet·NA	2.0	0.39	competitive
Formestin B	fMet-AP	fMet·NA	2.0	1.23	competitive
Ebelactone A	fMet-AP	fMet·NA	2.0	1.73	noncompetitive
Ebelactone B	fMet-AP	fMet·NA	2.0	0.63	noncompetitive
Diprotin A	DAP-IV	Gly-Pro·NA	4.0	22.0	competitive
Diprotin B	DAP-IV	Gly-Pro·NA	4.0	76.0	competitive

Glu·NA = glutamic acid β-naphthylamide, other abbreviations defined in text.

Table 2

Kinetic constants of carboxypeptidase inhibitors

Inhibitor	Enzyme	Substrate	K_m ($\times 10^{-4}$ M)	K_i ($\times 10^{-7}$ M)	Type of inhibition
(S)-α-Benzylmalic acid	CP-A	Hip-Phe	10.0	6.7	competitive
Histargin	CP-B	Hip-Lys	62.0	320.0	competitive
Foroxymithine	ACE	Hip-His-Leu	0.5	–	uncompetitive

Hip-Phe = hippuryl-L-phenylalanine, other abbreviations defined in text.

an esterase inhibitor which suppresses immune responses.

Forphenicine strongly inhibits alkaline phosphatase prepared from chicken intestine [15]. The formyl group is essential for the molecule to develop its inhibitory activity. Esterastin, discovered as an inhibitor of esterase, shows strong inhibitory activity against esterase, lipase, and cholesterol esterase, and weakly inhibits fMet-AP [28]. Ebelactones A and B, discovered as inhibitors of esterase, strongly inhibit not only esterase, lipase, and cholesterol esterase, but also fMet-AP [38]. These compounds are of great interest in the study of the mechanism of chemotaxis.

Therapeutic applications of enzyme inhibitors

A summary of the biological and therapeutic effects of enzyme inhibitors discovered in our laboratory is given in Fig. 2. Immunopotentiation was found to be a property of actinonin, amastatin, arphamenines A and B, benzylmalic acid, bestatin, diprotins A and B, esterastin, ebelactones A and B, forphenicinol, forphenicine, foroxymithine, and histargin. Fertilization is suppressed by antipain, chymostatin, and leupeptin. Analgesic action is exerted by actinonin, amastatin, arphamenines A and B, and bestatin. Carrageenin edema is suppressed by antipain, chymostatin, elastatinal, esterastin, leupeptin, phosphoramidon and pepstatin, and ascites and pleural fluid by pepstatin. Blister forma-

tion after a burn is suppressed by leupeptin. Leupeptin inhibits the serine proteinases released by pancreatitis. Renal vascular hypertension is suppressed by bestatin, foroxymithine, histargin, and pepstatin. Therapeutic effects in muscular dystrophy were suggested by the use of antipain, bestatin, forphenicinol, or leupeptin. Demyelinative diseases can be suppressed by leupeptin, forphenicine, arphamenine B, and esterastin. Chemical carcinogenesis can be suppressed by leupeptin and antipain. Malignant diseases in man can be suppressed by bestatin, forphenicinol, and forphenicine. Autoimmune diseases, including systemic lupus erythematosus, can be suppressed by arphamenine A, esterastin, forphenicine, and leupeptin.

We would like to close this discussion by expressing hope that the application of these enzyme inhibitors will, some day, lead to elucidation of the cause of diseases and even to their therapeutic treatment.

ACKNOWLEDGEMENTS

We wish to express our heartfelt gratitude to the late Professor Hamao Umezawa. Also, it is needless to say that this work was done with the cooperation of many collaborators. We sincerely hope that this work, started by the late Professor Umezawa, will bear fruit in many areas of medicine, pharmacology and biochemistry.

Immunopotentiation:	Ac, Am, Ar(A,B), Bm, Bs, Dp(A,B), Es, Eb(A,B), Fl, Fn, Fo, Hs
Fertilization:	Ap, Cs, Lp
Analgesic action:	Ac, Am, Ar(A,B), Bs
Inflammation:	Ap, Cs, El, Es, Lp, Ph, Ps
Ascites and pleural fluid:	Ps
Chemical carcinogenesis:	Ap, Lp
Burn:	Lp
Pancreatitis:	Lp
Hypertension:	Bs, Fo, Hs, Ps
Muscular dystrophy:	Ap, Bs, Fl, Lp
Malignant diseases:	Bs, Fl, Fn
Autoimmune diseases:	Ar-A, Es, Fn, Lp

Fig. 2. Biological and therapeutic effects of enzyme inhibitors. Am = amastatin; Ac = actinonin; AP = antipain; Ar = arphamenine; Bm = (*S*)-α-benzylmalic acid; Bs = bestatin; Cs = chymostatin; Dp = diprotin; Eb = ebelactone; El = elastatinal; Es = esterastin; Fl = forphenicinol; Fn = forphenicine; Fo = foroxymithine; Lp = leupeptin; Hs = histargin; Ph = phosphoramidon; Pr = probestin; Ps = pepstatin.

REFERENCES

1 Aoyagi, T. 1978. Structure and activities of proteinase inhibitors of microbial origin. In: Bioactive Peptides Produced by Microorganisms (Umezawa, H., T. Takita and T. Shiba, eds.), pp. 129–151, Kodansha Ltd., Tokyo/John Wiley and Sons, New York.

2 Aoyagi, T. 1986. Biological significance of proteases and their inhibitors. Proc. Jpn. Soc. Invest. Dermatol. 10: 77–82.

3 Aoyagi, T., T. Komiyama, K. Nerome, T. Takeuchi and H. Umezawa. 1975. Characterization of myxovirus sialidase. Experientia 31: 896–898.

4 Aoyagi, T., S. Kunimoto, H. Morishima, T. Takeuchi and H. Umezawa. 1971. Effect of pepstatin on acid protease. J. Antibiot. 24: 687–694.

5 Aoyagi, T., H. Morishima, R. Nishizawa, S. Kunimoto, T. Takeuchi and H. Umezawa. 1972. Biological activity of pepstatins, pepstanone A and partial peptides on pepsin, cathepsin D and renin. J. Antibiot. 25: 689–694.

6 Aoyagi, T., M. Nagai, M. Iwabuchi, W.S. Liaw, T. Andoh and H. Umezawa. 1978. Aminopeptidase activities on the surface of mammalian cells and their alterations associated with transformation. Cancer Res. 38: 3505–3508.

7 Aoyagi, T., K. Nerome, J. Suzuki, T. Takeuchi and H. Umezawa. 1974. Change of enzyme activities during the early stage of influenza virus infection. Biochem. Biophys. Res. Commun. 60: 1178–1184.

8 Aoyagi, T., K. Ogawa, H. Iinuma, H. Naganawa, M. Hamada and T. Takeuchi. 1989. J. Antibiot., in press.

9 Aoyagi, T., H. Suda, M. Nagai, K. Ogawa, J. Suzuki, T. Takeuchi and H. Umezawa. 1976. Aminopeptidase activities on the surface of mammalian cells. Biochim. Biophys. Acta 452: 131–143.

10 Aoyagi, T., J. Suzuki, K. Nerome, R. Nishizawa, T. Takeuchi and H. Umezawa. 1974. Sialic acid residues exposed on mammalian cell surface: the effect of adsorption of denatured virus particles. Biochem. Biophys. Res. Commun. 57: 271–278.

11 Aoyagi, T., T. Takeuchi, A. Matsuzaki, K. Kawamura, S. Kondo, M. Hamada, K. Maeda and H. Umezawa. 1969. Leupeptins, new proteinase inhibitors from actinomycetes. J. Antibiot. 22: 283–286.

12 Aoyagi, T., H. Tobe, F. Kojima, M. Hamada, T. Takeuchi and H. Umezawa. 1978. Amastatin, an inhibitor of aminopeptidase A, produced by actinomycetes. J. Antibiot. 31: 636–638.

13 Aoyagi, T. and H. Umezawa. 1975. Structures and activities of protease inhibitors of microbial origin. In: Proteases and Biological Control (Reich, E., D.B. Riffkin and E. Show, eds.), pp. 429–454, Cold Spring Harbor Laboratory, Cold Spring Harbor, NY.

14 Aoyagi, T. and H. Umezawa. 1981. The relationships between enzyme inhibitors and function of mammalian cells. Acta Biol. Med. Germ. 40: 1523–1529.

15 Aoyagi, T., T. Yamamoto, K. Kojiri, F. Kojima, M. Hamada, T. Takeuchi and H. Umezawa. 1978. Forphenicine, an inhibitor of alkaline phosphatase, produced by actinomycetes. J. Antibiot. 31: 244–246.

16 Miyano, T., M. Tomiyasu, H. Iizuka, S. Tomisaka, T. Takita, T. Aoyagi and H. Umezawa. 1972. New pepstatins, pepstatins B and C, and pepstanone A, produced by streptomycetes. J. Antibiot. 25: 489–491.

17 Nishikiori, T., F. Kawahara, H. Naganawa, Y. Muraoka, T. Aoyagi and H. Umezawa. 1984. Production of acetyl-L-leucyl-L-argininal, inhibitor of dipeptidyl aminopeptidase III by bacteria. J. Antibiot. 37: 680–681.

18 Nishizawa, R., T. Saino, T. Takita, H. Suda, T. Aoyagi and H. Umezawa. 1977. Synthesis and structure-activity relationships of bestatin analogues, inhibitors of aminopeptidase. J. Med. Chem. 20: 510–515.

19 Okuyama, A., S. Ohuchi, T. Tanaka, T. Aoyagi and H. Umezawa. 1986. Cell-free biosynthesis of arphamenine A. Biochem. Int. 12: 485–491.

20 Ollis, W.D., A.J. East, J.J. Gordon and I.O. Sutherland. 1964. The constitution of actinonin – structural and synthetic studies. In: I.A.M. Symposia on Microbiology No. 6, Chemistry of Microbial Products, pp. 204–214, The Microbial Research Foundation, Tokyo.

21 Suda, H., T. Aoyagi, M. Hamada, T. Takeuchi and H. Umezawa. 1972. Antipain, a new protease inhibitor isolated from actinomycetes. J. Antibiot. 25: 263–266.

22 Suda, H., T. Aoyagi, T. Takeuchi and H. Umezawa. 1973. A thermolysin inhibitor produced by actinomycetes: phosphoramidon. J. Antibiot. 26: 621–623.

23 Tanaka, T., H. Suda, H. Naganawa, T. Takeuchi, T. Aoyagi and H. Umezawa. 1984. Production of (S)-α-benzylmalic acid, inhibitor of carboxypeptidase A by actinomycetes. J. Antibiot. 37: 682–684.

24 Umezawa, H. 1972. Enzyme Inhibitors of Microbial Origin, University of Tokyo Press, Tokyo.

25 Umezawa, H. 1976. Structures and activities of protease inhibitors of microbial origin. Methods Enzymol. 45: 678–695.

26 Umezawa, H. (ed.) 1980. Small molecular weight immunomodifiers produced by microorganisms: their screening and discoveries, and the genetics of microbial secondary metabolites. In: Small Molecular Immunomodifiers of Microbial Origin – Fundamental and Clinical Studies of Bestatin, pp. 1–16, Japan Scientific Societies Press, Tokyo/Pergamon Press, Oxford.

27 Umezawa, H. and T. Aoyagi. 1977. Activities of proteinase inhibitors of microbial origin. In: Proteinases in Mammalian Cells and Tissues (Barrett, A.J., ed.), pp. 637–662, North-Holland, Amsterdam.

28 Umezawa, H., T. Aoyagi, T. Hazato, K. Uotani, F. Kojima, M. Hamada and T. Takeuchi. 1978. Esterastin, an inhibitor of esterase, produced by actinomycetes. J. Antibiot. 31: 639–641.

29 Umezawa, H., T. Aoyagi, H. Morishima, S. Kunimoto, M.

Matsuzaki, M. Hamada and T. Takeuchi. 1970. Chymostatin, a new chymotrypsin inhibitor produced by actinomycetes. J. Antibiot. 23: 425–428.

30 Umezawa, H., T. Aoyagi, H. Morishima, M. Matsuzaki, M. Hamada and T. Takeuchi. 1970. Pepstatin, a new pepsin inhibitor produced by actinomycetes. J. Antibiot. 23: 259–262.

31 Umezawa, H., T. Aoyagi, K. Ogawa, H. Iinuma, H. Naganawa, M. Hamada and T. Takeuchi. 1984. Histargin, a new inhibitor of carboxypeptidase B produced by actinomycetes. J. Antibiot. 37: 1088–1090.

32 Umezawa, H., T. Aoyagi, K. Ogawa, H. Naganawa, M. Hamada and T. Takeuchi. 1984. Diprotins A and B, inhibitors of dipeptidyl aminopeptidase IV, produced by bacteria. J. Antibiot. 37: 422–425.

33 Umezawa, H., T. Aoyagi, K. Ogawa, T. Obata, H. Iinuma, H. Naganawa, M. Hamada and T. Takeuchi. 1985. Foroxymithine, a new inhibitor of angiotensin-converting enzyme, produced by actinomycetes. J. Antibiot. 38: 1813–1815.

34 Umezawa, H., T. Aoyagi, S. Ohuchi, A. Okuyama, H. Suda, T. Takita, M. Hamada and T. Takeuchi. 1983. Arphamenine A and B, new inhibitors of aminopeptidase B, produced by bacteria. J. Antibiot. 36: 1572–1575.

35 Umezawa, H., T. Aoyagi, A. Okura, H. Morishima, T. Takeuchi and Y. Okami. 1973. Elastatinal, a new elastase inhibitor produced by actinomycetes. J. Antibiot. 26: 787–789.

36 Umezawa, H., T. Aoyagi, H. Suda, M. Hamada and T. Takeuchi. 1976. Bestatin, an inhibitor of aminopeptidase B, produced by actinomycetes. J. Antibiot. 29: 97–99.

37 Umezawa, H., T. Aoyagi, T. Tanaka, H. Suda, A. Okuyama, H. Naganawa, M. Hamada and T. Takeuchi. 1985. Production of actinonin, an inhibitor of aminopeptidase M, by actinomycetes. J. Antibiot. 38: 1629–1630.

38 Umezawa, H., T. Aoyagi, K. Uotani, M. Hamada, T. Takeuchi and S. Takahashi. 1980. Ebelactone, an inhibitor of esterase, produced by actinomycetes. J. Antibiot. 33: 1594–1596.

39 Umezawa, H., T. Miyano, T. Murakami, T. Takita, T. Aoyagi, T. Takeuchi, H. Naganawa and H. Morishima. 1973. Hydroxypepstatin, a new pepstatin produced by streptomycetes. J. Antibiot. 26: 615–617.

40 Yamamoto, K., H. Suda, M. Ishizuka, T. Takeuchi, T. Aoyagi and H. Umezawa. 1980. Isolation of α-aminoacyl arginines in screening of aminopeptidase B inhibitors. J. Antibiot. 33: 1597–1599.

Novel Microbial Products for Medicine and Agriculture

Editors: A.L. Demain, G.A. Somkuti, J.C. Hunter-Cevera and H.W. Rossmoore

© 1989, Society for Industrial Microbiology

CHAPTER 13

Chemistry, biochemistry and therapeutic potential of microbial α-glucosidase inhibitors

Lutz Mueller

Pharma Corporate Project Management, Bayer AG, Leverkusen, F.R.G.

SUMMARY

The search for α-glucosidase inhibitors to reduce the rate of the intestinal digestion of oligo- and polysaccharides in the diet has yielded a number of chemically distinct inhibitory substances of microbial origin with different pharmacological and pharmacodynamic properties. More than 20 inhibitors (or groups of structurally related inhibitors) have, to date, been reported in scientific and patent literature. There is, however, enormous variation regarding structural elucidation, biochemical characterization, standards of fermentation and isolation procedures, and exploration of pharmacological potential. In all of these aspects, two projects today are the most advanced, i.e. acarbose and tendamistat (the latter having recently been discontinued). Studies in animals and man conducted mainly with acarbose and the two deoxynojirimycin derivatives, miglitol and emiglitate, showed α-glucosidase inhibitors not to have hypoglycemic activity like insulin or sulfonylureas. Rather they lower the postprandial rise in blood glucose in healthy and diabetic individuals after intake of food containing carbohydrates, reduce postprandial insulin secretion and lessen diabetic glucosuria. In addition, α-glucosidase inhibitors reduce the carbohydrate-driven synthesis of very low density lipoproteins and, in contrast to insulin and sulfonylureas, have no lipogenic potential. Because of these properties, α-glucosidase inhibitors are to be regarded as a new therapeutic principle for the treatment of diabetes with potential applications in the prevention of late diabetic complications.

INTRODUCTION

It has been recognized for some time that enzyme inhibitors have a rational place in the complex field of drug therapy. Aprotinin, for instance, a polypeptide isolated from bovine lung tissue, has been in clinical use for the last 25 years for controlling the excessive activities of trypsin, plasmin and kallikrein in certain pathological conditions. Increased insight into the mechanisms and regulation underlying the interplay of enzymatic reactions has greatly stimulated the systematic research and development of enzyme inhibitors in various areas of regulatory and metabolic disorders. For example, drugs for controlling elevated blood pressure, i.e. angiotensin converting enzyme (ACE) inhibitors, and for reducing endogenous cholesterol synthesis, i.e. a hydroxymethylglutaryl-CoA (HMG-CoA) reductase inhibitor, have been developed, approved and recently launched in major markets.

Like hypertension and hypercholesterolemia, diabetes is a disease with growing prevalence, affecting a sizeable proportion of the (generally elderly) population with Western lifestyles, and is held to be very serious in view of the grave late complications resulting from this metabolic disorder.

Today, two forms of drug therapy are essentially available for controlling a diabetic patient's elevated blood glucose levels. Injection of exogenous insulin will make up for the failing production of the hormone in type I (insulin-dependent) diabetic patients for whom this treatment is an absolutely necessary and life-saving measure. On the other hand, oral administration of sulfonylureas stimulates the secretion of insulin by the pancreas in type II (maturity-onset) diabetic patients, who are generally still able to produce the hormone but do not adequately respond to stimulation by increased blood glucose concentrations. Clearly, both approaches – insulin and sulfonylureas – are targeted at the lowering of elevated blood glucose levels by means of their hypoglycemic action.

Both antidiabetic drug regimens have to be based on optimal patient compliance with dietary rules regarding total caloric intake, distribution of meals and nutrient composition. However, in spite of the heavy use of insulin and sulfonylureas and notwithstanding the significant progress over the past decade in the areas of dietary advice, patient education and metabolic self-monitoring, many diabetic patients – of both types I and II – are by no means in satisfactory control. Obviously, a novel comprehensive approach is needed here.

Conceptionally, the new idea put forward in the late sixties [11] was to prevent or at least effectively reduce postprandial hyperglycemia by slowing down the digestion of nutrient carbohydrates and, consequently, the absorption of monosaccharides, essentially that of glucose. For that purpose, the activities of intestinal α-glucosidases were to be modified by inhibitors of distinct specificity and potency.

In the last 20 years, research and development of α-glucosidase inhibitors has mainly been carried out by West European and Japanese pharmaceutical companies [7]. In vitro test methods employing commercially available (porcine pancreatic α-amylase) or partially purified (porcine intestinal brush border α-glucosidase complex) enzyme preparations and defined substrates (starch and various disaccharides) were used for the detection, purification and characterization of α-glucosidase inhibitors. Microorganisms proved to be a yielding source for such active compounds. Originally, the family of Actinoplanaceae, above all the genera *Actinoplanes*, *Ampullariella* and *Streptosporangium*, were found to produce a variety of compounds active against intestinal α-glucosidases. Later on, a whole range of *Streptomyces* strains, but also *Bacillus* strains and even fungi such as *Aspergillus* and *Cladosporium*, were added to the growing list of producers.

Upon isolation and more detailed characterization, though in many cases rather preliminary, it was recognized that microbial α-glucosidase inhibitors exhibit a remarkable variation in their chemical nature [7]. Many of them are carbohydrates, mostly complex pseudo-oligosaccharides; others were shown to be polypeptides or glycopeptides. Applying the yardstick of at least basic structural elucidation, the lengthy list is reduced to a dozen different entities or series of homologs (Table 1). Of these, only few have reached the stage of clinical development as antidiabetic drugs: the pseudo-oligosaccharides acarbose (BAY g 5421) and trestatin, the polypeptide tendamistat (HOE 467), and certain monosaccharide derivatives of 1-deoxynojirimycin (BAY m 1099 = miglitol and BAY o 1248 = emiglitate) and of valiolamine (AO-128).

ACARBOSE AND HOMOLOGS

Acarbose and its homologs (Fig. 1) were isolated from fermentations of various *Actinoplanes* strains in the early seventies. The characteristic feature of their structure is the core – essential for inhibitory activity – composed of an unsaturated cyclitol unit (hydroxymethyl conduritol residue) and a 4,6-dideoxy-4-amino-D-glucopyranose unit (4-deoxy-4-amino-D-quinovose residue). This pseudo-disaccharide core structure, which was named acarviosine

Table 1

Structural variation in microbial α-glucosidase inhibitors [7, 14]

Pseudo-oligosaccharides

Actinoplanes sp.	acarbose and homologs	1972
Streptomyces diastaticus	amylostatins	1974
Streptomyces sp.	'amino sugars'	1977
Streptomyces calvus	adiposins	1978
Streptomyces dimorphogenes	trestatins	1978
Streptomyces myxogenes	oligostatins	1979
Streptomyces flavochromogenes	'amino-oligosaccharides'	1982
Streptomyces sp.	AI-5662 and homologs	1984

Monosaccharides

Bacilli, *Streptomyces lavendulae*	1-deoxynojirimycin	1978
Streptomyces hygroscopicus	valiolamine	1982

Polypeptides

Streptomyces tendae	tendamistat	1977
Streptomyces griseosporeus	Haim I and II	1979
Streptomyces corchorushii	Paim I and II	1983

Glycopeptides

Cladosporium cladosporioides	tomastachin	1981

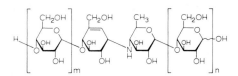

Fig. 1. General structural formula of the acarbose series.

and is not stable in the free form, is linked to a varying number of glucose residues. All glycosidically connected elements are bound by 1,4-linkages; in the cyclitol unit the arrangement of substituents is stereochemically similar to that of an α-D-glucopyranose unit [13].

The most important member of this homologous series is acarbose, a pseudo-tetrasaccharide formed from one acarviosine and one maltose unit (Fig. 2). No other microbial α-glucosidase inhibitor to date has been so thoroughly researched and developed with respect to fermentation conditions, isolation procedures, chemical and biochemical characterization and modification, pharmacology, safety profile and clinical efficacy. Since several publications have presented and summarized these findings and results [7, 14], this review focuses on those properties of acarbose which demonstrate its pharmacological potential and form the basis for successful clinical development.

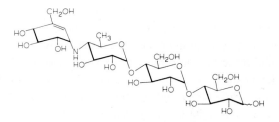

Fig. 2. Structural formula of acarbose.

In vitro, acarbose and its homologs display a characteristic pattern of inhibitory potency against various mammalian intestinal and pancreatic α-glucosidases (Table 2). Obviously, there is considerable dependence on molecular weight in the case of sucrase, maltase and glucoamylase, but scarcely for dextrinase. In any case, acarbose is – in vitro – for these enzymes by far the most potent inhibitor in the homologous series. α-Amylase inhibition is fairly poor with the first three members of the series (including acarbose) but increases dramatically with four or five glucose units attached to the acarviosine core structure [8].

Test tube enzyme inhibition assays are not necessarily indicative of in vivo efficacy since several parameters cannot properly be controlled or assessed under in vitro conditions. Metabolic stability, pharmacokinetic properties and involvement in the degradation of oligo- and polysaccharides of enzymes which are not available for in vitro testing may strongly influence the in vivo activity and the clinical efficacy of an α-glucosidase inhibitor.

This is clearly shown by comparing the activities

Table 2

Amounts (in ng) of acarbose and homologs required for 50% inhibition of intestinal and pancreatic α-glucosidases [8]

| | Number of glucose units | | Sucrase | Maltase | Isomaltase | Dextrinase | Glucoamylase | α-Amylase |
	n	$m+n$	10 mU	10 mU	10 mU	29 mU	10 mU	100 mU
Acarbose:	1		560	100	43500	205	83	895
	2		74	15	42000	64	9.3	680
		3	455	80	54500	93	39	1135
		4	700	236	>100000	100	110	4.7
		5	700	1000	>>100000	93	410	2.8

of homologs of the acarbose series *in vitro* and *in vivo*, i.e. inhibition of sucrase *vs.* efficacy in sucrose loading tests, and inhibition of α-amylase *vs.* efficacy in starch loading tests (Table 3; ED_{50} is defined as the dose which reduces postprandial blood glucose increments by 50%). While *in vitro* inhibition of sucrase generally corresponds to *in vivo* effects on sucrose digestion, the first three members of the series (including acarbose) were strikingly more potent in reducing *in vivo* starch digestion than could be expected from the *in vitro* results [12]. It is assumed that these inhibitors act upon enzymes involved in the later steps of intestinal starch degradation rather than on the amylolysis of the native starch substrates.

Sucrose and starch are essential carbohydrate components in food consumed by man. Therefore, a well balanced *in vivo* efficacy for delaying both starch and sucrose digestion is very important for a drug with the mode of action of an α-glucosidase inhibitor.

Since the mechanism of action of an intestinal α-glucosidase, i.e. the active sucrase-isomaltase complex isolated from rabbit small intestine, has been studied in detail [4], there is a fairly clear perception of how acarbose works as a potent, specific, reversible and competitive inhibitor for α-glucosidases. Due to its high structural similarity to the substrate, acarbose binds to the active site of the enzyme with an affinity exceeding that of the substrate (sucrose) by a factor of $10^4 - 10^5$. While the nitrogen in the acarviosine unit still lends itself to protonation by a proton donor group (just like the glucosidic oxygen in the sucrose molecule), splitting of

Table 3

Inhibition of α-glucosidase activity *in vitro* and *in vivo* by acarbose and homologs [12]

| | Number of glucose units | | *In vitro* 50% inhibition of 10 mU sucrase | *In vivo* ED_{50} in sucrose loading tests | *In vitro* 50% inhibition of 100 mU α-amylase | *In vivo* ED_{50} in starch loading tests |
	n	$m+n$				
Acarbose:	1		560	1.0	895	1.1
	2		74	1.1	680	1.5
		3	455	3.3	1135	1.4
		4	700	10.0	4.7	1.0
		5	700	≈25.5	2.8	0.4

The amounts of acarbose and homologs required for the in vitro and in vivo tests are given in ng and mg/kg rat respectively.

the C-N linkage is impossible and, as a result, the enzymatic reaction is brought to a halt. Consequently, the enzyme will not take part in the process of digesting carbohydrates as long as acarbose remains bound to its active site.

OTHER PSEUDO-OLIGOSACCHARIDE INHIBITORS

During the last 15 years, acarbose and its homologs have not remained the only series of microbial pseudo-oligosaccharide inhibitors. By reviewing today at least seven additional discoveries of such inhibitors (Table 1), the following summary can be made regarding structural variations observed in pseudo-oligosaccharide inhibitors [7, 14]:

(a) Amylostatins comply with the same structural elements as the acarbose series and probably are not structurally different; specifically, several β-amylase degradation products of amylostatins are identical to certain homologs of the acarbose series.

(b) There are three distinct natural variations known to affect the acarviosine core structure (Fig. 3): first, an additional hydroxy group at C-6 of the amino sugar leads to the adiposins and the so-called 'amino sugars' which are of identical structure; second, hydration (formally seen) of the double bond in the cyclitol residue is a characteristic feature of oligostatins; and third, replacement of the same

double bond by an epoxy function results in the series of 'amino-oligosaccharides'.

(c) Two additional series of inhibitors were shown to have the – unmodified– acarviosine core structure embodied in their molecules not only once but also in multiples. Trestatins, as a typical structural element, have nonreducing trehalose in place of the reducing end found in all other pseudo-oligosaccharide inhibitors; they may contain one, two or even three acarviosine units [17]. The one member of another series which has been structurally characterized and designated AI-5662, contains two acarviosine units and, in contrast to trestatins, exhibits a reducing end in the form of maltose [15].

Though several reports on the pharmacological properties of these inhibitors have been published in patent and scientific literature, only trestatin has, as yet, reached the stage of clinical development.

TENDAMISTAT

Among several polypeptide and glycopeptide inhibitors, tendamistat is clearly the most advanced in its development, including clinical trials. One component was obtained in homogeneous, crystalline form (HOE 467A) and found to be a single-chain polypeptide consisting of 74 amino acid residues. It is composed of naturally occurring amino acids with the exception of methionine and phenylalanine and contains two disulfide bridges [2]. A fairly compact spatial structure is assumed to be one of the factors contributing to the remarkable stability of this inhibitor with respect to heat treatment and enzymatic degradation.

Tendamistat exhibits a high inhibitory specificity for mammalian α-amylases from pancreas and saliva. Results of kinetic measurements are indicative of irreversible, largely pH-independent inactivation of α-amylase, probably through the formation of a very stable 1:1 complex of enzyme and inhibitor [16].

In 1984, clinical trials with tendamistat were discontinued due to adverse side effects which are definitely not related to the therapeutic principle.

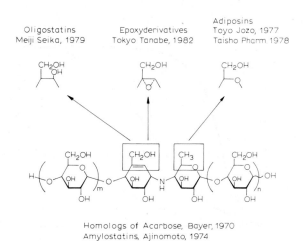

Fig. 3. Structural variations in microbial pseudo-oligosaccharide inhibitors.

MONOSACCHARIDE INHIBITORS

1-Deoxynojirimycin and valiolamine are two monosaccharide α-glucosidase inhibitors of microbial origin. Though they exhibit potent activity *in vitro*, they are not useful *in vivo* because of their rapid removal from the small intestine by absorption. Modification of the two parent molecules by attaching suitable substituents, however, has led to improved pharmacokinetic properties with a concomitant increase in inhibitory potency. Two 1-deoxynojirimycin derivatives (Fig. 4) are currently in clinical development: BAY m 1099 (miglitol) and BAY o 1248 (emiglitate) [5]. This is also the case for the *N*-bishydroxyisopropyl derivative of valiolamine, designated AO-128.

It is suggested that the mechanism of action of the N-containing monosaccharide inhibitors is, as with acarbose, of a highly specific, reversible and competitive nature. After binding to the active site and subsequent protonation of the nitrogen atom the resulting stable ion pair complex prevents the enzyme from binding and cleaving natural substrates for as long as the inhibitor stays bound.

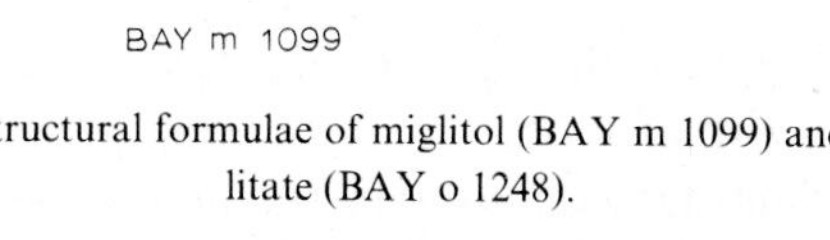

BAY o 1248

BAY m 1099

Fig. 4. Structural formulae of miglitol (BAY m 1099) and emiglitate (BAY o 1248).

α-GLUCOSIDASE INHIBITION AS A NEW THERAPEUTIC PRINCIPLE

α-Glucosidases are absolutely essential in the intestinal digestion of practically all food carbohydrates. Since only monosaccharides are readily taken up from the intestine, all other carbohydrates (disaccharides and polysaccharides) have to be broken down enzymatically before they can be absorbed. With the refined types of food so typical of Western societies, this usually takes place very quickly in the uppermost parts of the small intestine with the lower segments becoming idle due to lack of substrate in spite of considerable enzymatic activities being present also in this part of the digestive tract (Fig. 5). Consequently, postprandial rise in blood glucose is generally rapid and high following ingestion of nutrient carbohydrates.

While this poses no problem for the healthy individual, diabetic patients find themselves in a difficult position in dealing with markedly elevated postprandial blood glucose levels due to either lack of insulin (type I patients) or impairment of insulin action (generally type II patients). In a diabetic condition, blood glucose levels tend to remain rather high for prolonged periods of time, thereby creating a decisive risk factor for late diabetic complications.

Diabetic patients would obviously be helped if the postprandial blood glucose response could be smoothed and therefore reduced. This is exactly what acarbose and other suitable α-glucosidase inhibitors are capable of effecting by modifying the activity of intestinal carbohydrate-splitting enzymes. Retardation in time and spatial displacement into the lower small intestine of carbohydrate digestion and, consequently, glucose absorption re-

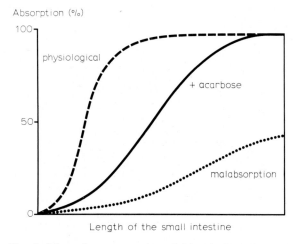

Fig. 5. Schematic representation of delayed absorption as a therapeutic principle.

sults in the lowering of postprandial blood glucose peaks with concomitant reduction in postprandial insulin requirements. This effect has been shown with acarbose in a large number of diabetic patients to be of major clinical benefit [3,5].

Efficacy and side effects of an α-glucosidase inhibitor like acarbose depend on certain factors, some of which can be controlled by the doctor and his patient and others which are beyond exercise of influence, such as the individual pattern of intestinal α-glucosidase activities or the quality of colonic flora (Fig. 6).

The amount and composition of nutrient carbohydrates are of special importance for securing optimal clinical efficacy and minimizing side effects. The diabetic patient's diet should include a sufficient amount of complex carbohydrates, essentially starch, in order to provide sufficient substrate for inhibitor action. Carbohydrates which are not digestible (like cellulose), not cleaved by an α-glucosidase (like lactose) or directly absorbed (monosaccharides like glucose, fructose and sorbitol) will obviously not contribute to drug efficacy. By choosing a well balanced combination of carbohydrates (in terms of quality and quantity) and acarbose dosage, digestion and absorption will be retarded and extended over the full length of the small intestine (Fig. 5). It is, however, of utmost importance that all carbohydrates which can be cleaved by α-glucosidases are fully digested and absorbed while still in the small intestinal tract. Otherwise they will enter the colon and give rise to side effects like meteorism, flatulence and even diarrhea as a consequence of colonic bacterial fermentation. From this, it becomes clear that α-glucosidase inhibitors, as antidiabetic drugs, are definitely not intended to promote loss of calories due to malabsorption. Their beneficial mode of action is the retardation of carbohydrate digestion and absorption without the spilling of such nutrients into the colon [6,9].

One of the alluring aspects of the new therapeutic principle is that, in bringing about optimal efficacy and avoiding side effects, it complies perfectly with the dietary rules currently recommended by national and international Diabetes and Health Associations [1,10].

Due to their antihyperglycemic mechanism of action, α-glucosidase inhibitors will not provoke hypoglycemia and not cause or intensify hyperinsulinemia but rather reduce the carbohydrate-driven, insulin-mediated synthesis of very low density lipoproteins. They lack the lipogenic potential of insulin and sulfonylureas which frequently creates a major problem in the treatment of type II diabetic patients. Because of these properties, α-glucosidase inhibitors such as acarbose are to be regarded as a promising new approach for the treatment of diabetes with potential benefits in the prevention of late diabetic complications.

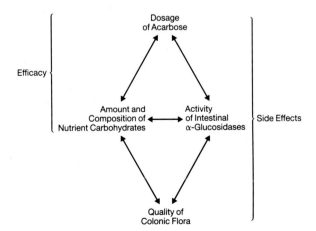

Fig. 6. Efficacy and side effects of acarbose.

REFERENCES

1 American Diabetes Association. 1987. Nutritional recommendations and principles for individuals with diabetes mellitus. 1986. Diabetes Care 10: 126–132.
2 Aschauer, H., L. Vértesy, G. Nesemann and G. Braunitzer. 1983. The primary structure of the α-amylase inhibitor Hoe 467A from *Streptomyces tendae* – a new class of inhibitors. Hoppe-Seyler's Z. Physiol. Chem. 364: 1347–1356.
3 Berchtold, P., T.R. Weihrauch and M. Berger. 1984. Food and drug interactions on digestive absorption. World Rev. Nutr. Diet 43: 10–33.
4 Cogoli, A. and G. Semenza. 1975. A probable oxocarbonium ion in the reaction mechanism of small intestinal sucrase and isomaltase. J. Biol. Chem. 250: 7802–7809.
5 Foelsch, U.R. and B. Lembcke. 1987. The clinical use of α-glucosidase inhibitors. In: Structure and Function of the Small Intestine (Caspary, W.F., ed.), pp. 301–318, Excerpta Medica, Amsterdam.

6 Lembcke, B. 1987. Control of absorption: delaying absorption as a therapeutic principle. In: Structure and Function of the Small Intestine (Caspary, W.F., ed.), pp. 263–280, Excerpta Medica, Amsterdam.

7 Mueller, L. 1986. Microbial glycosidase inhibitors. In: Biotechnology (Rehm, H.-J. and G. Reed, eds.), Vol. 4, pp. 531–567, VCH Verlagsgesellschaft, Weinheim.

8 Mueller, L., B. Junge, W. Frommer, D. Schmidt and E. Truscheit. 1980. Acarbose (Bay g 5421) and homologous α-glucosidase inhibitors from Actinoplanaceae. In: Enzyme Inhibitors (Brodbeck, U., ed.), pp. 109–122, Verlag Chemie, Weinheim.

9 Mueller, L. and W. Puls. 1987. Pharmacology of α-glucosidase inhibitors. In: Structure and Function of the Small Intestine (Caspary, W.F., ed.), pp. 281–300, Excerpta Medica, Amsterdam.

10 National Institutes of Health. 1986. Diet and exercise in non-insulin-dependent diabetes mellitus. NIH Consensus Development Conference Statement 6: 1–7.

11 Puls, W. and U. Keup. 1973. Influence of an α-amylase inhibitor (Bay d 7791) on blood glucose, serum insulin and NEFA in starch loading tests in rats, dogs and man. Diabetologia 9: 97–101.

12 Puls, W., U. Keup, H.P. Krause, L. Mueller, D.D. Schmidt, G. Thomas and E. Truscheit. 1980. Pharmacology of a glucosidase inhibitor. Front. Hormone Res. 7: 235–247.

13 Schmidt, D.D., W. Frommer, B. Junge, L. Mueller, W. Wingender, E. Truscheit and D. Schaefer. 1977. α-Glucosidase inhibitors – new complex oligosaccharides of microbial origin. Naturwissenschaften 64: 535.

14 Truscheit, E., I. Hillebrand, B. Junge, L. Mueller, W. Puls and D. Schmidt. 1988. Microbial α-glucosidase inhibitors: chemistry, biochemistry and therapeutic potential. In: Progress in Clinical Biochemistry and Medicine, Vol. 7, pp. 17–99, Springer-Verlag, Berlin, Heidelberg.

15 Vértesy, L., R. Bender and H.-W. Fehlhaber. 1986. New α-glucosidase inhibitor. Eur. Pat. Appl. 0173950, Hoechst AG.

16 Vértesy, L., V. Oeding, R. Bender, K. Zepf and G. Nesemann. 1984. Tendamistat (Hoe 467), a tight-binding α-amylase inhibitor from *Streptomyces tendae* 4158. Eur. J. Biochem. 141: 505–512.

17 Yokose, K., K. Ogawa, Y. Suzuki, I. Umeda and Y. Suhara. 1983. New α-amylase inhibitor, trestatin – structure determination of trestatins A, B and C. J. Antibiot. 36: 1166–1175.

Novel Microbial Products for Medicine and Agriculture
Editors: A.L. Demain, G.A. Somkuti, J.C. Hunter-Cevera and H.W. Rossmoore
© 1989, Society for Industrial Microbiology

CHAPTER 14

Trestatin: α-amylase inhibitor

Kazuteru Yokose[1], Tamotsu Furumai[1], Yasuji Suhara[1] and Wolfgang Pirson[2]

[1]*Department of Microbiology and Chemistry, Nippon Roche Research Center, Kanagawa, Japan and* [2]*Department of PF/DO, F. Hoffmann-La Roche & Co. Ltd., Basel, Switzerland*

SUMMARY

The α-amylase inhibitor, trestatin, isolated from the culture filtrate of *Streptomyces dimorphogenes*, is a homologous mixture of oligosaccharides. The mixture contains three major components (trestatins A, B and C) and minor components (Ro 09-0765–8, Ro 09-0896–7, and others). The major components of trestatin have a nitrogen-containing pseudosaccharide, which is essential for α-amylase inhibition, and trehalose. Trestatin specifically inhibits porcine pancreas α-amylase (IC$_{50}$ 6×10^{-7}–8×10^{-9} M) and human saliva α-amylase. In rats and dogs, trestatin (0.1–1 mg/kg, p.o.) reduced the increase in blood glucose and insulin after a starch loading (1.6 g/kg). Trestatin also effectively reduced the increase in blood glucose and insulin after a meal containing starch both in healthy volunteers and in non-insulin-dependent diabetic patients (dose range 10–30 mg/meal). Therefore, trestatin may be used concurrently with other therapies to control diabetes.

INTRODUCTION

Starch, usually the predominant carbohydrate in the human diet, is digested in the gastrointestinal tract by α-amylase to maltose. Maltose is further hydrolyzed by intestinal maltase to glucose. Finally, glucose is absorbed by active transport into the blood. Starch digestion is a rapid process, which leads to a marked rise in blood glucose and insulin, shortly after a meal containing starch. This postprandial hyperglycemia and the concomitant insulin rise, however, are highly undesirable in diabetic or obese patients. The postprandial hyperglycemia and hyperinsulinemia can be reduced by decreasing the starch content of the diet and the meal size as generally recommended for diabetic and obese patients. Theoretically, these disorders can be improved by an appropriate diet. However, in practice, a therapeutic approach of this kind is not likely to work well due to lack of patient compliance. Therefore, a limitation on starch digestion by α-amylase or α-glucosidase could be useful in the treatment of these disorders. Several α-amylase inhibitors, and inhibitors of other α-glucosidases, have been investigated for this purpose [2, 5–14, 16, 18–20].

In the course of our screening program searching for α-amylase inhibitors, we discovered a series of novel homologous oligosaccharides in the culture filtrate of a *Streptomyces* strain isolated from soil, and designated it trestatin (Ro 09-0154). We named the organism *Streptomyces dimorphogenes* after identifying it as a new species.

Trestatin had potent inhibitory activity against

various α-amylases *in vitro*, and effectively reduced the increase in blood glucose and insulin when it was administered p.o. to animals, healthy volunteers and non-insulin-dependent diabetic patients after starch loading.

Trestatin (Ro 09-0154) contains trestatins A, B and C as major components, and Ro 09-0765–8, Ro 09-0896–7, and others as minor components. They are water-soluble basic oligosaccharides consisting of D-glucose and pseudo-disaccharide. In this report, we describe the taxonomy of the producing organism, the production of trestatin by fermentation, and the isolation, physicochemical characterization, structure determination and biological properties of trestatin (Ro 09-0154), major components A, B, C, and minor components.

TAXONOMIC STUDIES ON THE PRODUCING ORGANISM

We examined over 500 culture filtrates of streptomycetes isolated from soil samples during our screening program for α-amylase inhibitors, found a strain that produced a potent α-amylase inhibitor and designated it as NR-320-OM7HB. This strain was isolated from a soil sample collected in 1974 in Chichibu City, Saitama Prefecture, Japan. This strain had two types of spore chain morphology, flexuous (major) and spiral (minor). A morphovar with spiral spore chains was obtained by single spore selection. However, this morphovar also showed two types of morphology (flexuous and spiral) when cultivated at 37°C or above.

A comparative study of the parent strain with taxonomically related species within the *Streptomyces* genus indicated that *S. olivaceus* was the closest relative to this strain. However, the physiological characteristics of these two strains were different; i.e., their temperature range for growth, heat tolerance, sodium chloride tolerance of mycelia, and antibiotic sensitivity. In addition, the reciprocally hybridized DNA-DNA homology of the two strains was very low (<35%). Thus, we proposed to name it *S. dimorphogenes* nov. sp. Watanabe and Maruyama [21].

FERMENTATION

The seed culture was prepared in a medium containing 2.0% potato starch, 2.0% glucose, 2.0% soya meal, 0.5% yeast extract, 0.25% NaC1, 0.005% $ZnSO_4 \cdot 7H_2O$, 0.0005% $CuSO_4 \cdot 5H_2O$, 0.0005% $MnCl_2 \cdot 4H_2O$, 0.32% $CaCO_3$ (pH 7.0) by shaking for 48 h at 27°C, and transferring into a 50-liter fermentor containing 25 liters of the same medium as the seed culture. The culture was agitated (300 rpm) at 27°C for 43 h with an air flow rate of 25 l/min. The peak level of the α-amylase inhibitory activity was approximately 3.1×10^4 IU/ml* [23].

ISOLATION OF TRESTATIN

Isolation of trestatin complex (Ro 09-0154)

Activated charcoal was added to a 19-liter culture filtrate (3.1×10^4 IU/ml). Then, the mixture was stirred at room temperature for 20 min. The carbon cake was filtered and eluted with 50% aqueous acetone at pH 2.0. The eluate was adjusted to pH 7.0 and concentrated under reduced pressure. The concentrate was then put on a column of Dowex 50 (H^+ form). The column was eluted with 1 N NH_4OH. The active eluate was concentrated under reduced pressure and lyophilized. The lyophilized powder was suspended in methanol, stirred at room temperature for 2 h. The part that was insoluble in methanol was collected by filtration, applied to a column of Dowex 1 (acetate form), and eluted with water. The active eluate was concentrated under reduced pressure. The concentrate was then put on a column of Dowex 50 (ammonium form), and eluted with water. The active eluate was concentrated under reduced pressure and lyophilized to give 10.6 g trestatin complex (Ro 09-0154) as a pale yellow powder (3.6×10^7 IU/g) [23].

---

*α-Amylase inhibitory activity was determined by the method of Bernfeld [3]. The inhibition unit (IU) is defined as the amount of inhibitor which gives 50% inhibitory activity under assay conditions.

Isolation of trestatins A, B and C

Each component was purified by column chromatography using a weak cation exchange resin, Amberlite CG-50 [23]. Trestatin complex (Ro 09-0154) was dissolved in water, put on a column of Amberlite CG-50, type I (mixed bed consisting of 3.5 parts of ammonium form and 6.5 parts of H^+ form), and then was eluted with water, obtaining trestatin B first, followed by trestatin A and trestatin C. Each trestatin was further purified by chromatography using Amberlite CG-50, type II (mixed bed of ammonium form and H^+ form) or Sephadex G-25 to give trestatin A (7.1×10^7 IU/g), trestatin B (1.4×10^6 IU/g) and trestatin C (4.9×10^7 IU/g) as colorless amorphous powders.

Isolation of minor components (Ro 09-766, Ro 09-0767 and Ro 09-0768)

Ro 09-0766, Ro 09-0767 and Ro 09-0768 were isolated as minor components of trestatin complex (Ro 09-0154) by the following procedure. Thirty grams of trestatin complex (3.5×10^7 IU/g) was dissolved in water, put on a column of Amberlite CG-50, type I (mixed bed consisting of 1 part of ammonium form and 2 parts of H^+ form) and eluted with water. Each eluate containing Ro 09-0766, Ro 09-0767 or Ro 09-0768 was further purified by gel filtration using Sephadex G-25. The active fractions were concentrated under reduced pressure and lyophilized to give Ro 09-0766 (315 mg, 3.6×10^7 IU/g), Ro 09-0767 (710 mg, 4.7×10^7 IU/g), and Ro 09-0768 (188 mg, 3.8×10^7 IU/g) as colorless amorphous powders [22].

PHYSICO-CHEMICAL PROPERTIES OF TRESTATINS A, B AND C, Ro 09-0766, Ro 09-0767, AND Ro 09-0768

The physicochemical properties of trestatin components are summarized in Table 1.

The spectroscopic (IR, ^{1}H- and ^{13}C-NMR) and physico-chemical properties of trestatins A, B and C and Ro 09-0766–8 show that these components are basic oligosaccharide homologs possessing the same constituents. Upon hydrolysis (4 N HCl, 80°C, 3 h), trestatin complex (Ro 09-0154), trestatin A, trestatin B, and trestatin C each gave only two hydrolysis products, compound 1 (Fig. 1) and D-glucose [16]. Since compound 1 is derived from pseudo-disaccharide 2 (see Fig. 1 for structures), trestatin complex and each component were found to be composed of D-glucose and pseudo-disaccharide 2 [16]. (Methyl glycoside 3, which retained the pseudo-saccharide structure, was obtained from

Table 1

Physico-chemical properties of trestatin

	Trestatin A	Trestatin B	Trestatin C	Ro 09-0766	Ro 09-0767	Ro 09-0768
Appearance	colorless powder	colorless powder	colorless powder	colorless powder	colorless powder	colorless powder
Melting point (decomp.) (°C)	221–232	209–219	230–237	232–237	223–233	213–220
UV spectrum	end absorption	end absorption	end absorption	end absorption	end absorption	end absorption
$[\alpha]_D^{24}$ ($c = 1.0$, H_2O)	+177°	+187°	+169.5°	+168°	+172°	184°
FAB-MS m/z	1435 (MH$^+$)	970 (MH$^+$)	1900 (MH$^+$)	2224 (MH$^+$)	1759 (MH$^+$)	1294 (MH$^+$)
Molecular formula	$C_{56}H_{94}N_2O_{40}$	$C_{37}H_{63}NO_{28}$	$C_{75}H_{125}N_3O_{52}$	$C_{87}H_{145}N_3O_{62}$	$C_{68}H_{114}N_2O_{50}$	$C_{49}H_{83}NO_{38}$
Color reactions phenol-sulfuric acid	+	+	+	+	+	+
anthrone	+	+	+	+	+	+
red-tetrazolium	−	−	−	−	−	−

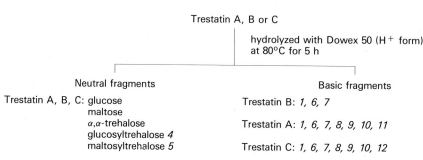

Fig. 1. Structures of compound 1, pseudo-disaccharide 2 and its methyl glycoside 3.

trestatin complex and trestatin A, B or C by methanolysis.)

The molar ratio of D-glucose to pseudo-disaccharide 2 of each component (Table 2) was determined by their ^{1}H-NMR spectra (ratio of integration of olefinic proton to anomeric proton) and FAB-MS spectra. Thus, we could determine the molecular formula of each component (Table 1) [22,23].

STRUCTURE DETERMINATION OF TRESTATINS A, B AND C

In order to determine the sugar sequence, each trestatin component (A, B and C) was partially hydrolyzed under the conditions shown in Fig. 2. The partial hydrolysis products were easily separated into neutral and basic fragments when Dowex 50 was used as the acid catalyst.

The neutral fragments of trestatin A, B or C were glucose, maltose, α,α-trehalose, glucotriose and glucotetraose. The structures of glucotriose and glucotetraose were determined to be glucosyltrehalose 4 and maltosyltrehalose 5 (Fig. 3) by analysis of ^{1}H- and ^{13}C-NMR data of their peracetates, respectively. Therefore, trestatins A, B and C contained the same partial structure, maltosyltrehalose 5.

Structure of trestatin B

The basic fragments obtained by partial hydrolysis of trestatin B (Fig. 2) were purified by chromatography using an Amberlite CG-50 (mixed bed consisting of the ammonium form and H+ form), which was eluted with water to give compound 1, pseudo-trisaccharide 6 and pseudo-tetrasaccharide 7. The structures of 6 and 7 (Fig. 4) were elucidated by ^{1}H-NMR, ^{13}C-NMR and mass spectroscopy. Pseudo-tetrasaccharide 7 was identical to Bayer's α-glucosidase inhibitor, acarbose. Since trestatin B was composed of 4 mol of D-glucose and 1 mol of pseudo-disaccharide 2 (Table 2), and maltosyltrehalose 5 was obtained from trestatin B by partial

Table 2

Molar ratios: D-glucose/pseudo-disaccharide 2

	Trestatin			Ro 09-0766	Ro 09-0767	Ro 09-0768
	A	B	C			
D-glucose	5	4	6	8	7	6
pseudo-disaccharide 2	2	1	3	3	2	1

Trestatin A, B or C

    hydrolyzed with Dowex 50 (H+ form)
    at 80°C for 5 h

Neutral fragments

Trestatin A, B, C: glucose
    maltose
    α,α-trehalose
    glucosyltrehalose *4*
    maltosyltrehalose *5*

Basic fragments

Trestatin B: *1, 6, 7*

Trestatin A: *1, 6, 7, 8, 9, 10, 11*

Trestatin C: *1, 6, 7, 8, 9, 10, 12*

Fig. 2. Partial hydrolysis of trestatins A, B and C.

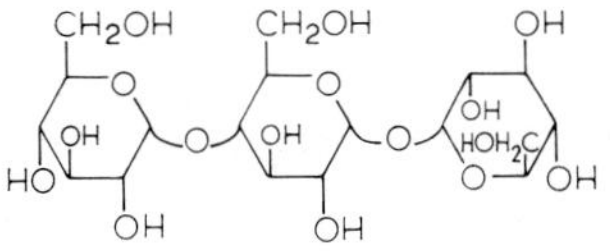

Fig. 3. Structures of glucosyltrehalose and maltosyltrehalose.

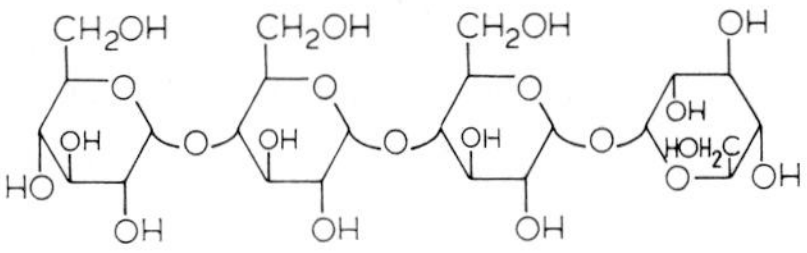

hydrolysis, we were able to determine the structure of trestatin B [24].

Structure of trestatins A and C

The basic fragments obtained by partial hydrolysis of trestatin A (Fig. 2) were also purified by chromatography using Amberlite CG-50 to give compounds 1, 6, 7, 8, 9, 10 and 11 (Fig. 5). The structures of compounds 8, 9, 10 and 11 were eluci-

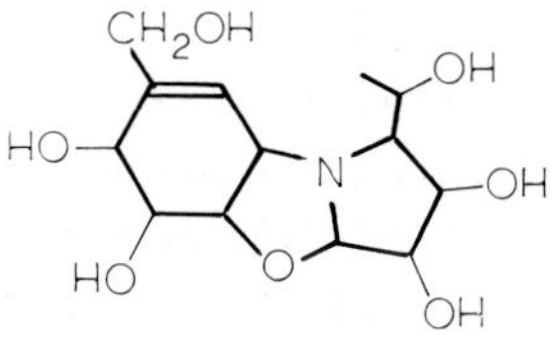

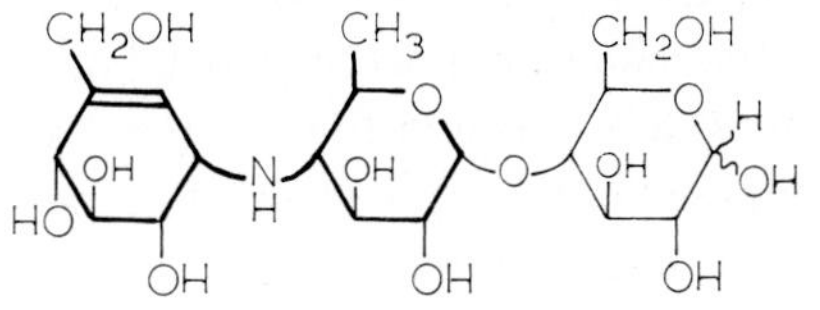

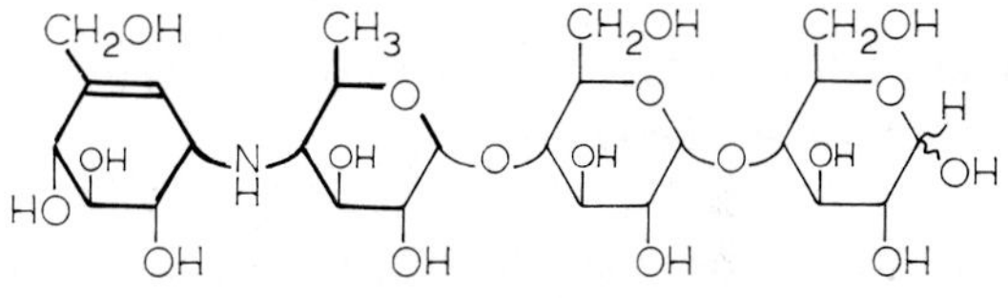

Fig. 4. Structures of basic fragments obtained by partial hydrolysis of trestatin B.

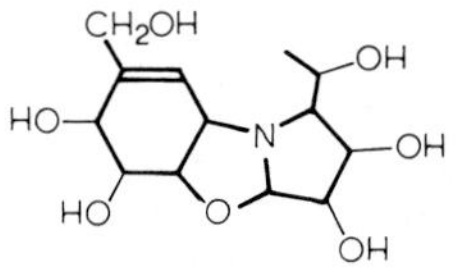

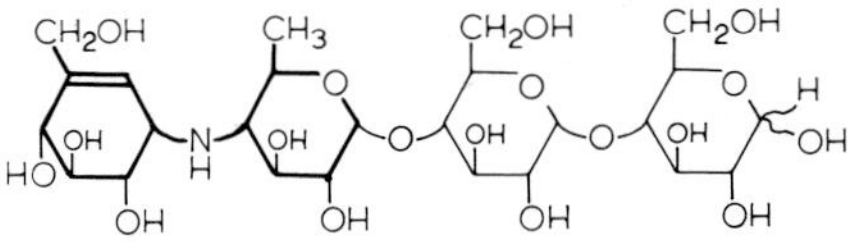

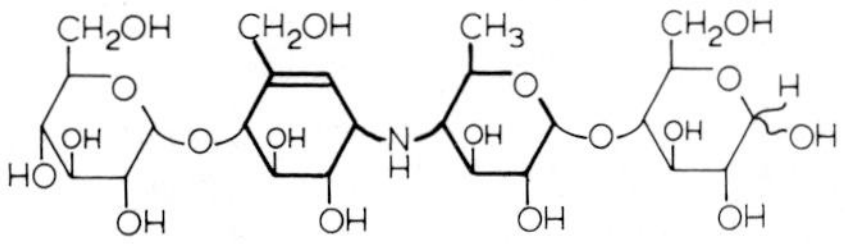

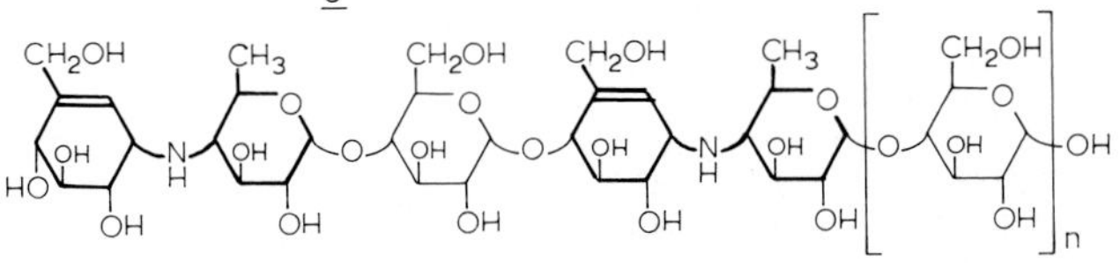

10 (n = 1)
11 (n = 2)

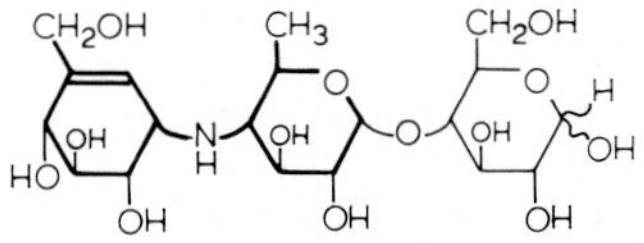

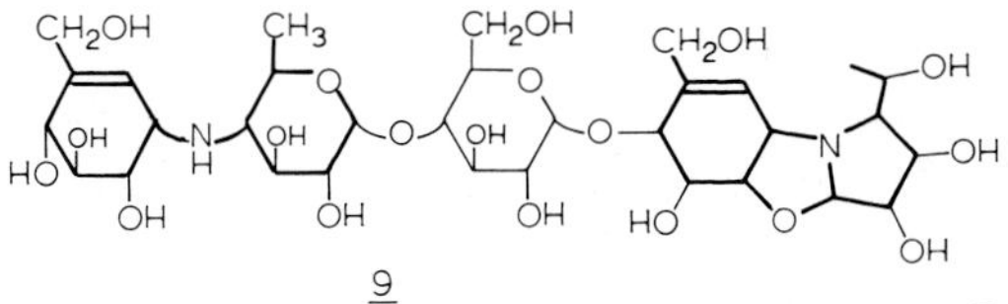

Fig. 5. Structures of basic fragments obtained by partial hydrolysis of trestatin A.

dated by ^{1}H-NMR, ^{13}C-NMR, and mass spectroscopy. Since trestatin A was composed of 5 mol of D-glucose and 2 mol of pseudo-disaccharide 2 (Table 2), and maltosyltrehalose 5 was also obtained from trestatin A by partial hydrolysis, the structure of trestatin A was determined.

The structure of trestatin C was determined in a similar way to that of trestatins B and A. The structures of basic fragments obtained by partial hydrolysis of trestatin C are shown in Fig. 6. Since trestatin C was composed of trestatins B and A as partial structures, the structures of these homologs (trestatins A, B and C) were thus depicted by the general formula as shown in Fig. 7 [24].

STRUCTURE DETERMINATION OF Ro 09-0766, Ro 09-0767 AND Ro 09-0768

The signals of the ^{13}C-NMR spectra of Ro

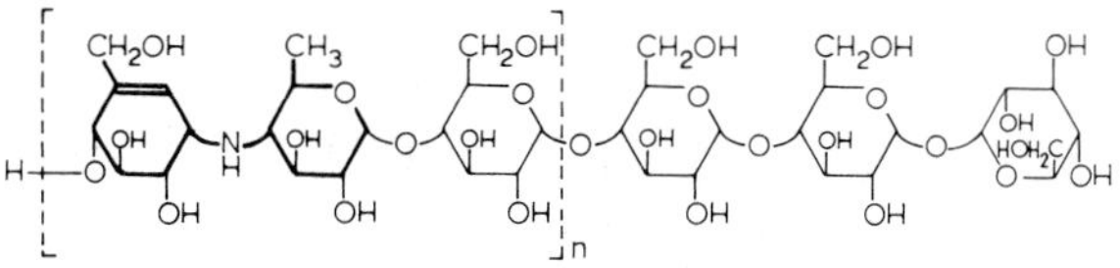

Trestatin A (n = 2)
Trestatin B (n = 1)
Trestatin C (n = 3)

Fig. 7. Structures of trestatins A, B and C.

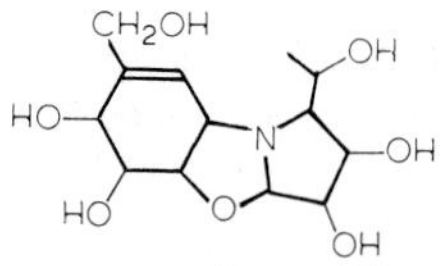

09-0766–8 at around δ55.8, 62.9, 65.0, 98.4, 127.1 and 137.3 were assigned to the corresponding carbons of the partial structure a (Fig. 8), but we did not observe the signals assigned to the corresponding carbons of partial structure b (Fig. 8) in the ^{13}C-NMR spectra of Ro 09-0766–8. However, we observed other signals of the ^{13}C-NMR spectra of these components at almost the same chemical shift as those of trestatins A, B and C. We concluded that these components possess a glucose oligomer

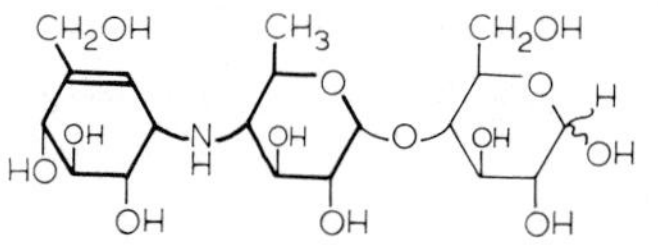

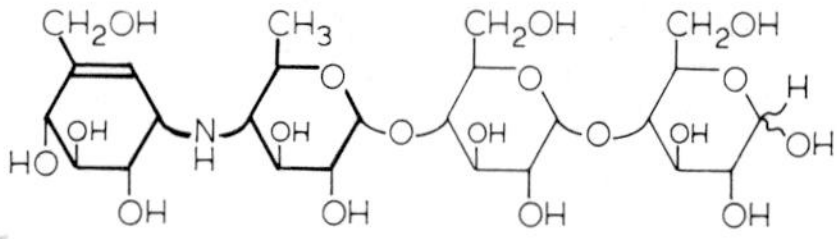

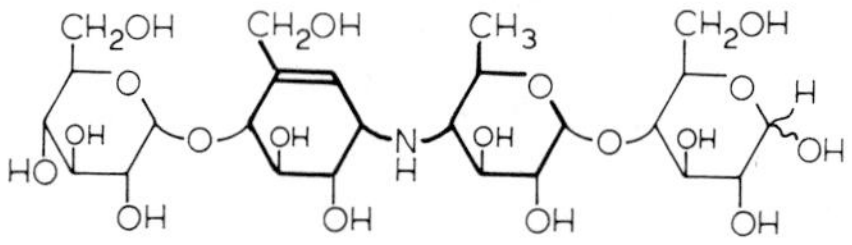

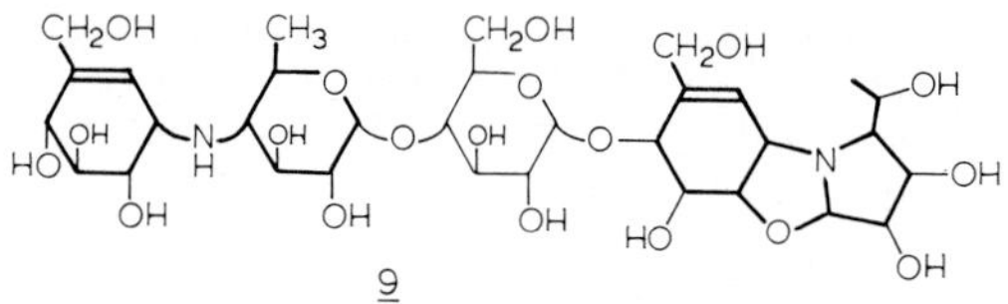

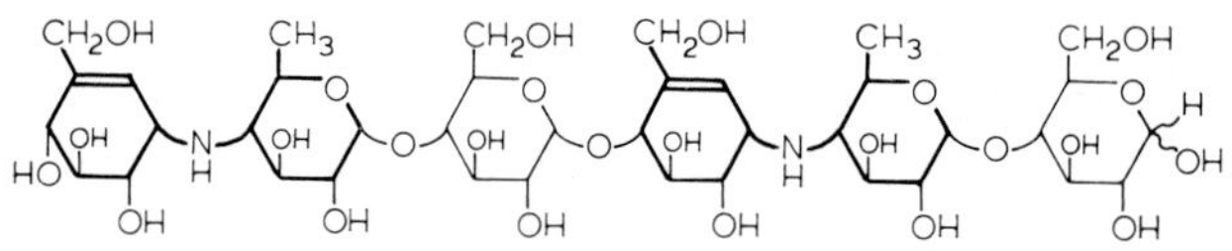

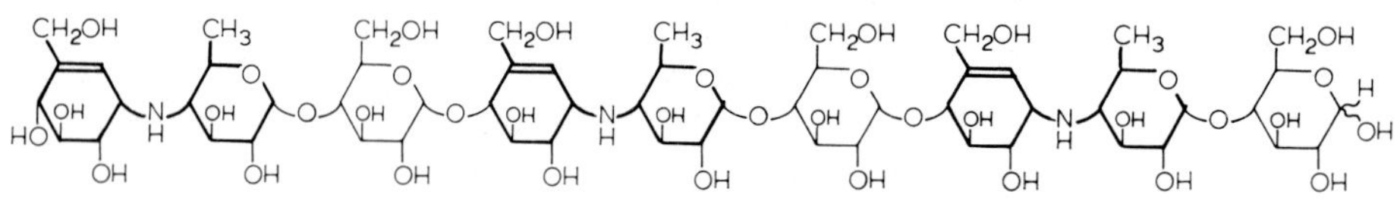

Fig. 6. Structures of basic fragments obtained by partial hydrolysis of trestatin C.

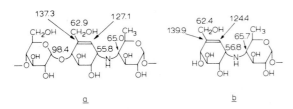

Fig. 8. ^{13}C-NMR chemical shifts (in ppm) for partial structures a and b.

at the secondary allylic hydroxy group of pseudo-disaccharide $\underline{2}$ through glycosidic linkage [22]. In order to determine the glucose oligomer linking through the allylic hydroxy group, each minor component was hydrogenated over Pd-C under hydrogen atmosphere to give maltose.

Since Ro 09-0766, Ro 09-0767 and Ro 09-0768 possess two more glucose molecules than trestatins C, A and B (Table 2), we assumed that Ro 09-0766, Ro 09-0767 and Ro 09-0768 might be maltosyl trestatin C, maltosyl trestatin A and maltosyl trestatin B, respectively.

This assignment was confirmed by enzymatic degradation. Each minor component was treated with β-amylase from barley in acetate buffer (pH 4.9) at 27°C. We found that Ro 09-0766, Ro 09-0767 and Ro 09-0768 were hydrolyzed into trestatin C and maltose, trestatin A and maltose, and trestatin B and maltose, respectively. Analysis of the ^{1}H- and ^{13}C-NMR data of each component indicated the α-glucoside linkage between maltose and pseudo-disaccharide $\underline{2}$. Thus, we determined the structures of Ro 09-0766, Ro 09-0767 and Ro 09-0768 to be maltosyl trestatin C, maltosyl trestatin A, and maltosyl trestatin B, respectively (Fig. 9) [22].

STRUCTURE DETERMINATION OF Ro 09-0765, Ro 09-0896 AND Ro 09-0897

Ro 09-0765 (300 mg), Ro 09-0896 (214 mg) and Ro 09-0897 (54 mg) were isolated as minor components from 10 g of trestatin complex (Ro 09-0154) by chromatography using Amberlite CG-50, Sephadex G-25 and preparative HPLC (μBondapak/CH). Their physicochemical properties are summarized in Table 3. We determined the structures shown in Fig. 10, based on the alkaline hydrolysis* and partial hydrolysis** results [1].

BIOLOGICAL PROPERTIES

Inhibition of α-amylase and other enzymes in vitro

Trestatins A, B and C, Ro 09-0766, Ro 09-0767 and Ro 09-0768 strongly inhibited pancreatic α-amylase (Table 4). These components also inhibited α-amylase from *Bacillus subtilis* and *Aspergillus oryzae*, and amylo-α-1,4-α-1,6-glucosidase of *A. niger*. They were inactive against β-amylase of sweet potato, sucrase or maltase of yeast, and β-glucosidase of sweet almond [22,23].

Characterization of α-amylase inhibition

Some kinetic studies were done with porcine pan-

---

*Ro 09-0765, Ro 09-0897 and Ro 09-0896 were treated with alkaline solution at pH 12.5 at 100°C for 1 h under nitrogen to give compound $\underline{9}$.
**Ro 09-0765, Ro 09-0897 and Ro 09-0896 were partially hydrolyzed with Dowex 50 (H$^+$ form) at 80°C for 5 h to give glucose, maltose, maltotriose and maltotetraose; glucose, maltose and maltotriose; glucose and maltose, respectively.

Ro 09-0766 (n = 3)
Ro 09-0767 (n = 2)
Ro 09 0768 (n = 1)

Fig. 9. Structures of Ro 09-0766, Ro 09-0767 and Ro 09-0768.

124

Table 3

Physico-chemical properties of Ro 09-0765, Ro 09-0897 and Ro 09-0896

Compound	Ro 09-0765	Ro 09-0897	Ro 09-0896
Appearance	colorless powder	colorless powder	colorless powder
Melting point (decomp.) (°C)	204–212	199–210	192–197
UV spectrum	end absorption	end absorption	end absorption
$[\alpha]_D^{24}$ (in H_2O)	$+166.3°$ (c 1.0)	$+151.3°$ (c 0.3)	$+113.8°$ (c 0.2)
FAB-MS m/z	1435 (MH^+)	1273 (MH^+)	1111 (MH^+)
Molecular formula	$C_{56}H_{94}N_2O_{40}$	$C_{50}H_{84}N_2O_{35}$	$C_{44}H_{74}N_2O_{30}$
Color reaction:			
red-tetrazolium	+	+	+

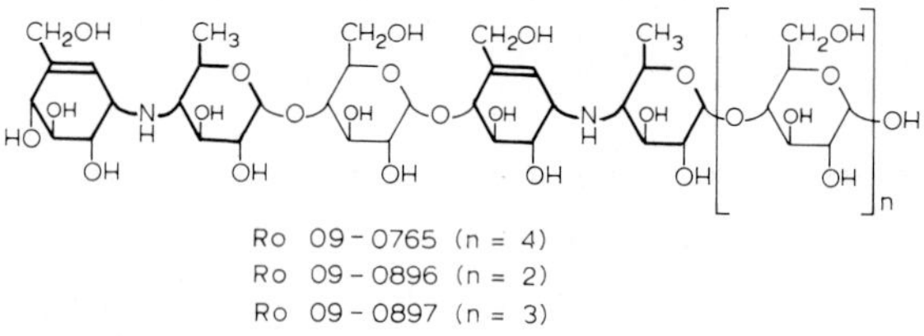

Ro 09-0765 (n = 4)
Ro 09-0896 (n = 2)
Ro 09-0897 (n = 3)

Fig. 10. Structures of Ro 09-0765, Ro 09-0896 and Ro 09-0897.

creatic α-amylase using trestatin complex (Ro 09-0154), trestatin A, B, or C. The results are summarized as follows: (i) trestatin uncompetitively inactivates α-amylase; (ii) inactivation of α-amylase occurs through rapid complex formation.

Toxicity

Trestatin (Ro 09-0154) had an acute toxicity (LD_{50}) greater than 8000 mg/kg after p.o. or i.p. administration in mice. Trestatin was well tolerated in the 13-week toxicological study in rats (daily doses of 36, 120, 360 mg/kg, p.o.).

ANTIDIABETIC PROPERTIES OF TRESTATIN (Ro 09-0154)

Animal studies

Trestatin (0.1, 0.3, and 1.0 mg/kg, p.o.) dose-dependently reduced the increase in blood glucose and insulin levels in rats and dogs after loading them with starch (1.6 g/kg). Oral glucose tolerance was not affected.

In diabetic rats, subchronic treatment with trestatin (doses of 0.03–0.5 mg/g diet) produced a reduction in postprandial hyperglycemia. During the treatment, urinary glucose excretion in diabetic rats was markedly reduced by trestatin [15].

Healthy volunteer studies

Trestatin at doses of 3 mg and 10 mg reduced the postprandial increase in blood glucose and plasma insulin after 75 g starch was given orally to each volunteer. Suprabasal glucose oxidation, measured by indirect calorimetry, was markedly decreased by trestatin [17].

Table 4

Molar concentration required for a 50% inhibition against various α-amylases

	Porcine pancreas	A. oryzae	B. subtilis
Trestatin A	8.1×10^{-9}	1.1×10^{-6}	2.1×10^{-5}
Trestatin B	6.1×10^{-7}	3.1×10^{-5}	5.4×10^{-5}
Trestatin C	8.8×10^{-9}	1.3×10^{-6}	1.8×10^{-6}
Ro 09-0766	1.0×10^{-8}		
Ro 09-0767	1.0×10^{-8}		
Ro 09-0768	1.7×10^{-8}		

Trestatin also reduced the increase in blood glucose and plasma insulin after breakfast (white bread containing 115 g starch) and lunch (mashed potatoes containing 67.5 g starch). Trestatin did not influence glucose and insulin profiles after oral glucose or sucrose loading [4].

Patient studies

In non-insulin-dependent diabetic patients, trestatin (10, 20, 30 and 50 mg) dose-dependently reduced the increase in glucose and insulin after breakfast (white bread containing 50 g starch). The 50 mg dose almost completely inhibited the post-prandial increase in blood glucose [4].

The inhibitory effect of trestatin (Ro 09-0154) on the increase in blood glucose and plasma insulin after starch loading was well demonstrated in animals, healthy volunteers and non-insulin-dependent diabetic patients. Therefore, trestatin can be used to control diabetes.

ACKNOWLEDGEMENTS

The authors thank Drs. J. Businger and A. Kaiser of F. Hoffmann-La Roche & Co. Ltd., Switzerland, and Messrs. K. Watanabe, K. Ogawa and M. Aoki, Ms. J. Watanabe and Dr. H.B. Maruyama of Nippon Roche Research Center for their collaboration.

REFERENCES

1 Aoki, M., H. Shirai, K. Yokose and H.B. Maruyama. 1985. α-Amylase inhibitor, Trestatin. IV. Isolation and structure determination of Ro 09-0765, Ro 09-0896 and Ro 09-0897. 105th Annual Meeting of the Pharmaceutical Society of Japan, Abstract 448, Kanazawa.

2 Belloc, A., J. Florent, J. Lunel, D. Mancy and J.C. Palla. 1977. Glycohydrolase inhibitor by fermentation with streptomycetes. Ger. Offen. 2,702,417.

3 Bernfeld, P. 1955. Amylases, α and β. Methods Enzymol. 1: 149–158.

4 Eichler, H.G., A. Korn, S. Gasic, W. Pirson and J. Businger. 1984. The effect of a new specific α-amylase inhibitor on post-prandial glucose and insulin excursions in normal subjects and Type 2 (non-insulin-dependent) diabetic patients. Diabetologia 26: 278–281.

5 Frommer, W., W. Puls, D. Schafer and D.D. Schmidt. 1972. Glycoside hydrolase inhibitors from actinomycetes. Ger. Offen. 2,064,092.

6 Goto, H., T. Inukai and M. Amano. 1975. Amylase inhibitor from *Streptomyces*. Japan Kokai 50–77,594.

7 Itoh, J., S. Omoto, T. Shomura, H. Ogino, K. Iwamatsu and S. Inouye. 1981. Oligostatins, new antibiotics with amylase inhibitory activity. I. Production, isolation and characterization. J. Antibiot. 34: 1424–1428.

8 Murao, S., A. Goto, Y. Matsui and K. Ohyama. 1980. New proteinous inhibitor (Haim) of animal α-amylase from *Streptomyces griseosporeus* YM-25. Agric. Biol. Chem. 44: 1679–1681.

9 Murao, S. and K. Ohyama. 1979. Chemical structure of an amylase inhibitor, S-AI. Agric. Biol. Chem. 43: 679–681.

10 Nakano, H., T. Tajiri, Y. Koba and S. Ueda. 1981. Some properties of amylase inhibitor A produced by *Streptomyces* sp. No. 280. Agric. Biol. Chem. 45: 1053–1060.

11 Namiki, S., K. Kangouri, T. Nagate, K. Sugita, H. Hara, E. Mori, S. Ohmura and M. Ohzeki. 1979. Amylase inhibitor TAI. Denpun Kagaku 26: 134–144.

12 Niwa, T., S. Inouye, T. Tsuruoka, Y. Koaze and T. Niida. 1970. Nojirimycin as a potent inhibitor of glucosidase. Agric. Biol. Chem. 34: 966–968.

13 Oeding, V., W. Pfaff, L. Vertesy and H.L. Weidemuller. 1978. α-Amylase inhibitor by fermentation with streptomycetes. Ger. Offen. 2,701,890.

14 Otani, M., T. Saito, S. Satoi, J. Mizoguchi and N. Muto. 1979. Amino sugars. Ger. Offen. 2,855,409.

15 Pirson, W. and P. Buchschacher. 1981. Pharmacological properties of Trestatin, a new α-amylase inhibitor (Ro 09-0154). Diabetologia 21: 315.

16 Schmidt, D.D., W. Frommer, B. Junge, L. Muller, W. Wingender, E. Truscheit and D. Schafer. 1977. α-Glucosidase inhibitors. New complex oligosaccharides of microbial origin. Naturwissenschaften 64: 535–536.

17 Tappy, L., A. Buckert, M. Griessen, A. Golay, E. Jequier and J. Felber. 1986. Effect of Trestatin, a new inhibitor of pancreatic α-amylase, on starch metabolism in man. Int. J. Obes. 10: 185–192.

18 Truscheit, E., W. Frommer, B. Junge, L. Muller, D.D. Schmidt and W. Wingender. 1981. Chemistry and biochemistry of microbial α-glucosidase inhibitors. Angew. Chem. Int. Ed. Engl. 20: 744–761.

19 Ueda, K. and S. Gochyo. 1976. Glucoamylase inhibitor. Japan Kokai 51–54,990.

20 Vertesy, L., R. Bender and H.W. Fehlhaber. 1986. α-Glucosidase inhibitor, its use and pharmaceutical compositions. Eur. Pat. Appl. EP 173,950.

21 Watanabe, K., T. Furumai, M. Sudoh, K. Yokose and H.B. Maruyama. 1984. New α-amylase inhibitor, Trestatins. IV. Taxonomy of the producing strains and fermentation of Trestatin A. J. Antibiot. 37: 479–486.

22 Yokose, K., M. Ogawa and K. Ogawa. 1984. New α-amylase inhibitor, Trestatins. III. Structure determination of new

Trestatin components, Ro 09-0766, Ro 09-0767 and Ro 09-0768. J. Antibiot. 37: 182–186.

23 Yokose, K., K. Ogawa, T. Sano, K. Watanabe, H.B. Maruyama and Y. Suhara. 1983. New α-amylase inhibitor, Trestatins. I. Isolation, characterization and biological activities of Trestatins A, B and C. J. Antibiot. 36: 1157–1165.

24 Yokose, K., K. Ogawa, Y. Suzuki, I. Umeda and Y. Suhara. 1983. New α-amylase inhibitor, Trestatins. II. Structure determination of Trestatins A, B and C. J. Antibiot. 36: 1166–1175.

Novel Microbial Products for Medicine and Agriculture
Editors: A.L. Demain, G.A. Somkuti, J.C. Hunter-Cevera and H.W. Rossmoore

CHAPTER 15

Aldostatin, a novel aldose reductase inhibitor

Satoshi Yaginuma, Akira Asahi, Masaki Takada, Mitsuo Hayashi, Masatoshi Tsujino and Kimio Mizuno

Medicinal Research Laboratory, Toyo Jozo Co., Ltd., Shizuoka, Japan

SUMMARY

Aldostatin was isolated from a culture filtrate of *Pseudeurotium zonatum* as a novel inhibitor of aldose reductase. The substance was purified by high porous resins, aluminum oxide, Sephadex G-15 column chromatography procedures and finally by preparative reverse phase high performance liquid chromatography (HPLC). Its molecular formula was determined by elemental analysis and fast atom bombardment (FAB) mass spectrometry (FAB-MS) to be $C_{20}H_{20}N_2O_8$. The chemical structure was determined from its physico-chemical properties to be (−)2,2′-dihydroxy-5,5′-bis(β-carboxy-β-formamidoethyl)diphenyl. The IC_{50} of aldostatin was 1.2×10^{-6} M for partially purified aldose reductase of calf lens. In a rat lens culture with a high glucose concentration, aldostatin suppressed sorbitol accumulation.

INTRODUCTION

Insulin therapy can greatly improve the lifespan of diabetic patients, yet they can still suffer from complications associated with diabetes, such as cataracts [10], retinopathy [6], neuropathy [1] and nephropathy [5]. Increased synthesis of intracellular polyols, such as sorbitol and fructose, has been proposed to play a critical pathophysiological role in the development of diabetic complications [6].

Aldose reductase inhibitors, such as sorbinil, tolrestat, ONO-2,235, M-79,175 and ICI-105,552, have been shown to reduce tissue sorbitol content in diabetic animals [9].

Aldose reductase (EC 1.1.1.21), which catalyzes the conversion of glucose to sorbitol, is a key enzyme of the polyol pathway in tissues such as lens, retina, nerve and kidney, causing diabetic complications [6].

It is possible that cell functions in diabetics can be maintained normally by inhibition of aldose reductase activity.

In screening for inhibitors of aldose reductase from microbial products, a new inhibitor named aldostatin was isolated. In this paper, the fermentation and isolation procedures, physico-chemical and biological properties, and structure determination of aldostatin are described.

MATERIALS AND METHODS

Materials

Reduced nicotinamide adenine dinucleotide phosphate (NADPH), nicotinamide adenine dinucleotide (NAD^+), sorbitol dehydrogenase and horseradish peroxidase (Boehringer Mannheim GmbH), and L-tyrosine and DL-glyceraldehyde (Wako Pure Chemical Industries Ltd.) were purchased for this work. Sorbinil was synthesized in our laboratories according to its patent [15].

Microorganism

The aldostatin-producing strain M4109 was isolated from a soil sample collected in Shizuoka Prefecture, Japan. It was identified as *Pseudeurotium zonatum*, from its culture characteristics and microscopic observation.

Aldose reductase preparation

Aldose reductase was isolated by methods similar to those employed by Hayman and Kinoshita [8]. Calf eyes were obtained from a local abattoir soon after slaughtering. The lenses were removed and homogenized in 3 volumes of cold distilled water in a Teflon homogenizer and centrifuged at $10\,000 \times g$ for 15 min to remove insoluble material. Saturated ammonium sulfate was added to the supernatant to 40% saturation. After allowing to stand with stirring for 15 min, the supernatant was centrifuged and the resulting supernatant was recovered. Additional protein was removed by increasing the ammonium sulfate concentration to 50% saturation and recentrifuging. Aldose reductase was precipitated from the 50% saturated solution by the addition of powdered ammonium sulfate to 75% saturation, and was isolated by centrifugation. The precipitated enzyme was dissolved in 0.05 M sodium chloride, and was used in the enzymatic reaction as a partially purified aldose reductase. All procedures for enzyme preparation were carried out at 4°C.

Enzymatic activity

Aldose reductase activity was measured according to the method of Hayman and Kinoshita [8]. Oxidation of NADPH (a cofactor for aldose reductase) to $NADP^+$ was assayed by following the UV absorbance at 340 nm with a Hitachi 220A spectrophotometer attached to a recorder. The reaction mixture contained 100 mM phosphate buffer (pH 6.0), 0.04 mM NADPH, enzyme solution and 0.5 mM DL-glyceraldehyde as a substrate, in a total volume of 3 ml. The reaction was started by the addition of DL-glyceraldehyde into the cuvette and was followed by the determination of loss of absorbance at 340 nm for 3 min at 37°C.

Rat lens preparation and incubation

Lenses were quickly removed from anesthetized rats (Sprague-Dawley male rats, 180–200 g). The lenses were incubated in 5 ml of medium equilibrated with 95% air and 5% CO_2 at 37°C for 18 h. The medium contained NaCl 6.87 g, $NaHCO_3$ 1.19 g, KCl 281.8 mg, $MgSO_4$ 65.1 mg, NaH_2PO_4 32.4 mg, KH_2PO_4 30.6 mg, $KHCO_3$ 90.1 mg, $CaCl_2$ 138.7 mg, glucose 9.0 g, and aldostatin 0–10 mg, in 1 liter distilled water [14].

Determination of sorbitol content in lens

To remove adherent fluid, lenses were placed on filter paper, weighed and then homogenized in 1.0 ml of cold 8% perchloric acid. The homogenate was centrifuged at $5500 \times g$ for 10 min and the supernatant neutralized at 4°C with 2 N KOH. The neutralized extract was recentrifuged and the supernatant used for the assay of sorbitol. Sorbitol content was measured using the method of Bergmeyer et al. [3].

Production of aldostatin

The first seed culture was prepared by inoculating the growth from an agar slant (14 days, 26°C) of the strain *P. zonatum* M4109 into 100 ml of seed medium in a 500 ml Erlenmeyer flask. This was incubated at 26°C for 3 days on a rotary shaker at 200 rpm and 5 cm throw, and then transferred to a 30-liter jar fermentor containing 10 liters of the same seed medium. The seed medium consisted of glucose 1%, dextrin 1%, yeast extract 0.5%, casein hydrolyzate 0.5%, and $CaCO_3$ 0.1% (pH 6.5 before sterilization).

The second seed was grown at 26°C for 2 days with aeration (10 l/min) and agitation (200 rpm). The second seed culture was transferred to 200 liters of fermentation medium in a 250-liter fermentor. The fermentation medium consisted of glucose 2.0%, yeast extract 1.0%, $MgSO_4 \cdot 7H_2O$ 0.1%, and

K$_2$HPO$_4$ 0.2% (pH 6.5 before sterilization). Fermentation was carried out at 26°C with aeration (160 l/min) and agitation (180 rpm).

Assay of aldostatin

The titers of aldostatin in the fermentation broth and various fractions obtained during the purification procedure were determined by high performance liquid chromatography (HPLC). This assay was performed using a Hitachi Model 655 HPLC instrument equipped with a Hitachi gel No. 3056 column (4.5 mm i.d. × 15 cm) with UV detection at 285 nm. The mobile phase was 8% methanol solution containing 1% ammonium acetate at a flow rate of 0.8 ml/min.

Hydrolysis of aldostatin

Aldostatin (100 mg) was refluxed with 1 N HCl (6 ml) for 1 h and concentrated under reduced pressure. The concentrated material was dissolved in water (2 ml), followed by the addition of 10 volumes of acetone, and held at room temperature. It yielded a solid, white powder (75 mg), named compound A.

Preparation of LL-bityrosine

LL-Bityrosine was synthesized by oxidation of L-tyrosine with horseradish peroxidase according to Amado et al. [2], and purified by carbon, alumina and Sephadex G-15 column chromatography.

RESULTS

Production

The maximum titer of aldostatin reached about 18 μg/ml after 72 h in the production medium. Production of aldostatin began after the first 40 h, by which time the glucose concentration was markedly decreased, just before cessation of cell growth. Production continued throughout the stationary phase.

Isolation procedure

The fermentation broth was adjusted to pH 4.0 with 6 N HCl and filtered with the aid of diatomaceous earth. The filtrate (180 liters) was passed through a Diaion HP-20 column (15 liters, Mitsubishi Chemical Industries Ltd.). After the column was washed with water, the active material was eluted with 50% methanol, adjusted to pH 6.5, concentrated in vacuo, and added to a 10-fold volume of methanol. The methanol-soluble fraction was put on an alumina column (2 liters, Wako Pure Chemical Industries Ltd.) which was washed with methanol and acetonitrile, and then developed with acetonitrile/1 N aqueous ammonia (2:1). The active fractions were pooled, concentrated in vacuo and applied to a Sephadex G-15 column (4 liters, Pharmacia). They were then eluted with water, combined and freeze-dried. The freeze-dried powder was dissolved in water and applied to a Lichroprep RP-18 reverse phase column (1.98 liters, Merck). The active fractions, eluted with 0.5% ammonium acetate/methanol (97:3), were combined, adjusted to pH 4.0, and passed through a Diaion HP-20 column (300 ml). After washing the column with water, the active material was eluted with 50% methanol and the active aqueous methanol fractions concentrated in vacuo and then freeze-dried to give 950 mg of pure aldostatin (29% recovery).

Physico-chemical properties

Aldostatin behaved as an acidic substance, and was stable at neutral or alkaline pH. It was soluble in water, methanol and dimethyl sulfoxide (DMSO), and insoluble in benzene, chloroform and n-hexane. The other physico-chemical properties, ^{1}H-NMR, and ^{13}C-NMR spectra are summarized in Tables 1, 2, and 3, respectively. Acid hydrolysis of aldostatin yielded a ninhydrin-positive substance, named compound A, as the dihydrochloride, $C_{18}H_{20}N_2O_6 \cdot 2HCl$. The physico-chemical properties, ^{1}H-NMR and ^{13}C-NMR spectra of compound A are also summarized in Tables 1, 2, and 3, respectively. The UV, ^{1}H-NMR, and ^{13}C-NMR spectra of compound A are closely related to those of aldostatin. On the amino acid autoanalyser, compound A eluted between phenylalanine and histidine.

Biological properties

Aldostatin inhibited aldose reductase with an

Table 1

Physico-chemical properties of aldostatin and compound A

	Aldostatin (free acid)	Compound A (HCl salt)
Appearance	white powder	white powder
m.p. (°C)	144–146	258–260 (decomp.)
$[\alpha]_D^{26}$ (c 0.5, H_2O)	$+59.0°$	$-51.9°$
Molecular formula	$C_{20}H_{20}N_2O_8$	$C_{18}H_{20}N_2O_6 \cdot 2HCl$
Elemental analysis		
found	C 57.20, H 4.70, N 6.97	C 49.75, H 5.36, N 6.51, Cl 16.10
calcd.	C 57.69, H 4.84, N 6.73	C 49.90, H 5.12, N 6.47, Cl 16.37
FAB-MS	MH^+ 417	MH^+ 361
UV		
$\lambda_{max}^{H_2O}$ nm ($\varepsilon_{1cm}^{1\%}$)	285 (135)	285 (134)
$\lambda_{max}^{0-1N\ NaOH}$ nm ($\varepsilon_{1cm}^{1\%}$)	316 (195)	315 (198)
IR (KBr) cm^{-1}	3400–2300, 1725, 1660	3400–2300, 1620, 1500
Color reaction		
positive	ferric chloride	ferric chloride, ninhydrin
negative	ninhydrin, Molisch	Molisch
TLC[a] (R_f)		
BuOH/AcOH/H_2O (4:1:1)	0.63	0.19
CHCl$_3$/MeOH/H_2O (5:5:1)	0.31	0.11
CHCl$_3$/MeOH/AcOH/H_2O (10:5:1:1)	0.36	0.05

[a] TLC: silicagel-f spotfilm (Tokyo Kasei Kogyo Co.).

Table 2

^{1}H-NMR data for aldostatin and compound A (400 MHz)

Assignment	Aldostatin (free acid)			Compound A (HCl salt)		
	ppm	multiplicity	J (Hz)	ppm	multiplicity	J (Hz)
H-7α	2.82 (1H × 2)	dd	8.3, 14.2	3.10 (1H × 2)	dd	7.8, 14.7
H-7β	3.02 (1H × 2)	dd	4.9, 14.2	3.25 (1H × 2)	dd	4.9, 14.7
H-8	4.51 (1H × 2)	ddd	4.9, 7.8, 8.3	3.98 (1H × 2)	dd	4.9, 7.8
H-3	6.81 (1H × 2)	d	7.8	7.01 (1H × 2)	d	8.3
H-4	7.00 (1H × 2)	dd	2.4, 7.8	7.23 (1H × 2)	dd	2.2, 8.3
H-6	7.04 (1H × 2)	d	2.4	7.14 (1H × 2)	d	2.2
H-10	8.00 (1H × 2)	s				
NH	8.05 (1H × 2)	d	7.8			

^{1}H-NMR spectra of aldostatin and compound A taken in d_6DMSO (at 70°C, standard: TMS = 0.00 ppm) and D_2O (at 30°C, standard: TSP = 0.00 ppm), respectively.

IC$_{50}$ of 1.2×10^{-6} M (Table 4). Aldostatin did not inhibit lactate dehydrogenase, glutamate dehydrogenase, sorbitol dehydrogenase, glucose-6-phosphate dehydrogenase, β-D-glucosidase, α-amylase, hexokinase, trypsin, α-chymotrypsin and papain (IC$_{50}$ > 4.8×10^{-4}M). A kinetic study of aldostatin was performed in a Lineweaver-Burk plot for aldose reductase. Aldostatin inhibited aldose reduc-

Table 3

^{13}C-NMR data for aldostatin and compound A (100 MHz)

Assignment	Aldostatin (free acid)		Compound A (HC1 salt)	
	δ(ppm)	multiplicity	δ(ppm)	multiplicity
C-9	171.7	s	174.7	s
C-10	160.1	d		
C-2	152.1	s	153.3	s
C-6	131.7	d	133.0	d
C-4	128.2	d	131.2	d
C-5	127.1	s	127.9	s
C-1	125.1	s	126.4	s
C-3	115.3	d	117.2	d
C-8	52.1	d	56.9	d
C-7	35.9	t	36.3	t

^{13}C-NMR spectra of aldostatin and compound A taken in d_6DMSO (at 27°C, standard: TMS = 0.00 ppm) and D$_2$O (at 27°C, standard: dioxane = 67.40 ppm), respectively.

Table 4

Inhibition of calf lens aldose reductase by aldostatin, compound A and sorbinil

Inhibitor	IC$_{50}$ value (M)
Aldostatin	1.2×10^{-6}
Compound A	$> 4.8 \times 10^{-4}$
Sorbinil	1.0×10^{-6}

tase uncompetitively with DL-glyceraldehyde as the substrate. The K_i of aldostatin was 1.3×10^{-6} M. When rat lens was incubated in the presence of 50 mM glucose, aldostatin suppressed sorbitol accumulation in a dose-dependent manner (Fig. 1).

Aldostatin showed no antimicrobial activity at 3 mg/ml concentration, using the paper disc assay method against *Bacillus subtilis*, *Sarcina lutea*, *Staphylococcus aureus*, *Escherichia coli*, *Pseudomonas aeruginosa*, *Vibrio percolans* and *Candida albicans*. Aldostatin showed no toxic effect in ddy mice at an intravenous dose of 200 mg/kg.

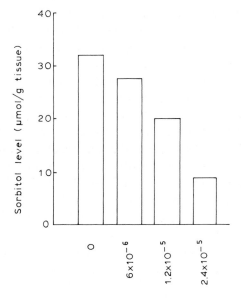

Fig. 1. Effect of aldostatin on sorbitol accumulation in isolated rat lenses. The procedures for rat lens preparation, incubation, and assay of sorbitol concentration are described in Materials and Methods.

DISCUSSION

Aldose reductase has been shown to play a critical pathophysiological role in the development of dia-

betic complications. Several chemically synthesized aldose reductase inhibitors, such as sorbinil, tolrestat, ONO-2,235, ICI-105,552 and M-79,175, have been developed and evaluated *in vivo* [9].

There have been few reports of aldose reductase inhibitor production by microbes. The aldose reductase inhibitor WF-3681, from the culture filtrate of *Chaetomella raphigera*, was recently reported [13].

In screening for aldose reductase inhibitors in microbial cultures, we have obtained a novel aldose reductase inhibitor, named aldostatin, from the culture broth of *P. zonatum*.

The molecular formula of aldostatin was determined to be $C_{20}H_{20}N_2O_8$ from elemental analysis and FAB-MS. The IR spectrum showed characteristic bands at 3400–3200 (phenolic OH, NH, and COOH), 1725 (COOH), and 1660 (CONH) cm^{-1}. Aldostatin was positive in a color reaction with ferric chloride, indicating the presence of phenolic hydroxy groups in its structure. The ^{1}H-NMR spectrum of aldostatin (Table 2) showed formyl protons at $\delta 8.00$ (2H, s), and NH protons at $\delta 8.05$ (2H, d, $J = 7.8$ Hz) which disappeared on the addition of deuterium oxide. These results suggest that there may be N-formyl groups. In addition, the ^{1}H-NMR spectrum indicated the presence of aromatic protons at $\delta 6.81$ (2H, d, $J = 7.8$Hz), $\delta 7.00$ (2H, dd, $J = 2.4$ and 7.8 Hz), and $\delta 7.04$ (2H, d, $J = 2.4$ Hz). The ^{1}H-NMR spectrum indicates that aldostatin is a symmetric dimer in which a 1,2,4-trisubstituted benzene ring and an ABX type three spin system are present in one half of the molecule. The aliphatic part of the spectrum is very similar to that of tyrosine.

The ^{13}C-NMR spectrum of aldostatin (Table 3) showed six carbons of the aromatic moiety at $\delta 152.1$ (s), $\delta 131.7$ (d), $\delta 128.2$ (d), $\delta 127.1$ (s), $\delta 125.1$ (s) and $\delta 115.3$ (d). The carbon signal at $\delta 152.1$ was assigned to the carbon of the phenolic hydroxy group. Three carbon signals at $\delta 127.1$, $\delta 125.1$, and $\delta 115.3$ showed high-field shifts under the influence of the phenolic hydroxy group, and were assigned a position *ortho*- or *para*- to the phenolic hydroxy group. Two carbon signals at $\delta 131.7$ and $\delta 128.2$ showed low-field shifts, indicating the *meta* position.

A long-range ^{1}H-^{13}C COSY NMR experiment was performed. The carbon of the phenolic hy-

droxy group at $\delta 152.1$ was coupled to the aromatic proton at $\delta 7.04$, which was further coupled to the two carbons at $\delta 125.1$ and $\delta 128.2$. Furthermore, the carbon at $\delta 152.1$ was coupled to the two aromatic protons at $\delta 6.81$ and 7.00. The methylene protons at $\delta 2.82$ and 3.02 were coupled to the three carbons at $\delta 128.2$, $\delta 127.1$, and $\delta 131.7$.

That the coupling position of the symmetric dimer is *ortho* and not *meta* to the phenolic hydroxy group was apparent from the chemical shifts of the aromatic constituents in ^{1}H-NMR and ^{13}C-NMR spectral data.

From the overall characteristics, the structure of aldostatin was shown to be *N,N*-diformylbityrosine.

Next we tried acid hydrolysis of aldostatin and isolation of the hydrolysis product, compound A. The molecular formula of compound A ($C_{18}H_{20}N_2O_6$·2HCl) was established by elemental analysis and FAB-MS (Table 1). It was optically active and gave a positive ninhydrin test.

The molecular formula, UV maximum, ^{1}H-NMR and ^{13}C-NMR spectra data of compound A (Tables 1, 2, 3) suggested that it was bityrosine [4,16]. The following experiments supported that conclusion. LL-Bityrosine was synthesized by the method of Amado *et al.* [2] and was identical to compound A in spectral analysis (UV, IR, ^{1}H-NMR, ^{13}C-NMR and FAB-MS), and in specific rotation.

The ^{1}H-NMR spectrum of aldostatin showed a formyl signal at $\delta 8.00$, but that of compound A did not. Also, in the ^{13}C-NMR spectrum, the formyl carbon ($\delta 160.1$) of aldostatin disappeared in compound A (Tables 2, 3).

Based on the data, we propose the structure for aldostatin shown in Fig. 2, *N,N*-diformyl-LL-bityrosine. The absolute structure of aldostatin was assumed to be $(-)2,2'$-dihydroxy-5,5'-bis(β-carboxy-β-formamidoethyl)diphenyl. The chemical structure of aldostatin is novel for an aldose reductase inhibitor.

The results (Table 4) indicate that aldostatin has about the same inhibitory potency on calf lens aldose reductase as sorbinil, although aldostatin did not inhibit a number of enzymes related to carbo-

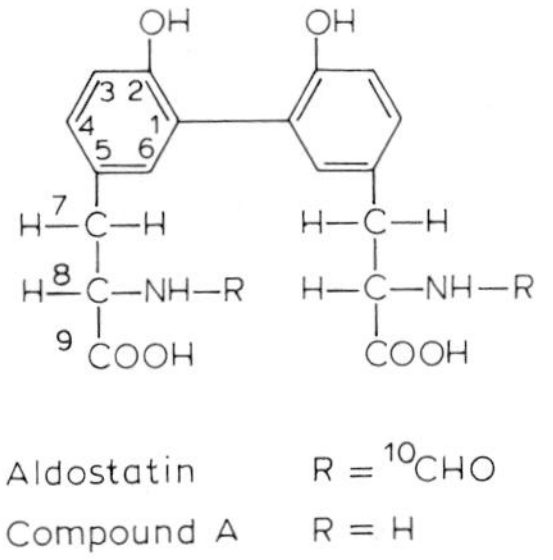

Fig. 2. Structure of aldostatin and compound A.

hydrate and protein metabolism.

In kinetic studies, Peterson *et al.* [14] reported that sorbinil uncompetitively inhibited calf lens aldose reductase. In our study aldostatin produced the same result as sorbinil.

In tissue culture studies, aldostatin suppressed sorbital accumulation in isolated rat lens. These results from both cell-free and tissue studies prove that aldostatin is a selective and potent inhibitor of aldose reductase. Bityrosine itself did not inhibit aldose reductase.

Bityrosine had previously been found only in connective tissue proteins [12], such as collagen [17], but recently it has been isolated from the insoluble protein of human cataractous lenses [7]. It is interesting that aldostatin, *N*,*N*-diformyl-LL-bityrosine, is expected to be useful as a new aid in the treatment of diabetic cataracts, while bityrosine is contained in cataractous lens.

In vivo activities of aldostatin are now being tested in diabetic animal models and the results will be reported in due course.

REFERENCES

1 Akagi, Y., P.F. Kador, T. Kuwabara and J.H. Kinoshita. 1983. Aldose reductase in human retinal mural cell. Invest. Ophthalmol. Vis. Sci. 24: 1516–1519.

2 Amado, R., R. Aeschbach and H. Neukom. 1984. Dityrosine: in vivo production and characterization. Methods Enzymol. 107: 377–388.

3 Bergmeyer, H.U., W. Gruber and I. Gutmann. 1974. Method for determination of metabolites; D-sorbitol. In: Methods of Enzymatic Analysis (Bergmeyer, H.U., ed.), pp. 1323–1326. Academic Press, New York.

4 Briza, P., G. Winkler, H. Kalchhauser and M. Breitenbach. 1986. Dityrosine is a prominent component of the yeast ascospore wall. J. Biol. Chem. 261: 4288–4294.

5 Corder, C.N., J.H. Braughler and P.A. Culp. 1979. Quantitative histochemistry of the sorbitol pathway in glomeruli and small arteries of human diabetic kidney. Folia Histochem. Cytochem. 17: 137–146.

6 Gabbay, K.H. 1973. The sorbitol pathway and the complications of diabetes. N. Engl. J. Med. 288: 831–836.

7 Garcia-Castineiras, S., J. Dillon and A. Spector. 1978. The detection of bityrosine in cataractous human lens proteins. Science 199: 897–899.

8 Hayman, S. and J.H. Kinoshita. 1965. Isolation and properties of lens aldose reductase. J. Biol. Chem. 240: 877–882.

9 Kador, P.F. and J.H. Kinoshita. 1984. Diabetic and galactosaemic cataracts. In: Human Cataract Formation; Ciba Foundation Symposium No. 106, pp. 110–131, Pitman Publishing, London.

10 Kinoshita, J.H. 1974. Mechanism initiating cataract formation. Proctor Lect. Invest. Ophthalmol. 13: 713–724.

11 Kinoshita, J.H., L.O. Merola and S. Hayman. 1965. Osmotic effect on the amino acid-concentrating mechanism in the rabbit lens. J. Biol. Chem. 240: 310–315.

12 LaBella, F., P. Waykole and G. Queen. 1968. Formation of insoluble gels and dityrosine by the action of peroxidase on soluble collagens. Biochem. Biophys. Res. Commun. 30: 333–338.

13 Nishikawa, M., Y. Tsurumi, T. Namiki, K. Yoshida and M. Okuhara. 1987. Studies on WF-3681, a novel aldose reductase inhibitor. I. Taxonomy, fermentation, isolation and characterization. J. Antibiot. 40: 1394–1399.

14 Peterson, M.J., S. Sarges, C.E. Aldinger and D.P. MacDonald. 1979. CP-45,634: a novel aldose reductase inhibitor that inhibits polyol pathway activity in diabetic and galactosemic rats. Metabolism 28: 456–461.

15 Reinhardt, S. 1978. Hydantoin derivatives. Japan Patent Appl. 1978-53,653, pp. 385–405, published May 16, 1978.

16 Ushijima, Y., M. Nakano and T. Goto. 1984. Production and identification of bityrosine in horseradish peroxidase-H₂O₂-tyrosine system. Biochem. Biophys. Res. Commun. 125: 916–918.

17 Waykole, P. and E. Heidemann. 1976. Dityrosine in collagen. Connect. Tissue Res. 4: 219–222.

Novel Microbial Products for Medicine and Agriculture
Editors: A.L. Demain, G.A. Somkuti, J.C. Hunter-Cevera and H.W. Rossmoore

CHAPTER 16

Emeriamine: a new inhibitor of long chain fatty acid oxidation and its antidiabetic activity

Tsuneo Kanamaru and Hisayoshi Okazaki

Applied Microbiology Laboratories, Central Research Division, Takeda Chemical Industries, Ltd., Osaka, Japan

SUMMARY

A new convenient agar-plate method using *Candida albicans* IFO 0583 was devised to detect inhibitors of long chain fatty acid oxidation. By this method, inhibitors were found in a culture filtrate of *Emericella quadrilineata* IFO 5859 and emericedins A, B, and C, new betaines, were isolated and their structures were elucidated as (*R*)-3-acylamino-4-(trimethylammonio)butyric acid (acyl: A, acetyl-; B, propionyl-; C, *n*-butyryl-). Emeriamine, a desacylderivative of the emericedins, (*R*)-3-amino-4-(trimethylammonio)butyric acid, proved to be a strong and specific inhibitor of long chain fatty acid oxidation in rat liver mitochondria (IC$_{50}$ 3.2×10^{-6} M). Carnitine palmitoyltransferase I is the main inhibition site of emeriamine. Emeriamine also inhibits gluconeogenesis in hepatocytes. In liver mitochondria, emeriamine and palmitoyl-CoA react and form palmitoylemeriamine, which is a stronger inhibitor than emeriamine itself *in vitro*. These findings suggest that the inhibition of fatty acid oxidation by emeriamine *in vivo* occurs by a complex mechanism. Emeriamine, when administered orally to fasted normal and diabetic animals, shows dose-dependent hypoglycemic and antiketogenic activities (1–10 mg/kg). Among homogenates of liver, muscle, heart, and diaphragm, emeriamine most effectively inhibits long chain fatty acid oxidation in the liver homogenates. Emeriamine may provide a tool for analyzing the relation between glucose and fatty acid metabolism and may have potential utility as a therapeutic agent for treating diabetes.

INTRODUCTION

Since Randle and his associates initially proposed the glucose-fatty acid cycle [10–12], it has been suggested that the interaction of glucose and fatty acid metabolism might be a key factor in diabetes. The metabolic disorders in diabetes mellitus are shown in Fig. 1. An increase in fatty acid oxidation is one of the characteristic features of diabetes. Insulin deficiency leads to enhanced lipolysis and the released free fatty acids are available for oxidation in many tissues, especially in the liver. As the result of the acceleration of acyl-CoA synthetase and β-oxidation and ketone body formation, the concentration of ketone bodies in the blood is abnormally increased and ketonemia develops. In contrast, glucose utilization is lowered and gluconeogenesis, that is, glucose formation, is accelerated. Consequently, the concentration of glucose in the blood is abnormally increased and hyperglycemia develops. It is said that fatty acid oxidation and gluconeogenesis occur by coupling with each other. It

136

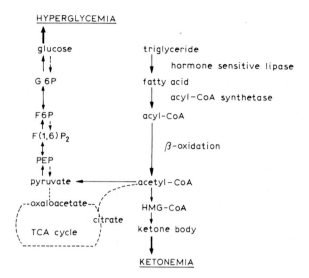

HYPERGLYCEMIA

KETONEMIA

Fig. 1. Metabolic disorders in diabetes mellitus. HMG-CoA = hydroxymethylglutaryl-CoA; PEP = phospho*enol*pyruvate; F(1,6)P$_2$ = fructose 1,6-diphosphate; F6P = fructose 6-phosphate; G6P = glucose 6-phosphate.

might be possible to correct these metabolic disorders by inhibiting the abnormally increased free fatty acid oxidation.

Based on this hypothesis, many compounds, such as hypoglycin, 4-pentenoic acid, (+)decanoylcarnitine and α-bromo-fatty acid, which inhibit free fatty acid oxidation, have been tested to treat diabetes and induced hypoglycemia. However, none have been used clinically because they were either not specific for the fatty acid oxidation, or were toxic, or both [16–18]. Thus, we began to search for specific inhibitors of long chain fatty acid oxidation among microbial metabolites [8, 15].

MATERIALS AND METHODS

Materials

[1-^{14}C]Palmitic acid, L-[*palmitoyl*-1-^{14}C]palmitoylcarnitine and [1-^{14}C]octanoic acid were purchased from New England Nuclear and L-[*methyl*-^{3}H]carnitine from Amersham. Carnitine acetyltransferase from pigeon breast muscle was purchased from Sigma. Emeriamine was prepared by hydrolyzing emericedin using 6 N HCl at 95°C for

16 h. Acetylemeriamine and palmitoylemeriamine were prepared according to the method of Shinagawa et al. [15].

Microorganisms

Candida albicans IFO 0583 was used as screening microorganism and *Emericella quadrilineata* IFO 5859 as producer of emericedins.

Assay of mitochondrial oxidation of long chain fatty acids

Rat liver mitochondria were prepared as described previously [8]. The activity of L-carnitine-dependent oxidation of long chain fatty acids was assayed by measuring $^{14}CO_2$ released from ^{14}C-labeled substrate in the presence or absence of L-carnitine [4, 14]. Percent inhibition of carnitine-dependent oxidation activity was calculated as follows: Inhibition (%) = $[1 - (A_i - B_i)/(A_o - B_o)]$ where A_o and B_o represent $^{14}CO_2$ released (dpm) with and without L-carnitine, respectively, in the absence of inhibitor, and A_i and B_i represent $^{14}CO_2$ released (dpm) with and without L-carnitine, respectively, in the presence of inhibitor.

Assay of carnitine palmitoyltransferase I

The activity of carnitine palmitoyltransferase I was measured as the rate of conversion of palmitoyl-CoA and L-[^{3}H]carnitine into palmitoyl-L-[^{3}H]carnitine within 3 min, according to the method of Bremer [3]. The reaction mixture was the same as that for the mitochondrial oxidation of long chain fatty acids mentioned above except that 0.6 μmol of palmitoyl-CoA was used as a substrate instead of 0.6 μmol of CoA and palmitic acid. To investigate the formation of *N*-palmitoylemeriamine from emeriamine and palmitoyl-CoA by hepatic mitochondria, 50 μM [1-^{14}C]palmitoyl-CoA (0.5 μCi) and 250 μM L-carnitine or emeriamine were used, and the reaction was carried out according to the methods of Tutwiler et al. [16] and Bremer [3].

Assay of carnitine acetyltransferase

The activity of carnitine acetyltransferase was measured according to the method of Bieber and Lewin [1]. To investigate the formation of *N*-acetylemeriamine from emeriamine and acetyl-CoA by carnitine acetyltransferase, 12.3 μM [1-^{14}C]acetyl-CoA (0.1 μCi) and 9.1 μM L-carnitine or emeriamine were used.

Measurements of hypoglycemic and antiketogenic activities in rats

After they were fasted for 20 h, male Sprague-Dawley rats (7 or 10 weeks old) were given emeriamine (0.3–30 mg/kg) orally. Blood samples were taken from the tail vein 2 h later and blood glucose and ketone bodies were measured according to the method of Werner et al. [19] and the modified method of Williamson and Mallanby [20], respectively.

Determination of protein

The protein concentration of the mitochondrial fraction was determined by the method of Markwell et al. [9] using bovine serum albumin as a standard and protein concentration in the buffer was blanked out.

Statistics

The data were statistically evaluated using the Student's t-test.

RESULTS

Screening for inhibitors of long chain fatty acid oxidation in culture filtrates of microorganisms

A new screening method was devised to detect inhibitors of long chain fatty acid oxidation using two agar plates of glucose or oleic acid as sole carbon source and C. albicans IFO 0583. Transparent oleate and glucose plates were prepared using the components shown in Table 1; the important factors in preparing the transparent oleate plate were the concentration of oleic acid and the ratios of oleic acid and the surfactant Brij 58 (data not shown). After it has been incubated at 30°C overnight, the oleate plate becomes grayish white as a result of the growth of C. albicans but a transparent growth inhibition zone is obtained if inhibitors of fatty acid oxidation are present.

Table 1

Preparation of oleate and glucose plates

	Oleate plate	Glucose plate
Oleic acid	0.2%	–
Brij 58	0.25	–
Glucose	–	2.0%
NH$_4$NO$_3$	0.2	0.2
NH$_4$H$_2$PO$_4$	0.5	0.5
MgSO$_4$·7H$_2$O	0.1	0.1
Yeast extract	0.05	0.05
Trace metals	+	+
Agar	1.5	1.5
	pH 6.5	pH 6.5
C. albicans suspension	0.4%	0.4%

Incubation at 30°C overnight.

The screening for inhibitors of fatty acid oxidation was performed as follows. The first screening was done using C. albicans on both types of agar plate. When a microorganism produced a growth inhibition zone only on the oleate plate, it was selected as an inhibitor of fatty acid oxidation, but when a microorganism produced a growth inhibition zone only on the glucose plate or on both plates, it was discarded. The second screening was done by incubating culture broths with rat whole blood at 37°C for 60 min. Culture broths that were not inactivated by incubation were selected to isolate the inhibitors.

As the result of screening of many actinomycetes, bacteria and fungi, inhibitors were found in the culture filtrate of the genus Emericella. These strains were shown to produce the same two or three components when examined by thin layer chromatography. The isolation of the inhibitors of fatty acid oxidation from the culture filtrate of E. quadrilineata IFO 5859 was undertaken.

Fermentation, isolation, and structures of emericedins A, B and C

Fermentation. The fermentation medium for the production of inhibitors by E. quadrilineata IFO 5859 is shown in Table 2. Using oleic acid as a carbon source, fermentation was carried out at 28°C

138

Table 2

Fermentation medium for the production of emericedins by *E. quadrilineata* IFO 5859

Oleic acid	3.0%
Soybean flour	0.5
Malt extract	0.5
Polypeptone	0.5
Yeast extract	0.2
KH_2PO_4	0.1
$FeSO_4 \cdot 7H_2O$	0.05
$MnSO_4 \cdot nH_2O$	0.05
$MgSO_4 . 7H_2O$	0.05
	pH 4.5

Fermentation was carried out at 28°C for 5 days.

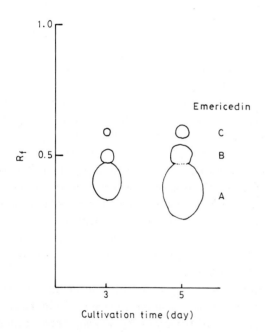

Fig. 2. Bioautogram of culture filtrate of *E. quadrilineata*. Cellulose TLC: solvent, *n*-Pro/H_2O/NH_4OH (70:28:2); detection, growth inhibition of *C. albicans* on oleate plate.

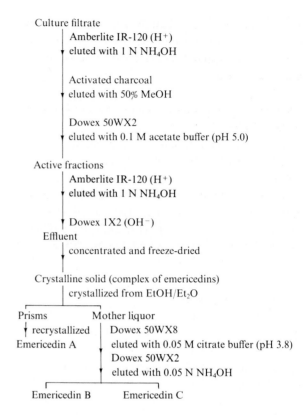

Fig. 3. Isolation procedure for emericedins.

for 5 days. Fig. 2 shows a typical thin layer chromatogram of the inhibitors, produced in a culture filtrate and detected on an oleate agar plate. Three components were detected and labeled A, B, and C; A is the main component.

Isolation and structures. The inhibitors in the culture filtrate were isolated according to the procedure shown in Fig. 3 [15]. Based on physico-chemi-

cal and chemical synthesis, the structures of inhibitors A, B, and C were elucidated and proved to be novel *N*-acylated *β*-aminobetaines as shown in Fig. 4, i.e. (*R*)-3-acylamino-4-(trimethylammonio)-butyric acid. The inhibitors were named emericedins A, B, and C. With respect to the acyl group, A has acetyl, B has propionyl, and C has *n*-butyryl [15]. These emericedins weakly inhibited fatty acid oxidation in rat liver mitochondria. However, a des-

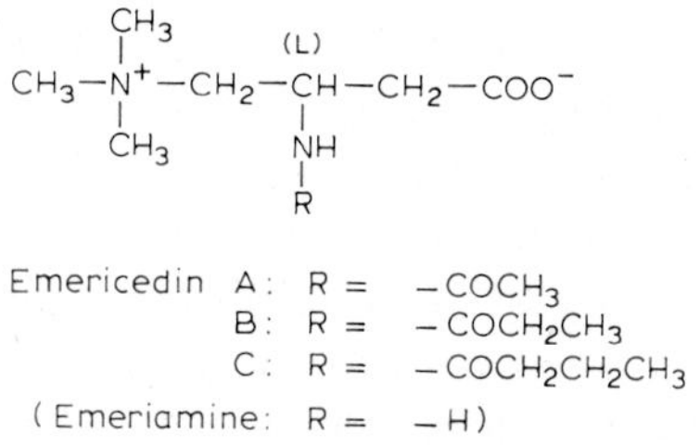

Fig. 4. Inhibitors of long chain fatty acid oxidation produced by *E. quadrilineata* IFO 5859.

acylderivative of the emericedins, named emeriamine, (*R*)-3-amino-4-(trimethylammonio)butyric acid, was a strong inhibitor. The activity of emeriamine *in vitro* and *in vivo* will be presented below. It is significant that the compound in which a hydroxy group replaces an amino group at the 3-position is L-carnitine, which is essential for transporting long chain fatty acids into the mitochondrial membrane.

Inhibition of long chain fatty acid oxidation in rat liver mitochondria by emeriamine and the inhibition site

Emeriamine dose-dependently inhibited the carnitine-dependent oxidation of [1-^{14}C]palmitate to $^{14}CO_2$ in the hepatic mitochondria of Sprague-Dawley rats fasted for 20 h. The activity of carnitine-dependent oxidation in mitochondria was almost completely inhibited by emeriamine at a concentration of 5×10^{-5} M, with a half-maximal inhibitory concentration (IC_{50}) as low as 3.2×10^{-6} M (Fig. 5). However, emeriamine did not affect the carnitine-independent oxidation of palmitate in the same mitochondria (Table 3).

The mitochondrial oxidation of [1-^{14}C]palmitoyl-carnitine to $^{14}CO_2$ was slightly inhibited by emeriamine in the presence or absence of L-carnitine (Table 3), suggesting that emeriamine may slightly inhibit carnitine palmitoyltransferase II. On the

Table 3

Effect of emeriamine on oxidation of palmitate, palmitoyl-L-carnitine and octanoate in rat liver mitochondria

Substrate	Emeriamine added (μM)	$^{14}CO_2$ formation (dpm/mg protein/20 min)	
		with carnitine	without carnitine
[1-^{14}C]Palmitate	0	1959 ± 57	1081 ± 20
	3.2	1467 ± 7	1033 ± 17
	12.5	1181 ± 19	1024 ± 29
	50	1056 ± 2	1026 ± 27
[1-^{14}C]Palmitoyl-L-carnitine	0	2577 ± 56	2593 ± 74
	3.2	2255 ± 61	2158 ± 24
	12.5	2065 ± 42	1948 ± 53
	50	1802 ± 61	1861 ± 7
[1-^{14}C]Octanoate[a]	0	1727 ± 76	1384 ± 93
	3.2	1902 ± 142	1373 ± 81
	12.5	1952 ± 191	1533 ± 89
	50	1879 ± 154	1551 ± 158

Values represent the mean of triplicate assay ± S.E.
[a] dpm/mg protein/10 min.

other hand, mitochondrial oxidation of [1-^{14}C]-octanoate to $^{14}CO_2$ was not affected by emeriamine at a concentration of 5×10^{-5} M (Table 3), suggesting that emeriamine may specifically inhibit the carnitine-dependent oxidation of long chain fatty acids. Thus, the inhibitory effect of emeriamine on carnitine palmitoyltransferase I was tested. Emeriamine strongly inhibited carnitine palmitoyltransferase I activity with an IC_{50} as low as 6.2×10^{-5} M (Fig. 6). These findings indicate that emeriamine specifically inhibits the carnitine-dependent transport of long chain fatty acid into the inner parts of mitochondria by inhibiting mainly carnitine palmitoyltransferase I.

Effect of emeriamine, acetylemeriamine and palmitoylemeriamine on carnitine acetyltransferase and carnitine palmitoyltransferase

Inhibitory effect of emeriamine, acetylemeriamine, and palmitoylemeriamine on carnitine acetyltransferase and carnitine palmitoyltransferase. Fatty acids are metabolized by different metabolic path-

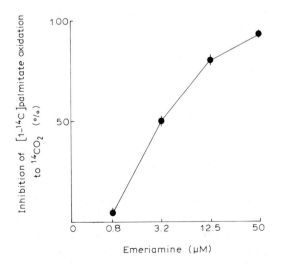

Fig. 5. Inhibition by emeriamine of carnitine-dependent oxidation of [1-^{14}C]palmitate to $^{14}CO_2$ in rat liver mitochondria.

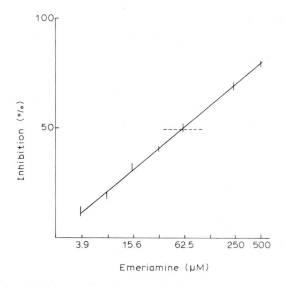

Fig. 6. Inhibition of carnitine palmitoyltransferase I by emeriamine.

ways depending on their chain length. Thus, the effect of emeriamine on (1) the oxidation of [1-^{14}C]palmitate to ^{14}CO$_2$, (2) carnitine acetyltransferase, and (3) carnitine palmitoyltransferase I was investigated. Carnitine acetyltransferase is said to be involved in the metabolism of short chain fatty acids and carnitine palmitoyltransferase I is involved in the metabolism of long chain fatty acids.

Table 4

In vitro inhibitory activity of emeriamine, acetylemeriamine and palmitoylemeriamine

	IC$_{50}$ (M)		
	emeriamine	acetyl-emeriamine	palmitoyl-emeriamine
Carnitine-dependent oxidation of long chain fatty acid	2.9×10^{-6}	8.0×10^{-3}	2.6×10^{-7}
Carnitine acetyltransferase	no inhibition	4.3×10^{-4}	$> 10^{-3}$
Carnitine palmitoyl-transferase I	1.3×10^{-4}	no inhibition	2.2×10^{-6}

Table 4 shows the inhibitory activity, that is, the IC$_{50}$ value, of emeriamine, acetylemeriamine, and palmitoylemeriamine. Carnitine-dependent oxidation of long chain fatty acids in mitochondria was inhibited most strongly by palmitoylemeriamine, IC$_{50}$ 2.6×10^{-7} M, followed by emeriamine, IC$_{50}$ 2.9×10^{-6} M. Acetylemeriamine inhibited very weakly. Carnitine acetyltransferase from pigeon breast muscle was inhibited most strongly by acetylemeriamine, IC$_{50}$ 4.3×10^{-4} M. Palmitoylemeriamine inhibited very weakly, IC$_{50}$ $> 10^{-3}$ M, and emeriamine did not inhibit, because, as will be shown later, emeriamine becomes a substrate of this enzyme. Carnitine palmitoyltransferase I in rat liver mitochondria was inhibited most strongly by palmitoylemeriamine, IC$_{50}$ 2.2×10^{-6} M, followed by emeriamine, IC$_{50}$ 1.3×10^{-5} M. Acetylemeriamine did not inhibit this enzyme.

The formation of N-acetylemeriamine from emeriamine and acetyl-CoA by carnitine acetyltransferase. The formation of N-acetylemeriamine from emeriamine and acetyl-CoA by carnitine acetyltransferase was investigated. Normally L-carnitine and [1-^{14}C]acetyl-CoA are converted into [^{14}C]acetylcarnitine by carnitine acetyltransferase. Emeriamine as a substrate was used in place of L-carnitine in the same reaction mixture and the formation of [^{14}C]acetylemeriamine was detected. The substrate concentration and formation of acetylcarnitine and acetylemeriamine are shown in Fig. 7. Acetylcarnitine and acetylemeriamine were formed from L-carnitine and emeriamine, respectively. The production rate of acetylemeriamine by carnitine acetyltransferase is about one-fiftieth that of L-carnitine. Emeriamine does not inhibit carnitine acetyltransferase but a product of the action of this enzyme becomes an inhibitor. N-acylated emeriamines were not substrates of this enzyme.

The formation of N-palmitoylemeriamine from emeriamine and palmitoyl-CoA by hepatic mitochondria. Normally, L-carnitine and [1-^{14}C]palmitoyl-CoA are converted into N-[^{14}C]palmitoylcarnitine by hepatic mitochondria. Emeriamine was used in place of L-carnitine as a substrate in the same reaction mixture and the formation of [^{14}C]palmitoylemeriamine was detected. The results of thin layer

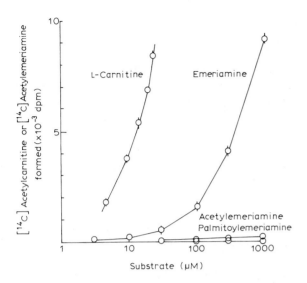

Fig. 7. Formation of acetylemeriamine from acetyl-CoA and emeriamine by carnitine acetyltransferase.

iamine was detected slightly after 3 min of incubation and was detected clearly after 10 min.

In hepatic mitochondria, palmitoyl-CoA reacts not only with the normal substrate carnitine, but also with emeriamine to form a stronger inhibitor, palmitoylemeriamine.

These findings suggest that the inhibition of long chain fatty acid oxidation by emeriamine *in vivo* may occur by a complex mechanism.

Effect of emeriamine on gluconeogenesis in hepatocytes

The effect of emeriamine on gluconeogenesis in hepatocytes was investigated by Harano *et al.* [5]. Hepatocytes were isolated from normal rats fasted for 2 days. After 10 mM lactate was added, glucose production was measured as gluconeogenesis with or without glucagon. Emeriamine effectively inhibited gluconeogenesis with or without glucagon (Fig. 9).

In vivo hypoglycemic and antiketogenic activity of emeriamine

The effect of emeriamine on glucose and fatty acid metabolism was examined in various animal models. Emeriamine produced a dose-dependent hypoglycemic effect when administered orally to

chromatography and radiochromatography are shown in Fig. 8. The two spots on the thin layer chromatograms are unlabeled palmitoylcarnitine and palmitoylemeriamine added as carriers. When L-carnitine was used as a substrate, palmitoylcarnitine was formed after 3 min of incubation. When emeriamine was used as a substrate, palmitoylemer-

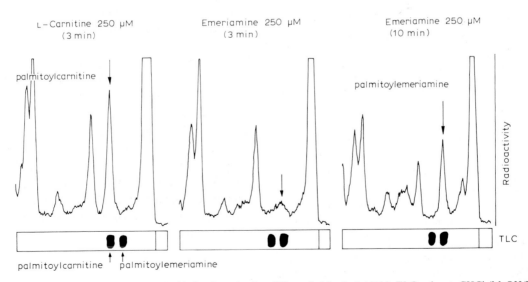

Fig. 8. Formation of palmitoylcarnitine and palmitoylemeriamine. Silica gel, Merck Art5715; TLC solvent, CHCl$_3$/MeOH/NH$_4$OH (60:25:4)

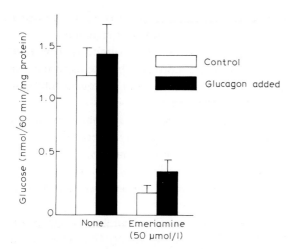

Fig. 9. Inhibitory effect of emeriamine on gluconeogenesis in isolated hepatocytes. From Ref. 5.

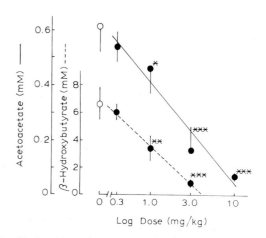

Fig. 11. Dose-dependent decrease of blood ketone bodies in fasted rats after oral administration of emeriamine. After 20 h fasting, male Sprague-Dawley rats (10 weeks old) were given emeriamine orally. Blood samples were taken 2 h later. Values are mean ± S.D. ($n = 5$). $^*P < 0.05$, $^{**}P < 0.01$, $^{***}P < 0.001$ vs. control.

fasted rats (Fig. 10). In addition, it had a more pronounced lowering effect on blood ketone bodies (Fig. 11): the minimal dose for lowering blood glucose significantly was 3 mg/kg, whereas the corresponding dose for ketone bodies was less than 1 mg/kg. The hypoglycemic and antiketogenic effects of emeriamine, at a dose of 10 mg/kg, lasted for more than 6 h. The hypoglycemic and antiketogenic effects of emeriamine were also observed in strepto-

zotocin-diabetic rats in a fasted state as well as in obese diabetic animals, such as Zucker-fatty rats and yellow KK mice (data not shown).

Tissue specificity of inhibition of fatty acid oxidation by emeriamine

Homogenates of liver, muscle, heart, and diaphragm were prepared and the inhibitory effect of emeriamine on the carnitine-dependent oxidation of long chain fatty acid was investigated by measuring [1-^{14}C]palmitate oxidation to $^{14}CO_2$. In liver homogenates, fatty acid oxidation was markedly inhibited by emeriamine (Fig. 12); liver is about 10-fold more sensitive than the other tissues.

Harano et al. [5] used hepatocytes and cardiomyocytes to investigate the effect of emeriamine on fatty acid oxidation. Fatty acid oxidation in hepatocytes was more sensitive and cardiomyocytes were less sensitive to inhibition by emeriamine. The fact that emeriamine acts most effectively in the liver is an important feature for its development as a drug to treat diabetes.

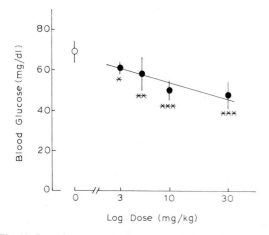

Fig. 10. Dose-dependent decrease of blood glucose in fasted rats after oral administration of emeriamine. After 20 h fasting, male Sprague-Dawley rats (7 weeks old) were given emeriamine orally. Blood samples were taken 2 h later. Values are mean ± S.D. ($n = 5$). $^*P < 0.05$, $^{**}P < 0.02$, $^{***}P < 0.01$ vs. control.

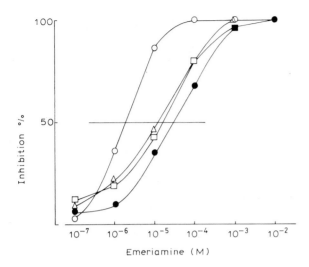

Fig. 12. Inhibitory effect of emeriamine on the carnitine-dependent fatty acid oxidation in various tissue homogenates. ○, liver; ●, muscle; △, heart; □, diaphragm.

DISCUSSION

The inhibitory activities of emeriamine on long chain fatty acid oxidation and carnitine palmitoyltransferase I *in vitro* were weaker than those of palmitoylemeriamine. However, the hypoglycemic and antiketogenic activities of emeriamine *in vivo* were more effective than those of palmitoylemeriamine (data not shown). This discrepancy between results obtained *in vitro* and those obtained *in vivo* may arise from differences in the absorption or transport ability of these compounds.

Some compounds, such as methyl-2-tetradecylglycidate (McN-3716), 2-tetradecylglycidate (McN-3802) [16–18] and 2-[5-(4-chlorophenyl)pentyl]-oxirane-2-carboxylate (B807-27) [2, 13, 21], were reported to selectively inhibit long chain fatty acid oxidation and show a hypoglycemic effect. The CoA esters of the first two are active-site-directed, irreversible inhibitors of carnitine palmitoyltransferase I [16]. The inhibitory mechanism of the third is thought to be the same as that of the other two, because its CoA ester is a strong inhibitor of carnitine palmitoyltransferase I [2] and these compounds are also oxiran derivatives. However, in our assay method for carnitine palmitoyltransferase I, inhibi-

tion by McN-3716 and McN-3802 could not be detected and preincubation of the enzyme with these compounds for more than 5 min was essential to obtain complete inhibition; but to obtain an inhibitory action of emeriamine did not require any preincubation with the enzyme (Fig. 5). These facts indicate that the inhibitory mechanism of the oxidation of long chain fatty acids by emeriamine is different from that of these compounds.

Recently, Jenkins and Griffith [6, 7] reported the synthesis and the inhibitory activity of fatty acid oxidation and carnitine acyltransferase of racemic emeriamine and racemic acylemeriamine (racemic aminocarnitine and racemic acylaminocarnitine) and described results similar to those obtained by us.

ACKNOWLEDGEMENTS

The authors wish to thank Drs. Y. Sugino and Y. Nakao for their encouragement during this work and also thank Dr. S. Shinagawa for preparation of emeriamine and *N*-acylemeriamine, and Dr. T. Fujita for *in vivo* evaluation of these compounds.

REFERENCES

1 Bieber, L.L. and L.M. Lewin. 1981. Measurement of carnitine and *O*-acylcarnitine. Methods Enzymol. 72: 276–287.

2 Bone, A.J., D.M. Turnbull, P.P. Koundakjian and H.S.A. Sherratt. 1981. Inhibition of carnitine palmitoyltransferase I by ethyl 2-[5-(4-chlorophenyl)pentyl]oxiran-2-carboxylate (CPOC): a new hypoglycaemic compound. Diabetologia 21: 504.

3 Bremer, J. 1963. Carnitine in intermediary metabolism, the biosynthesis of palmitoylcarnitine by cell subfractions. J. Biol. Chem. 238: 2774–2779.

4 Fritz, I.B. and N.R. Marquis. 1965. The role of acylcarnitine esters and carnitine palmitoyltransferase in the transport of fatty acyl groups across mitochondrial membranes. Proc. Natl. Acad. Sci. USA 54: 1226–1233.

5 Harano, Y., H. Kojima, A. Kashiwagi, Y. Tanaka, T. Nakamura, T. Fujita and Y. Shigeta. 1987. A new carnitine analogue for the correction of metabolic derangements in diabetes. In: Recent Trends in Management of Diabetes Mellitus. (Sakamoto, N., K.G.M.M. Alberti and N. Hotta, eds.), pp. 567–571, Excerpta Medica, Amsterdam.

144

6 Jenkins, D.L. and O.W. Griffith. 1985. DL-Aminocarnitine and acetyl-DL-aminocarnitine. J. Biol. Chem. 260: 14748–14755.

7 Jenkins, D.L. and O.W. Griffith. 1986. Antiketogenic and hypoglycemic effects of aminocarnitine and acylaminocarnitines. Proc. Natl. Acad. Sci. USA 83: 290–294.

8 Kanamaru, T., S. Shinagawa, M. Asai, H. Okazaki, Y. Sugiyama, T. Fujita, H. Iwatsuka and M. Yoneda. 1985. Emeriamine, an antidiabetic β-aminobetaine derived from a novel fungal metabolite. Life Sci. 37: 217–223.

9 Markwell, M.A.K., S.M. Haas, N.E. Tolbert and L.L. Bieber. 1981. Protein determination in membrane and lipoprotein samples: manual and automated procedures. Methods Enzymol. 72: 296–303.

10 Randle, P.J., P.B. Garland, C.N. Hales and E.A. Newsholme. 1963. The glucose-fatty acid cycle, its role in insulin sensitivity and the metabolic disturbances of diabetes mellitus. Lancet i: 785–789.

11 Randle, P.J., P.B. Garland, C.N. Hales, E.A. Newsholme, R.M. Denton and C.I. Pogson. 1966. Interactions of metabolism and the physiological role of insulin. Recent Horm. Res. 22: 1–48.

12 Randle, P.J., E.A. Newsholme and P.B. Garland. 1964. Regulation of glucose uptake by muscle. Biochem. J. 93: 652–665.

13 Rosen, P. and H. Reinauer. 1984. Inhibition of carnitine palmitoyltransferase I by phenylalkyloxiranecarboxylic acid and its influence on lipolysis and glucose metabolism in isolated, perfused hearts of streptozotocin-diabetic rats. Metab. Clin. Exp. 33: 177–185.

14 Seikagaku Zikken Koza. 1975. β-Oxidation of Fatty Acid. (Nozima, S. and T. Yamakawa, eds.), Vol. 9, pp. 74–77, Tokyo Kagaku Dojin, Japan.

15 Shinagawa, S., T. Kanamaru, S. Harada, M. Asai and H. Okazaki. 1987. Chemistry and inhibitory activity of long chain fatty acid oxidation of emeriamine and its analogues. J. Med. Chem. 30: 1458–1463.

16 Tutwiler, G.F., W. Ho and R.J. Mohrbacher. 1981. 2-Tetradecylglycidic Acid. Methods Enzymol. 72: 533–551.

17 Tutwiler, G.F., T. Kirsch, R.J. Mohrbacher and W. Ho. 1978. Pharmacologic profile of methyl 2-tetradecylglycidate (MCN-3716) – an orally effective hypoglycemic agent. Metab. Clin. Exp. 27: 1539–1556.

18 Tutwiler, G.F., R.J. Mohrbacher and W. Ho. 1979. Methyl 2-tetradecylglycidate, an orally effective hypoglycemic agent that inhibits long chain fatty acid oxidation selectively. Diabetes: 28: 242–248.

19 Werner, W., H.G. Rey and H. Wielinger. 1970. Über die Eigenschaften eines neuen Chromogens für die Blutzuckerbestimmung nach der GOD/POD-Methode. Z. Anal. Chem. 252: 224–228.

20 Williamson, D.H. and J. Mallanby. 1974. D-(−)-3-Hydroxybutyrate, acetoacetate. In: Methods of Enzymatic Analysis, 2nd Ed., Vol. III, pp. 1836–1843, Academic Press, New York.

21 Wolf, H.P.O., K. Eistetter and G. Ludwig. 1982. Phenylalkyloxirane carboxylic acids, a new class of hypoglycaemic substances: hypoglycaemic and hypoketonaemic effects of sodium 2-[5-(4-chlorophenyl)-pentyl]oxirane-2-carboxylate (B 807-27) in fasted animals. Diabetologia 22: 456–463.

Novel Microbial Products for Medicine and Agriculture
Editors: A.L. Demain, G.A. Somkuti, J.C. Hunter-Cevera and H.W. Rossmoore
© 1989, Society for Industrial Microbiology

CHAPTER 17

Lipoxygenase inhibitors

Shigeto Kitamura[1], Kazuko Hashizume[1], Takao Iida[1], Kenji Ohmori[2] and Hiroshi Kase[1]

[1]Tokyo Research Laboratories, Kyowa Hakko Kogyo Co., Ltd., Tokyo, and [2]Pharmaceutical Research Laboratory, Kyowa Hakko Kogyo Co., Ltd., Shuzuoka, Japan

SUMMARY

In screening for lipoxygenase inhibitors from microbial metabolites several compounds were isolated. Among them, KF8940 (2-*n*-heptyl-4-hydroxyquinoline-*N*-oxide), isolated from *Pseudomonas methanica*, is a potent and selective inhibitor of 5-lipoxygenase. The IC_{50} values of the compound for 5- and 12-lipoxygenases and cyclooxygenase are 0.15 μM, 35 μM, and 170 μM, respectively. In rat peritoneal cells and mouse myéloma cells (PB-3c cells), KF8940 inhibited the biosynthesis of leukotrienes, which are 5-lipoxygenase metabolites implicated as important mediators in hypersensitivity and inflammation. The compound, administered orally, showed suppressive activity for passive anaphylactic bronchoconstriction in guinea pigs. MY3-469 (3-methoxytropolone) was isolated from *Streptoverticillium hadanonense* as a selective inhibitor of 12-lipoxygenase. The IC_{50} values for 12- and 5-lipoxygenase are 1.8 μM and 280 μM, respectively.

INTRODUCTION

In mammalian tissues arachidonic acid is converted into numerous physiologically active mediators. There are two major enzymatic pathways in these reactions. One is the cyclooxygenase pathway, leading to prostaglandins, prostacyclin and thromboxane A_2. The second is the lipoxygenase pathway. Lipoxygenase catalyzes the oxidation of those lipids containing a *cis,cis*-1,4-pentadiene system with a molecular oxygen, to form hydroperoxides. In the case of arachidonic acid, hydroperoxyeicosatetraenoic acid (HPETE) is formed. At least six arachidonate lipoxygenases have been proposed in mammalian tissues. Three of them, 5-, 12-, and 15-lipoxygenases, have been studied. There has been increased interest in 5-lipoxygenase in recent years, since leukotrienes C_4, D_4, and E_4, metabolites of the 5-lipoxygenase pathway, collectively account for the biological activity known as slow reacting substance of anaphylaxis (SRS-A), a key mediator of immediate hypersensitivity reactions [12, 16]. Leukotriene B_4 has also been found to be in the 5-lipoxygenase pathway.

Leukotrienes C_4, D_4, and E_4 are potent bronchoconstrictors and vasoconstrictors with the ability to increase vascular permeability [18, 19]. Leukotriene B_4 has potent effects on neutrophils, related to their adhesion to venules, and extravasation as well as chemotaxis and degranulation [22]. Thus, leukotrienes have been considered to be important mediators in inflammation and immunological responses. From these observations, it is likely that a 5-lipoxygenase inhibitor would be a useful antiasthmatic and antiinflammatory drug.

The physiological significance of 12- and 15-

lipoxygenase is obscure. Development of selective inhibitors of these lipoxygenases may help clarify the physiological function of the enzymes.

In this paper we describe the work that led to the discovery of KF8940, a potent and orally active inhibitor of 5-lipoxygenase, and MY3-469, a selective inhibitor of 12-lipoxygenase.

MATERIALS AND METHODS

5-Lipoxygenase inhibitors from microbial metabolites

Production, isolation and identification. Precise assay procedures of lipoxygenases and cyclooxygenase were described by us in 1986 [7]. Briefly, 5-lipoxygenase was prepared from rat basophilic leukemia cells (RBL-1 cells). The homogenate of RBL-1 cells was used as 5-lipoxygenase. 12-Lipoxygenase and cyclooxygenase were prepared from bovine platelets. The ammonium sulfate precipitate of the cytosolic fraction was used as 12-lipoxygenase, and the microsomal fraction was used as cyclooxygenase. Each enzyme was incubated with [1-^{14}C]arachidonic acid. Under our assay conditions, the end products of 5-lipoxygenase, 12-lipoxygenase, and cyclooxygenase were 5-hydroxyeicosatetraenoic acid (5-HETE), 12-hydroxyeicosatetraenoic acid (12-HETE), and thromboxane B_2, respectively. After acidification and extraction, each radioactive product was chromatographed on a silica gel TLC plate and detected by autoradiography. The radioactivities of the products were counted by a liquid scintillation counter, after scraping off each corresponding spot.

Screening for 5-lipoxygenase inhibitors, we found that the fermentation broth of *Pseudomonas methanica* KY4634 showed potent inhibitory activity for 5-lipoxygenase. The typical time curve of production by this strain of 5-lipoxygenase inhibitors in a 30-liter jar fermentor is shown in Fig. 1. Inhibitory activity reached its maximum on the fifth day, then gradually decreased.

The inhibitors were isolated from the fermentation broth by the following procedure (Fig. 2). The filtered broth was acidified and extracted with ethyl

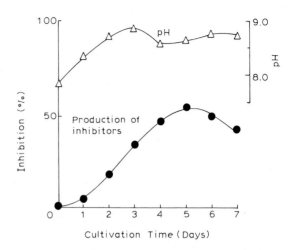

Fig. 1. Production of 5-lipoxygenase inhibitors by *P. methanica* KY4634 in a 30-liter jar fermentor. The production medium consisted of glucose 1%, glycerol 0.25%, soybean meal 1%, peptone 0.5%, NaCl 0.3%, KCl 0.03%, MgSO·7H$_2$O 0.05% and CaCO$_3$ 0.3%, pH 7.8. The thawed homogenate of RBL-1 cells was used as 5-lipoxygenase [7].

acetate. After evaporation, the aqueous solution was adsorbed onto Diaion HP-20. The eluate, with methanol, was put on a silica gel column. Two active fractions were obtained. MY12-62a was isolated from the F-1 fraction by rechromatography, and KF8940 and MY12-62c were isolated from the F-2 fraction by reversed phase column chromatography. Further purification was achieved by crystallization.

The structure of each compound (Fig. 3) was determined by ^{13}C-NMR, ^{1}H-NMR, and other physico-chemical analyses. All three compounds have previously been reported as antibiotic substances produced by *P. aeruginosa* [5, 6]. Lightbown and Jackson and Neuenhaux *et al.* reported KF8940 to be an inhibitor of electron transport through the cytochrome b-c_1 segment of the respiratory chain [11, 14]. However, there have been no reports that these compounds possess lipoxygenase inhibitory activity.

Characterization of 5-lipoxygenase inhibitors KF8940 inhibits 5-lipoxygenase in a dose-dependent manner. Fifty percent inhibition (IC$_{50}$) occurs at 0.15 μM concentration. Bovine platelet 12-lipoxygenase and cyclooxygenase were not inhibit-

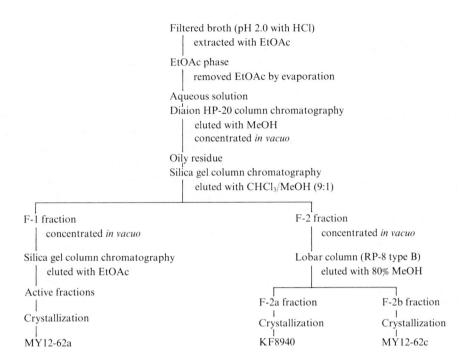

Fig. 2. Isolation procedures for KF8940, MY12-62a and MY12-62c.

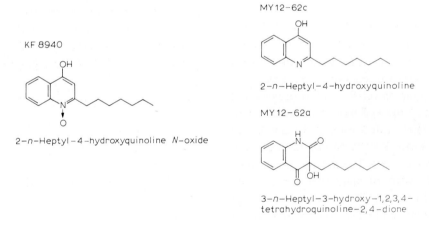

Fig. 3. Structures of KF8940, MY12-62a and MY12-62c.

ed by KF8940 at 10 μM, the concentration at which 5-lipoxygenase was inhibited completely. At higher concentrations, KF8940 inhibited 12-lipoxygenase and cyclooxygenase. The IC$_{50}$ values for 12-lipoxygenase and cyclooxygenase were 35 μM and 170 μM, respectively.

The IC$_{50}$ values of inhibitors from KY4634 for 5- and 12-lipoxygenases and cyclooxygenase are listed

in Table 1, together with representative 5-lipoxygenase inhibitors [9, 21, 23, 24]. The selectivity ratio for 5-lipoxygenase (IC$_{50}$ 12-lipoxygenase/IC$_{50}$ 5-lipoxygenase) is also given in Table 1. The inhibitory activity of MY12-62c against 5-lipoxygenase was less potent than that of KF8940, but MY12-62c inhibited 5-lipoxygenase selectively. The inhibitory activity of MY12-62a for these enzymes was

Table 1

Inhibitory activities of KF8940, MY12-62a, MY12-62c and representative 5-lipoxygenase inhibitors

Inhibitors	IC_{50} (M)			Selectivity ratio
	5-LO	12-LO	cyclo-oxygenase	
KF8940	1.5×10^{-7}	3.5×10^{-5}	1.7×10^{-4}	233
MY12-62a	8.0×10^{-5}	1.4×10^{-4}	2.7×10^{-4}	1.7
MY12-62c	1.9×10^{-5}	5.1×10^{-4}	2.8×10^{-4}	26.8
Cirsiliol [23]	1.0×10^{-7}	1.0×10^{-6}	–	10
Caffeic acid [9]	3.7×10^{-6}	3.0×10^{-5}	2.0×10^{-4}	81
AA-861 [24]	8.0×10^{-7}	$> 10^{-4}$	$> 10^{-4}$	> 125
U-60,257 [21]	2.1×10^{-6}	$> 10^{-4}$	–	> 48

5-LO = 5-lipoxygenase (10000 $\times$ g supernatant of RBL-1); 12-LO = 12-lipoxygenase; CO = cyclooxygenase; AA-861 = 2,3,5-trimethyl-6-(12-hydroxy-5,10-dodecadienyl)-1,4-benzoquinone); U-60,257 = 6,9-deepoxy-6,9-(phenylimino)-$\Delta^{6,8}$-prostaglandin I_1. Selectivity ratio is IC_{50} 12-LO/IC_{50} 5-LO.

rather weak and lacking in selectivity for 5-lipoxygenase.

The mode of inhibition of KF8940 for 5-lipoxygenase was studied. KF8940 at concentrations ranging from 0.1 μM to 1 μM was incubated with 5-lipoxygenase, with varying concentrations of arachidonic acid. Lineweaver-Burk plots showed that KF8940 inhibits 5-lipoxygenase in a noncompetitive manner. The K_i value, estimated from Dixon plots, was 0.35 μM. FK8940 inhibits 12-lipoxygenase noncompetitively also. The K_i value was 60 μM, more than two orders of magnitude greater than that for 5-lipoxygenase. These results show that KF8940 is a potent and highly selective inhibitor of 5-lipoxygenase.

Effects of KF8940 on leukotriene generation using intact cells. To examine the effect of KF8940 on leukotriene generation, we first used rat peritoneal exudate cells. The leukotriene generated was measured by biological methods using isolated guinea pig ileum. KF8940 inhibited leukotriene formation completely at 1 μM. The IC_{50} value was 0.2 μM.

Recently we have developed more convenient and accurate methods to measure leukotriene generation, using cultured PB-3c cells and an HPLC sys-

tem. The PB-3c cell line, originally described from mouse bone marrow as interleukin 3-dependent [1], was found by Shimizu *et al.* to have very high activities of 5-lipoxygenase, and leukotriene C_4 and B_4 biosynthesis [20]. Precise assay procedures for the system will be reported elsewhere. We can easily evaluate any type of inhibitor of leukotriene biosynthesis using this system, since the determination of 5-HPETE and leukotrienes C_4 and B_4 can be accomplished simultaneously. KF8940 inhibits the generation of these three compounds to a similar degree, indicating that KF8940 inhibits 5-lipoxygenase. Inhibitory activity for leukotriene C_4 generation by KF8940 is shown in Fig. 4. This is in good correlation with results using rat peritoneal exudate cells.

Effect on anaphylactic bronchoconstriction in guinea pigs. Pharmacological activities of KF8940 *in vivo* were examined in experimental allergic asthma in guinea pigs [15]. Guinea pigs, passively sensitized by anti-egg white albumin rabbit serum, were treated with egg white albumin to induce anaphylactic bronchoconstriction. Bronchoconstriction was monitored by air overflow volume under constant artificial respiration. When the guinea pigs were given KF8940 (10 mg/kg), orally administered

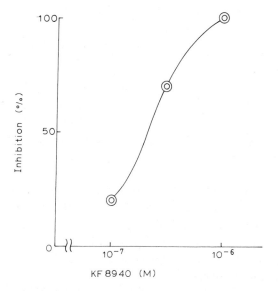

Fig. 4. Effect of KF8940 on leukotriene biosynthesis by PB-3c cells. Synthesized leukotriene C_4 was determined by HPLC.

1 h before the antigen challenge, bronchoconstriction was significantly reduced (55%). No acute toxicity was observed in rats orally administered KF8940 (400 mg/kg).

12-Lipoxygenase inhibitors from microbial metabolites

Isolation and characterization of a 12-lipoxygenase inhibitor. Streptoverticillium hadanonense KY11449 showed strong inhibitory activity for 12-lipoxygenase [8]. The structure of the inhibitor was determined to be 3-methoxytropolone, by ^{1}H-NMR and various physico-chemical properties.

MY3-469 inhibited bovine 12-lipoxygenase in a dose-dependent manner (Fig. 5). The IC_{50} value for this enzyme was 1.8 μM. Complete inhibition occurred at 10 μM. MY3-469 also inhibited 5-lipoxygenase, although the IC_{50} value was two orders of magnitude higher than that for 12-lipoxygenase. Cyclooxygenase and 15-lipoxygenase were not affected by MY3-469 at 1 mM. These results indicate that MY3-469 is a potent and highly selective inhibitor of 12-lipoxygenase. To our knowledge, this compound is the only one reported to be a selective inhibitor of 12-lipoxygenase.

Arachidonate 12-lipoxygenase was discovered in platelets by Hamberg and Samuelsson [3]. This enzyme is known to be widely distributed in various mammalian tissues [4]. Some biological activities have been reported, e.g., involvement of 12-lipoxygenase metabolites in platelet aggregation [2, 10], in

the genesis of atherosclerosis [13], and in the function of the sensory neurons [17]. Therefore, the newly developed 12-lipoxygenase inhibitor MY3-469 should facilitate studies on the various physiological roles of the enzyme.

CONCLUSION

We discovered two different types of lipoxygenase inhibitor from microbial metabolites. One, KF8940, is a specific inhibitor of 5-lipoxygenase. KF8940 and its synthetic derivatives are now being studied for their potential as antiasthmatic drugs. The other, MY3-469, is a selective 12-lipoxygenase inhibitor. The availability of a selective 12-lipoxygenase inhibitor should encourage research on 12-lipoxygenase.

REFERENCES

1 Ball, P.E., M.C. Conroy, C.H. Heusser, J.M. Davis and J.F. Conscience. 1983. Spontaneous, in vitro, malignant transformation of a basophil/mast cell line. Differentiation 24: 74–78.

2 Dutilh, C.F., E. Haddeman and F.T. Hoor. 1980. Role of arachidonate lipoxygenase pathway in blood platelet aggregation. In: Advances in Prostaglandins and Thromboxane Research, Vol. 6 (Samuelsson, B., ed.), pp. 101–105, Raven Press, New York.

3 Hamberg, M. and B. Samuelsson. 1974. Prostaglandin endoperoxides. Novel transformation of arachidonic acid in human platelets. Proc. Natl. Acad. Sci. USA 71: 3400–3404.

4 Hansson, G., C. Malmsten and O. Rådmark. 1983. The leukotrienes and other lipoxygenase products. In: Prostaglandins and Related Substances (Pace-Asciak, C.R. and E. Granström, eds.), pp. 127–169, Elsevier Science Publishers, Amsterdam.

5 Hays, E.E., I.C. Wells, P.A. Katzman, C.K. Cain, F.A. Jacobs, S.A. Thaye and E.A. Doisy. 1945. Antibiotic substances produced by *Pseudomonas aeruginosa*. J. Biol. Chem. 159: 725–749.

6 Jackson, F.L. and J.W. Lightbown. 1954. Observations on the inhibitory and growth-promoting activities of streptomycin and dihydrostreptomycin on bacteria. J. Gen. Microbiol. 11: iv.

7 Kitamura, S., K. Hashizume, T. Iida, E. Miyashita, K. Shirahata, and H. Kase. 1986. Studies on lipoxygenase inhibitors. II. KF8940, a potent and selective inhibitor of 5-lipoxygenase, produced by *Pseudomonas methanica*. J. Antibiot. 39: 1160–1166.

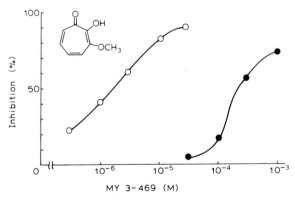

Fig. 5. Structure of 3-methoxytropolone (MY3-469), and inhibition of 12-lipoxygenase ($\bigcirc$, IC_{50} = 1.8 μM) and 5-lipoxygenase ($\bullet$, IC_{50} = 280 μM).

150

8 Kitamura, S., T. Iida, K. Shirahata, and H. Kase. 1986. Studies on lipoxygenase inhibitors. I. MY3-469, a potent and selective inhibitor of 12-lipoxygenase, produced by *Streptoverticillium hadanonense* KY11449. J. Antibiot. 39: 589–599.

9 Koshihara, Y., T. Neichi, S. Murota, A.-N. Lao, Y. Fujimoto and T. Tatsuno. 1984. Caffeic acid is a selective inhibitor for leukotriene biosynthesis. Biochim. Biophys. Acta 792: 92–97.

10 Laptina, E.G. and P. Cuatrecasas. 1979. Rapid inactivation of cyclooxygenase activity after stimulation of intact platelets. Proc. Natl. Acad. Sci. USA 76: 121–125.

11 Lightbown, J.W. and F.L. Jackson. 1956. Inhibition of the cytochrome systems of heart muscle and certain bacteria by the antagonists of dihydrostreptomycin: 2-alkyl-4-hydroxyquinoline-*N*-oxides. Biochem. J. 63: 130–137.

12 Murphy, R.C., S. Hammarström and B. Samuelsson. 1980. Leukotriene C: a slow-reacting substance from murine mastocytoma cells. Proc. Natl. Acad. Sci. USA 76: 4275–4279.

13 Nakao, J., T. Ooyama, W.C. Chang, S. Murota and H. Orimo. 1982. Comparative effect of lipoxygenase products of arachidonic acid on rat aortic smooth muscle cell migration. Atherosclerosis 44: 339–342.

14 Neuenhaux, W., H. Budzikiewicz, H. Korth and G. Pulveres. 1979. Bakterieninhyltsstoffe. III. 3-Alkyl-tetrahydrochinol-inderivate *Pseudomonas*. Z. Naturforsch. 34b: 313–315.

15 Ohmori, K., H. Ishii, Y. Takei, K. Shuto and N. Nakamizo. 1982. Pharmacological studies on oxatomide. (3) Effect of experimental asthma and Schultz-Dale response in rats and guinea pigs. Folia Pharmacol. Japon. 80: 481–493.

16 Örning, L., S. Hammarström and B. Samuelsson. 1980. Leukotriene D: a slow reacting substance from rat basophilic leukemia cells. Proc. Natl. Acad. Sci. USA 77: 2014–2017.

17 Piomelli, A., A. Volterra, N. Dale, S.A. Siegelbaum, E.R. Kandel, J.H. Schwartz and F. Belardetti. 1987. Lipoxygenase metabolites of arachidonic acid as second messengers for presynaptic inhibition of *Aplysia* sensory cells. Nature 328: 38–43.

18 Samuelsson, B. 1983. Leukotrienes: a new class of mediators of immediate hypersensitivity reactions and inflammation. In: Advances in Prostaglandin, Thromboxane, and Leukotriene Research (Samuelsson, B. *et al.*, eds.), Vol. 11, pp. 1–13, Raven Press, New York.

19 Samuelsson, B. 1983. Leukotrienes: mediators of immediate hypersensitivity reactions and inflammation. Science 220: 568–575.

20 Shimizu, T., T. Izumi, Y. Seyama, K. Tadokoro, O. Rådmark and B. Samuelsson. 1986. Characterization of leukotriene A_4 synthase from murine mast cells: evidence for its identity to arachidonate 5-lipoxygenase. Proc. Natl. Acad. Sci. USA 83: 4175–4179.

21 Sun, F.F. and J.C. McGuire. 1983. Inhibition of human neutrophil arachidonate 5-lipoxygenase by U-60,257. Prostaglandins 26: 211–221.

22 Yamamoto, S. 1983. Enzymes in the arachidonic acid cascades. In: Prostaglandins and Related Substances (Pace-Asciak, C.R. and E. Granström, eds.), pp. 171–202, Elsevier Science Publishers, Amsterdam.

23 Yoshimoto, T., M. Furukawa, S. Yamamoto, T. Horie and S. Kohno. 1983. Flavonoids: potent inhibitors of arachidonate 5-lipoxygenase. Biochem. Biophys. Res. Commun. 116: 612–618.

24 Yoshimoto, T., C. Yokoyama, K. Ochi, S. Yamamoto, Y. Maki, Y. Ashida, S. Terao and M. Shiraishi. 1982. 2,3,5-Trimethyl-6-(12-hydroxy-5,10-dodecadinyl)-1,4-benzoquinone (AA 861), a selective inhibitor of the 5-lipoxygenase reaction and the biosynthesis of slow-reacting substance of anaphylaxis. Biochim. Biophys. Acta 713: 470–473.

Novel Microbial Products for Medicine and Agriculture
Editors: A.L. Demain, G.A. Somkuti, J.C. Hunter-Cevera and H.W. Rossmoore

CHAPTER 18

A specific bacterial inhibitor of the extracellular polygalacturonase of *Geotrichum candidum*

Yair Aharonowitz[1], Shabtai Bauer[1], Shoshana Loya[1], Rachel Schreiber[1], Isaac Barash[2] and David L. Gutnick[1]

Departments of [1]Microbiology and [2]Botany, Tel Aviv University, The George S. Wise Faculty of Life Sciences, Ramat Aviv 69978, Israel

SUMMARY

Phytopathogenic fungi frequently infect fruits and vegetables, causing tissue maceration and soft rot disease. In many cases the enzymatic basis of tissue maceration can be attributed to the activity of extracellular polygalacturonases produced by the pathogen. In this report we describe the isolation and partial characterization of a specific polygalacturonase inhibitor produced by a streptomycete. The target enzyme was the polygalacturonase from the citrus sour rot pathogen *Geotrichum candidum*. Both enzyme-mediated polypectate hydrolysis and tissue maceration in a lemon peel disk assay were measured. The inhibition was also observed when tissue maceration was induced by spores of *G. candidum*. The inhibitor activity was found in the spent broth of the producer bacterium, *Streptomyces satsumaensis*, and purified some 24-fold using a combination of ion exchange and gel filtration chromatography followed by ethanol precipitation. The purified inhibitor consisted of about 95% by weight acid-labile phosphate, yet was specific for the target enzyme. Inhibition was observed in both an *in vitro* reducing sugar release assay and a tissue maceration assay. Preliminary studies using whole fruit suggest a possible potential application of such specific enzyme inhibitors in the control of postharvest plant diseases.

INTRODUCTION

Over the past 30 years, Umezawa and his colleagues have introduced a novel approach to the development of a new class of microbial products; specific inhibitors of eukaryotic enzymes. This approach involved the basic assumption that certain diseases and/or physiological conditions can be treated using an inhibitor of the specific enzymatic reaction involved. The efforts of the Umezawa group have been focused primarily on medical applications and have led to the development of a relatively large group of therapeutic agents currently on the market or in the late stages of development [17].

In principle, the approach of screening for microbial inhibitors of enzymes should be applicable to a variety of systems in which the enzymatic reaction is responsible for the pathogenic condition. Such is the case for many of the postharvest soft rot diseases prevalent in modern agriculture in which specific enzymatic reactions were shown to play a key role in the onset and spreading of the disease [13]. We have initiated a large-scale screening program to isolate specific enzyme inhibitors of microbial origin which can be applied in certain plant pathogenic situations. Citrus sour rot was chosen as our first model system for these studies.

Citrus sour rot has been shown to be caused by the fungus *Geotrichum candidum* Link ex Pers. This plant pathogen is a common saprophyte, which under appropriate conditions invades plant tissues [8]. On citrus fruits it produces a characteristic watery rot, which is the result of polygalacturonase released during spore germination and outgrowth [3]. Soft rot is characterized by extensive tissue maceration, a process involving cell separation due to enzymatic degradation of the middle lamella of the plant cell wall [5]. This maceration occurs as a result of the splitting of the α-1,4 linkages of the polygalacturonic acid in the pectic fraction of the middle lamella. Moreover, recent results on the molecular genetics of the bacterial soft rot pathogen *Erwinia* have provided unequivocal evidence for the role of pectate lyases as pathogenic determinants in certain soft rot diseases [13]. It appears likely, therefore, that the pectic enzymes from various soft rot pathogens could serve as useful targets for enzyme inhibitors of microbial origin.

In this report we describe our progress in the isolation, characterization and application of microbial inhibitors in the control of the postharvest soft rot disease, citrus sour rot.

MATERIALS AND METHODS

Microbial strains

The citrus sour rot pathogen *G. candidum* was isolated from a decayed lemon and used for the preparation of polygalacturonase. *Streptomyces satsumaensis* 1399 [9] was used throughout this study for the preparation of the polygalacturonase inhibitor.

Media

For growth and production of the polygalacturonase inhibitor, *S. satsumaensis* was routinely grown on a standard monosodium glutamate medium (MSG), containing per liter of distilled water: monosodium glutamate 2.5 g, glycerol 10 g,

$K_2HPO_4 \cdot 3H_2O$ 1 g, $MgSO_4 \cdot 7H_2O$ 0.5 g, 1 ml of $FeSO_4 \cdot 7H_2O$ (1%), and 2 ml of a trace metal solution consisting of $CuSO_4 \cdot 5H_2O$ 0.1%, $ZnSO_4$ 0.1% and $MnSO_4$ (0.1%). Semisolid medium was MSG supplemented with agar to a final concentration of 2%.

Culture conditions

Liquid cultures of *S. satsumaensis* were grown in 250 ml Erlenmeyer flasks containing 50 ml of MSG medium at 30°C on a rotary shaker at 250 rpm. Spores were scraped from petri plates, inoculated into 50 ml of MSG medium and incubated as described above for 3–4 days. The resulting seed culture was inoculated (5–20% volume) into either the shake flasks or fermentor and incubated for 6–8 days. Samples were taken at various times for analysis of pH, biomass and inhibitor activity. The fermentor used throughout this study was the model 19 bench-scale fermentor of New Brunswick Scientific Co. equipped with the 7.5 or 14 liter assembly. The fermentor was operated with water-saturated air flow of 1 liter per min. The pH was controlled automatically, and oxygen transfer rates routinely exceeded 0.2 μmol O_2 per ml per h. Either polypropylene glycol P-2000 or P-2050, at concentrations of 100–200 ppm, was used as antifoam.

Preparation of polygalacturonase from G. candidum culture broth

Two liters of culture medium containing 0.1% yeast extract, 0.1% glucose and 0.1% polypectate were inoculated with spores of *G. candidum* and incubated at 30°C for 72 h on a rotary shaker. Cells were removed by filtration. The crude culture filtrate was concentrated to dryness by lyophilization and the precipitate was dissolved in 45 ml of 0.01 M sodium acetate buffer pH 4.2 and dialyzed with the same buffer. Glycerol was added to the crude enzyme solution to a final concentration of 40% and the suspension was distributed into small portions and kept frozen at −20°C. One unit of the enzyme was that amount of enzyme which catalyzed the release of 1 mg of galacturonic acid per h. The specific activity of a typical preparation was 1650 U/mg protein. Protein was measured according to the procedure of Bradford using bovine serum albumin (Sigma) as a standard. The commercial preparation of polygalacturonase used was from *Aspergillus* (Sigma) with a specific activity of 1264 U/mg.

Phosphate determination

Inorganic phosphate (P_i) was measured according to Ames [2]. Polyphosphate was determined as acid-labile phosphate and was calculated as the difference in P_i before and after hydrolysis in the presence of boiling HCl (1 N, 20 min). The absorbance was read at 660 nm after addition of the molybdate reagent [2] and the microequivalents P_i determined from a standard calibration curve using potassium phosphate in the range of 0–0.2 μmol.

Reducing group determination

Polygalacturonase activity was determined by measuring the amount of reducing groups released by pectate hydrolysis with 3,5-dinitrosalicylic acid (DNS) reagent [15]. The standard assay system contained 20 μl of enzyme (4 μg protein) in 0.5 ml of 0.5% sodium polypectate dissolved in 0.1 M acetate buffer pH 4.2. The volume was brought to 1 ml with water in the control reaction or with different inhibitor concentrations as indicated in the text. The reaction was started by the addition of enzyme and allowed to proceed for about 5 min before the addition of 4 ml of DNS reagent to stop the hydrolysis. The color was developed by boiling for 15 min and absorbance was measured at 575 nm. About 0.5 μmol/min galacturonic acid was released in the control reaction under these conditions. One unit of inhibitor activity is defined as that amount required to reduce polygalacturonase activity in the standard assay by 50%.

Tissue maceration assay [4, 16]

Fresh, yellow lemon fruits were gently wiped with a moist sponge to remove dirt and the remnants of spray treatments from the orchard. They were soaked for 15 min in hypochlorite solution in order to destroy contaminating microorganisms, and finally washed several times with ample amounts of water. Disks of 6 mm diameter were excised at random from the peel with a cork borer to a depth of about 3–5 mm (about 100 mg per disk). If the albedo face of the disk was frayed, it was gently trimmed with a scalpel. The disks were rinsed twice in 0.01 M acetate buffer pH 4.2 and blotted with towel paper before use. In a standard assay, flasks containing five disks in 5 ml acetate buffer were incubated with shaking at 100 rpm at 30°C. Polygalacturonase was added at different concentrations ranging from 0.02 to 2.0 U/ml in the presence or absence of different inhibitor preparations. The time course as well as the velocity of both the maceration (absorbance at 540 nm) and reducing group release (DNS reaction) was determined. Maceration could be initiated by inoculating the assay vial with spores of the pathogen. The onset of maceration was dependent on the amount of spores added. Typically, between 2000 and 200 000 (1 μg– 1 mg) spores were added to the mixture. Both enzyme-mediated and spore-mediated maceration was expressed as the net turbidity measured at 540 nm (after correcting for the small amount of turbidity arising from spontaneous cell maceration).

RESULTS

In vitro assay for polygalacturonase inhibitor

The target enzyme used in these studies was a partially purified preparation of polygalacturonase isolated from cell-free broth of the citrus sour rot pathogen, *G. candidum*. In the first assay the enzymatic hydrolysis of sodium pectate was followed by determining the kinetics of reducing sugar release employing the colorimetric DNS test as described in Materials and Methods. The semi-*in vivo* tissue maceration assay will be described in a separate section. In order to test for inhibitor activity *in vitro* the target enzyme was preincubated with various dilutions of the inhibitor for 5 min prior to substrate addition. Control samples in the absence of the inhibitor preparation usually released about 0.5 μmol of galacturonic acid per min per standard reaction mixture. Fig. 1 shows the inhibition of polygalacturonase using a purified preparation from *S. satsumaensis* (see below). One unit of activity was

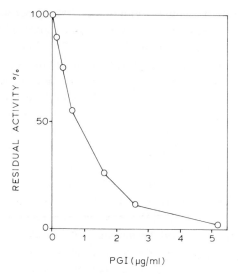

Fig. 1. Inhibition of polygalacturonase from *G. candidum* by the purified inhibitor preparation from *S. satsumaensis*. Polygalacturonase was prepared from a culture of *G. candidum*. The enzyme was assayed by the DNS assay as described in Materials and Methods. PGI = polygalacturonase inhibitor.

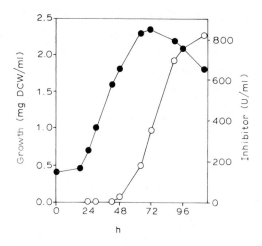

Fig. 2. Growth and production of the polygalacturonase inhibitor by *S. satsumaensis*. Cells were grown in a final volume of 7.5 liters MSG medium in a bench top fermentor as described in Materials and Methods. Samples were taken at the indicated time intervals, cells were removed by centrifugation and the pellet used for dry cell weight (DCW) measurements. The inhibitor in the supernatant was determined by the DNS assay. (●) growth; (○) inhibitor activity.

defined as that amount of material which inhibits the reaction by 50%, and corresponds to about 0.5 μg of this pure preparation. Complete inhibition was generally achieved in the presence of about 10 units of inhibitor.

Growth and production of polygalacturonase inhibitor by S. satsumaensis

Forty-five strains of *Streptomyces* from our collection in Tel Aviv University were grown for 120 h in shake flasks, and the filtrates screened for inhibitor activity as described above. One of the strains chosen for further study was *S. satsumaensis*. Growth and production of polygalacturonase inhibitor by *S. satsumaensis* was followed in a 7.5-liter bench top fermentor on a minimal salts medium containing glycerol as carbon source and monosodium glutamate as nitrogen source (Fig. 2). The kinetics of inhibitor accumulation in the culture filtrate exhibited a typical non-growth-associated profile. Maximum growth was achieved in about 55 h, whereas inhibitor concentrations reached maximum levels by about 4 days. Preliminary results indicated that inhibitor production was dependent on

the oxygen transfer rate. For example, when cells were grown at agitation rates lower than 400 rpm, no extracellular inhibitor was found, while at agitation rates above 700 rpm, cell-free concentrations of inhibitor higher than 400 U/ml were obtained. While both sucrose and soluble starch could replace glycerol in supporting normal growth, these carbon sources did not support inhibitor production. In addition, inhibitor production was observed in the presence of monosodium glutamate, asparagine or aspartate but not in the presence of ammonium salts. Typical inhibitor levels using the monosodium glutamate medium ranged between 500 and 1000 U/ml.

Purification of inhibitory activity

The inhibitor of the polygalacturonase produced by *S. satsumaensis* could be purified from the clarified cell-free supernatant using DEAE-Sephacel ion exchange chromatography. The DEAE-Sephacel slurry was preequilibrated with 1% NaCl solution, mixed with the culture fluid and poured onto a column. Inhibitory activity was eluted from the DEAE column with a NaCl gradient (1.5–3%) in

MOPS buffer (pH 7.2). A typical elution profile can be seen in Fig. 3. The inhibitory activity is eluted in the presence of about 2% NaCl. The pooled active fraction from the DEAE chromatography could be precipitated in the presence of NaCl with 1.75 volumes of absolute ethanol, resuspended in buffer and subjected to gel permeation chromatography on a Bio-Gel A-1.5 m (Bio-Rad) column. Table 1 summarizes the results for a typical purification. It can be seen that a specific activity of about 2000 U/mg was obtained for the purified inhibitor from *S. satsumaensis*. One of the most notable features of the purified polygalacturonase

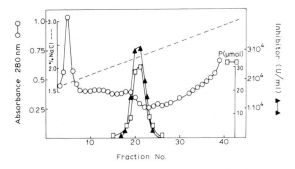

Fig. 3. DEAE-cellulose chromatography of the polygalacturonase inhibitor. Polygalacturonase inhibitor preparation was absorbed onto DEAE-cellulose and chromatographed as described in Materials and Methods. Inhibitory activity (▲) as well as the content of acid-labile phosphates (□) were determined for each fraction after elution in a NaCl gradient (dashed line).

Table 1

Purification of the polygalacturonase inhibitor from *S. satsumaensis*

Step	Total activity (U × 10^{-3})	Total phosphate (µEq. P$_i$)	Specific activity[a] (U/µEq. P$_i$)	Yield (%)
1. Culture supernatant (1 liter)	830	4380	189	100
2. DEAE-cellulose	500	1620	309	60
3. 1st ethanol ppt.	450	620	726	54
4. Bio-Gel A-1.5 m (pool)	240	353	680	29
5. 2nd ethanol ppt.	200	228	877	24

[a] Inhibitor activity was measured in the DNS assay.

inhibitor from *S. satsumaensis* was the fact that no proteinaceous material, nucleic acid or carbohydrate was detected in the final product. Since the product was readily bound to DEAE and was retained on gel permeation columns we considered the possibility that the inhibitor consisted primarily of polyphosphate.

Polyphosphate composition of the polygalacturonase inhibitor from S. satsumaensis.

The polygalacturonase inhibitor was found to consist of about 98% by weight acid-labile phosphate. As seen in Fig. 3, this peak of inhibition corresponded to a similar peak of acid-labile phosphate. Moreover, ^{31}P-NMR spectroscopy indicated (i) that the inhibitor consisted almost entirely (>95%) of polyphosphate, and (ii) that it had a molecular mass above 10 kDa. This latter observation supported similar conclusions based on the fact that the material was (i) non-dialyzable, (ii) retained by an ultrafilter with a 20 kDa cut-off, and (iii) showed less than 0.2% titratable phosphate groups prior to acid hydrolysis.

The tissue maceration assay

Polygalacturonase inhibition using the purified inhibitor preparation from *S. satsumaensis* was also analyzed using an assay more closely resembling the pathogenic effects of *G. candidum*. The basis of this assay is the enzyme-mediated hydrolysis of pectin present in the albedo of citrus fruit peels. It has been found that accompanying such hydrolysis is an increase of turbidity in the suspension resulting from polygalacturonase-catalyzed tissue maceration [4]. The kinetics of such maceration mediated by the polygalacturonase from *G. candidum* is illustrated in Fig. 4. Using enzyme concentrations in the range of 5 U/ml a linear increase in turbidity with time was observed during the first few hours of the reaction. When enzyme was added at concentrations of 0.01–0.05 U/ml the reaction was much slower but responded linearly to enzyme concentration at this range and could be followed for periods of up to 24 h (not shown). It was of interest to compare the increase in turbidity with enzyme-catalyzed release of reducing sugars on the same citrus

156

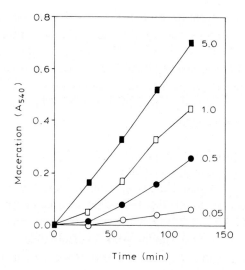

Fig. 4. Kinetics of lemon peel disk maceration by different concentrations of *G. candidum* polygalacturonase. The standard maceration assay was used. The number following each graph represents the amount of enzyme (U/ml) used in each assay.

peel disks. In the presence of low levels of enzyme (0.01–0.05 U/ml) both turbidity increase and reducing sugar accumulation showed the same dependence on enzyme concentration (Fig. 5A). This correlation was not observed at higher enzyme levels (Fig. 5B). Under these conditions turbidity increased to a much greater extent than reducing sugars for any given enzyme concentration. This may suggest that (i) additional tissue-associated enzymes which stimulated maceration were activated when larger amounts of polygalacturonase were used, or (ii) only a relatively small number of glycosidic bonds needed to be cleaved before maceration occurred.

The inhibition of polygalacturonase-mediated tissue maceration was studied in two experimental systems. In the first system the soluble polygalacturonase from *G. candidum* was used to catalyze the pathogenic reaction. In the second system the citrus peel disk suspension was infected with viable *G. candidum* spores themselves.

Inhibition of enzyme-mediated tissue maceration (Figs. 6 and 7)

In order to test the effect of the inhibitor on tissue maceration, increasing concentrations of

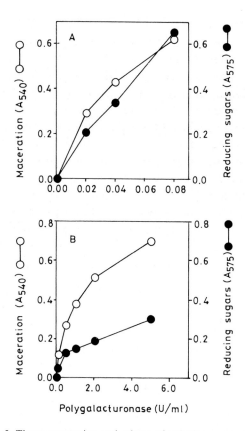

Fig. 5. Tissue maceration and release of reducing sugars from lemon peel disks by low (A) and high (B) levels of polygalacturonase from *G. candidum*. The results in panel A were obtained with low enzyme concentrations (0.02–0.08 U/ml) as measured 22 h after addition of enzyme. The results in panel B were obtained with high enzyme concentrations (0.1–5.0 U/ml) as measured 2 h after enzyme addition. (○) maceration; (●) reducing sugars.

polygalacturonase inhibitor (up to 800 U/ml) were added to lemon peel disks in the presence of 0.02 U/ml enzyme. The onset of maceration was delayed to a large extent at 200 U/ml and was inhibited almost completely at inhibitor concentrations above 500 U/ml. At enzyme concentrations of about 1–2 U/ml and polygalacturonase inhibitor concentrations of up to 500 U/ml, onset of maceration was delayed for several hours and then proceeded at a much slower rate (data not shown). This inhibition also appeared to depend on the time of inhibitor addition. Generally, preincubation of the disks for periods of up to 1 h prior to addition of 1 enzyme unit/ml gave rise to maximum inhibition.

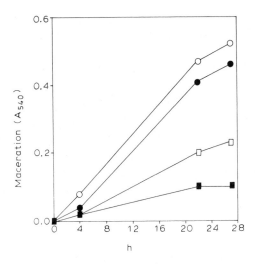

Fig. 6. Effect of purified inhibitor preparation from *S. satsumaensis* on enzyme-mediated maceration. Maceration was carried out with 0.02 U/ml polygalacturonase in the standard assay. Inhibitor was added at time zero and turbidity was measured at the indicated times. (○) control (in the absence of added inhibitor); (●) 200 U/ml; (□) 400 U/ml; (■) 800 U/ml.

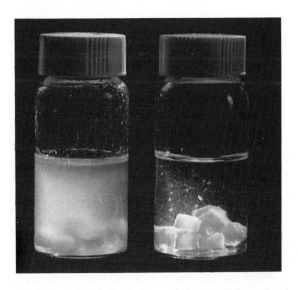

Fig. 7. Maceration of albedo tissue of lemon peel disks mediated by the endopolygalacturonase (0.05 U/ml) of *G. candidum* in the absence (left panel) and the presence (right panel) of purified inhibitor preparation from *S. satsumaensis* (500 U/ml).

Inhibition of spore-mediated maceration

As illustrated in Fig. 7, tissue maceration can also be catalyzed by the spores of *G. candidum* and inhibited by polygalacturonase inhibitor from *S. satsumaensis*. In this system the size of the spore inoculum determined the time of onset of maceration. In the presence of 1000 U/ml polygalacturonase inhibitor and 2×10^3 spores per ml (Fig. 8), the turbidity was only 30% of the control values at 20 h after infection. Between 20 and 24 h after infection there was a slight increase in turbidity. It was also of interest to note that when spores were first allowed to germinate, and inhibitor (1000 U/ml) was added 20 h after inoculation, the maceration rate was delayed significantly (not shown).

DISCUSSION

In this report we describe the isolation and characterization of a new class of microbial product; the inhibitors of pathogenic polygalacturonases from plant pathogens. The use of such materials in the control of soft rot diseases may have certain advan-

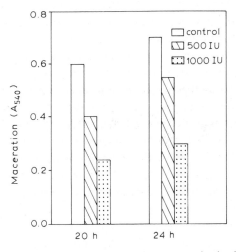

Fig. 8. Inhibition of spore-mediated tissue maceration by the polygalacturonase inhibitor. A series of standard maceration assay vials were inoculated with 1.8×10^4 *G. candidum* spores. Vials received equal volumes of either 500 or 1000 U/ml of the purified inhibitor preparation from *S. satsumaensis* and the maceration was measured at 20 and 24 h after infection.

tages including: (i) low likelihood of selecting resistant pathogens, (ii) low toxicity, (iii) the possibility of formulating the enzyme inhibitors together with other agents currently used in packing houses for enhancing shelf life, (iv) the possibility of finding other uses for the inhibitor in controlling pectinolytic processes in other industries (i.e. the food industry). Moreover, microbial metabolic inhibitors have already proven successful in a variety of pharmocological applications [7, 17]. It should be noted that the microbial inhibitors need not kill the invading pathogen, but simply control the tissue hydrolysis. In this regard, Maiti and Kolattukudy have shown that either specific antibodies raised against purified cutinase from *Fusarium solani pisi* or diisopropyl fluorophosphate, a potent inhibitor of this pathogenic enzyme, prevented infection of pea epicotyls without affecting the viability of the pathogenic *F. solani* spores [14].

While we know of no reported cases of bacterial products which inhibit pathogenic endopolygalacturonases, several cases have been reported in which host cell wall proteins and other substances inhibit polygalacturonases secreted by plant pathogens [1, 6, 10, 11]. In the case of the inhibitor from *S. satsumaensis*, the active material, found in supernatant fluid as a secondary metabolite, consisted largely of polyphosphate. It is of interest in this regard that even though polyphosphate is found in every living cell in one form or another [12], only a few of all the *Streptomyces* isolates that we examined yielded an extracellular product which inhibited the target polygalacturonase from *G. candidum*. This, coupled with the specificity of the inhibition, suggests that there may be a minor fraction associated with the biologically prepared polyphosphate which confers this specificity. Since the inhibitor first accumulates as an intracellular product prior to its release from the cells, the specificity for production may reside in the ability of the streptomycete to excrete the product in large amounts. Experiments are currently in progress to test the inhibitory capacity of polyphosphate-containing fractions from other prokaryotic and eukaryotic systems, as well as from chemical synthesis. Since polyphosphate has been shown to accumulate intracellularly in some systems in the form of large volutin granules [12] and in others as a nonaggregating polymer [12] we are using electron microscopy to investigate the physical form of intracellu-

lar polyphosphate prior to its secretion. Finally, while nothing is known about the mechanism of polygalacturonase inhibition, preliminary results from our laboratory suggest that for inhibition to occur the polyphosphate should have a molecular weight of at least 7500. This inhibitory activity appears to depend on the size of the molecule. Experiments designed to study the mechanism of inhibition and the basis for specificity are currently in progress.

The results of the spore-induced tissue maceration inhibition suggest that the inhibitor both delays the onset and slows down the rate of cell separation. This was also observed in the case of the enzyme-mediated maceration. It is to be expected that the inhibitor was more effective in the simple *in vitro* assay than in the maceration test, since tissue maceration in its later stages may involve additional hydrolytic activities of the host. In fact, when either enzyme or spore-mediated maceration was allowed to proceed for extended periods, there was a significant increase in turbidity even in the presence of the inhibitor. We are currently studying whether this resumption is due to inactivation of the inhibitor with time, or the release of additional enzymes.

Finally, we have begun a series of larger-scale storage tests on whole fruit. In a series of preliminary experiments the inhibitor was found to protect the fruit against sour rot induced either by virulent spores of *G. candidum* or by a spore-induced macerate itself (in preparation). The results presented in this report as well as the positive indications from the whole fruit studies suggest the possibility that microbial inhibitors of pathogenic tissue-degrading enzymes may find future uses as novel agents in the control of soft rot diseases.

ACKNOWLEDGEMENTS

The excellent technical assistance of Varda Kooper, Rina Avigad and Orna David is gratefully acknowledged. Thanks also to Wolfgang Minas for help in preparation of the figures.

REFERENCES

1 Albersheim, P. and A. J. Anderson. 1971. Proteins from plant cell walls inhibit polygalacturonases secreted by plant pathogens. Proc. Natl. Acad. Sci. USA 68: 1815–1819.

2 Ames, B.N. 1966. Assay of phosphate and phosphatases. Methods Enzymol. 8: 116.

3 Barash, I., E. Zilberman and L. Marcus. 1984. Purification of *Geotrichum candidum* endopolygalacturonase by affinity chromatography on cross-linked polypectate and its further characterization. Physiol. Plant Pathol. 25: 161–169.

4 Bateman, D.F. 1968. The enzymatic maceration of plant tissue. Neth. J. Plant Pathol. 74 (Suppl. 1): 67–80.

5 Bateman, D.F. and H.G. Basham. 1976. Degradation of plant cell walls and membranes by microbial enzymes. In: Encyclopedia of Plant Physiology, Vol. 4: Physiological Plant Pathology (Heitefuss, R. and P.H. Williams, eds.), pp. 316–355, Springer Verlag, New York.

6 Byrde, R.J.W. and S.A. Archer. 1977. Host inhibition or modification of extracellular enzymes of pathogens. In: Cell Wall Biochemistry (Solheim, B. and J. Raa, eds.), pp. 213–245, Tromso Universitetsforlaget, Tromso, Norway.

7 Demain, A.L. 1983. New applications of microbial products. Science 219: 709–714.

8 Eckert, J.M. 1978. Postharvest disease of citrus fruits. Outlook Agric. 9: 225–259.

9 Eveleigh, D.E., J.H. Sietsma, and R.H. Haskins. 1968. The involvement of cellulase and laminarinase in the formation of *Pithium* sp. protoplasts. J. Gen. Microbiol. 52: 89–97.

10 Fielding, A.H. 1981. Natural inhibitor of fungal polygalacturonase in infected fruit tissues. J. Gen. Microbiol. 123: 377–381.

11 Fisher, M.L., A.J. Anderson and P. Albersheim. 1973. A single plant protein efficiently inhibits endopolygalacturonases secreted by *Colletotrichum lindemuthianum* and *Aspergillus niger*. Plant Physiol. 51: 489–491.

12 Kulaev, I.S. and V.M. Vagabov. 1983. Polyphosphate metabolism in microorganisms. Adv. Microb. Physiol. 24: 83–171.

13 Lei, S.-P., H.-C. Lin, L. Heffernan and G. Wilcox. 1985. Evidence that polygalacturonase is a virulence determinant in *Erwinia carotovora*. J. Bacteriol. 164: 831–835.

14 Maiti, I.B. and P.E. Kolattukudy. 1979. Prevention of fungal infection of plants by specific inhibition of cutinase. Science 205: 507–508.

15 Miller, G.L. 1959. Use of dinitrosalicylic acid reagent for determination of reducing sugars. Anal. Biochem. 31: 426–428.

16 Mussell, H.W. and J.D. Morre. 1969. A quantitative bioassay for polygalacturonases. Anal. Biochem. 28: 353–360.

17 Umezawa, H. 1982. Enzyme inhibitors of microbial origin. Annu. Rev. Microbiol. 36: 75–99.

Novel Microbial Products for Medicine and Agriculture
Editors: A.L. Demain, G.A. Somkuti, J.C. Hunter-Cevera and H.W. Rossmoore
© 1989, Society for Industrial Microbiology

CHAPTER 19

Production of lovastatin, an inhibitor of cholesterol accumulation in humans

Barry Buckland, Kodzo Gbewonyo, Tom Hallada, Louis Kaplan and Prakash Masurekar*

Merck, Sharp & Dohme Research Laboratories, Merck & Co., Inc., Rahway, NJ, U.S.A.

SUMMARY

Lovastatin (MEVACOR®), produced by *Aspergillus terreus*, is a breakthrough drug for therapy of hypercholesterolemia, which is a risk factor for atherosclerosis and ischemic heart disease. Lovastatin is a member of a group of compounds which inhibit hydroxymethylglutaryl-coenzyme A (HMG-CoA) reductase which catalyzes a major rate-limiting step in the biosynthesis of cholesterol. In clinical studies at 40 mg b.i.d., a mean reduction of 33% was obtained in total plasma cholesterol. Fermentation process development studies in shake flasks showed that for high production, pH control and slow use of carbon source was essential. The yield was increased 5-fold by combination of culture reisolation and medium development. Scale-up studies from 800 liter to 19 000 liter scale involved comparisons of critical parameters such as carbon utilization rate, oxygen uptake rate and pH. These showed that the fermentation broths were very viscous and with such broths a novel axial flow impeller was more efficient at oxygen transfer than the Rushton radial flow impeller. Biosynthesis of lovastatin involves the polyketide pathway with acetate as a precursor of the carbon skeleton and methionine as a donor of the additional methyl groups.

INTRODUCTION

Lovastatin, also called mevinolin and MEVA-COR®, is the first compound of its kind to become available for the treatment of hypercholesterolemia [13]. It is produced by a filamentous fungus *Aspergillus terreus* [1]. Lovastatin and related compounds inhibit cholesterol synthesis by inhibiting the rate-limiting step in cholesterol biosynthesis, namely the conversion of hydroxymethylglutarylcoenzyme A (HMG-CoA) into mevalonate, catalyzed by HMG-CoA reductase [3, 7–9, 12]. The role of hypercholesterolemia as a risk factor for atherosclerosis and ischemic heart disease is indicated by clinical, epidemiologic and pathologic studies [13]; and therefore, this drug and those of similar types would be expected to help decrease the coronary event rates.

The structure of lovastatin and related compounds is shown in Fig. 1. It contains a naphthalene ring system, a β-hydroxylactone and methylbutyric acid. The active form of the drug is the corresponding β-hydroxy acid. In lovastatin R_1 is a methyl and R_2 is H. Simvastatin contains another methyl group at the 2′ position. Mevastatin lacks the methyl group at C-6. Eptastatin (Pravastatin)

---

* To whom correspondence should be addressed.

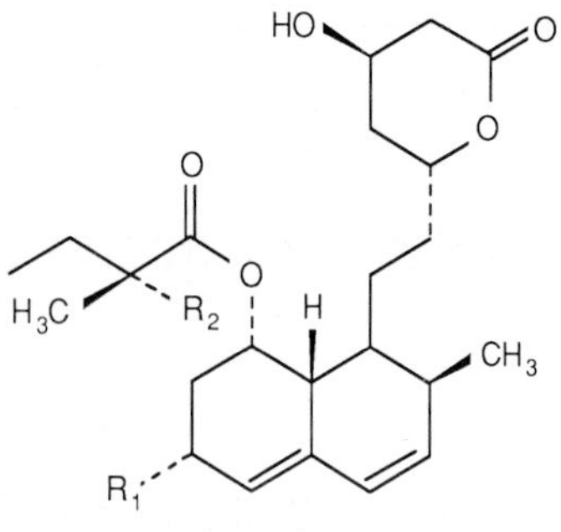

162

Lovastatin (Mevinolin, Mevacor®)	$R_1 = CH_3$	$R_2 = H$
Simvastatin (Synvinolin)	$R_1 = CH_3$	$R_2 = CH_3$
Mevastatin (Compactin)	$R_1 = H$	$R_2 = H$
Eptastatin (CS-514, Sq-31000)	$R_1 = OH$	$R_2 = H$

Fig. 1. Structure of lovastatin and related compounds.

has a hydroxy group in β-orientation at C-6. In addition, it is a sodium salt of the hydroxy acid.

Efficacy of lovastatin was demonstrated first in laboratory animals such as dogs and later in humans. In studies in humans [13] were measured total, low density lipoprotein (LDL), very low density lipoprotein (VLDL) and high density lipoprotein (HDL) cholesterol, plasma triglycerides and apolipoprotein B, which is the principal protein component of LDL. The results (Table 1) show a substantial decrease in total, LDL and VLDL cholesterol, in plasma triglycerides and in apolipoprotein B. A 10% increase was seen in HDL cholesterol.

Table 1

Summary of clinical studies

Parameter	% Change
Total plasma cholesterol	− 33
LDL cholesterol	− 40
VLDL cholesterol	− 35
Plasma triglycerides	− 25
HDL cholesterol	+ 10
Apolipoprotein B	− 20

Dose: 40 mg b.i.d.

Thus, the ratio of LDL cholesterol to HDL cholesterol, considered by some to be the best predictor of atherogenic risk, is reduced by almost 50% [13]. These results led to lovastatin being the first of the above-mentioned group of compounds to be approved by the FDA.

We describe in this paper the development of the process for the production of lovastatin.

MATERIALS AND METHODS

Organism

A. terreus ATCC 20542 or its reisolate 46-7 was used in these studies.

Media and fermentation conditions

The culture was maintained on agar slants of medium containing per liter: yeast extract 4 g, malt extract 10 g, dextrose 4 g and agar 20 g (pH 7.0) [1]. The slants were incubated at 28°C for 7 days and were stored at 4°C. The seed medium contained per liter: corn steep liquor 5 g, tomato paste 40 g, oat flour 10 g, glucose 10 g, and trace elements solution 10 ml [1]. The trace elements solution was composed of per liter: $FeSO_4 \cdot 7H_2O$ 1 g, $MnSO_4 \cdot 4H_2O$ 1 g, $CuCl_2 \cdot 2H_2O$ 25 mg, $CaCl_2 \cdot 2H_2O$ 100 mg, H_3BO_3 56 mg, $(NH_4)_6Mo_7O_{24} \cdot 4H_2O$ 19 mg and $ZnSO_4 \cdot 7H_2O$ 200 mg [1]. Forty milliliters of this medium in a 250 ml unbaffled Erlenmeyer flask was inoculated with 1 ml of spore suspension prepared by suspending the spores from a slant in 5 ml of water. The flasks were shaken at 220 rpm for 24 h. The production medium contained per liter: dextrose 45 g, peptonized milk 24 g, yeast extract 2.5 g, and polyethylene glycol P2000 2.5 ml (pH 7.4) [1]. The flasks were shaken at 220 rpm and 28°C for durations of up to 10 days.

Fermentor studies

The volume of the fermentors used for these experiments was 800 liters. These were instrumented to measure temperature, pH, dissolved oxygen, aeration and agitation rates and inlet and outlet oxygen and carbon dioxide concentrations [2]. Exhaust gas concentrations were measured by a Perkin Elmer

MGA-1200 mass spectrometer [5]. The control system was Honeywell TDC-2000 [4, 5]. The operating conditions were as those described in the Results section.

Analysis

Broth samples were centrifuged at 3000 rpm in Beckman Centrifuge Model TJ-6 (Beckman Instruments, Fullerton, CA) and the supernate was used for the analysis of the medium components. Glucose was measured using a Beckman Glucose Analyzer. Ammonia and inorganic phosphate were determined by a Technicon Autoanalyzer (Technicon). YSI Sugar Analyzer (Yellow Springs Instrument Co. Inc., Yellow Springs, OH) was used for the measurement of glycerol. For dry cell weight determination an aliquot of the broth was centrifuged. The pellet was washed with distilled water three times and resuspended in a small volume of distilled water. It was dried in a vacuum at 60°C to a constant weight. At the end of the fermentation, the flasks were harvested by adding 40 ml of methanol to the flasks and homogenizing the contents. Lovastatin was determined by HPLC in the supernate after centrifugation.

RESULTS AND DISCUSSION

Reisolation of the culture

Initial studies showed that while the culture was a pure culture, it was heterogeneous as far as the production was concerned (Table 2). In these population studies almost half of the reisolates produced very low levels of lovastatin, which can be seen from the very high coefficient of variation of the fer-

Table 2

Effect of culture reisolation

Culture	Lovastatin	
	mean U/l	%CV
ATCC 20542	91	54
Reisolate 46-7	207	12

mentation. One of the highest producing reisolates, 46-7, was found to be stable and more homogeneous. The results reported in this paper were obtained with either the original culture or the reisolate as indicated.

Medium optimization

Initial experiments demonstrated that the increase in glucose concentration from 45 g/l to 100 g/l improved the yield to 70–100 U/l, and therefore in all subsequent work the medium with 100 g of glucose/l was used.

Kinetics of fermentation

At the end of the preliminary medium development studies, we studied the kinetics of fermentation with culture *A. terreus* ATCC 20542 (Fig. 2). We believe that in order to carry out a rational process development, the knowledge of kinetics is essential. Fig. 2 shows growth, pH, glucose, lovasta-

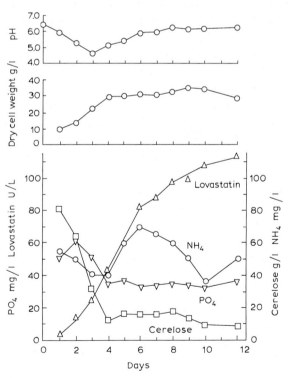

Fig. 2. Kinetics of fermentation of *A. terreus* ATCC 20542 in glucose medium. Dry cell weight, pH and NH_4 —○—, lovastatin —△—, PO_4 —▽—, cerelose —□—.

tin, ammonia and inorganic phosphate concentrations during the course of fermentation. The dry cell weight reached 30 g/l in 4 days and leveled off. At this point 90% of the glucose was used up and probably that was the reason for the cessation of the growth. The pH dropped to 4.5 on the third day and recovered when the glucose was used up. The rise in pH was accompanied by an increase in ammonia. These results suggested that the culture used the glucose metabolites and proteins as carbon sources in this phase. Lovastatin was produced at a rate of 0.8 U/l·h from the third to the sixth day, after which the rate slowed down considerably. These results suggested that one of the reasons for the reduction in the rate of synthesis was the exhaustion of the energy source. Another probable cause was that the pH decreased on the third day to too low a value to obtain optimal production.

Effect of additional glucose

We first examined the possibility that the production was limited by the energy source. For this purpose additional glucose, i.e. a glucose shot, was added on the fifth day. It was decided not to increase the initial glucose concentration of the medium so as not to allow the pH to go below 4.5. Control yield (without the shot) was 139 U/l (Table 3). It was increased by 25% or more upon addition of the shot. Interestingly, there was no advantage of adding more than 30 g/l as a shot. This could have been due to the fact that either the duration of the fermentation was not long enough to see the effect of more glucose, or the higher concentrations of

glucose led to undesirable pH changes and a shift in the metabolism. These results supported the inference that the production of lovastatin was limited by carbon source.

Effect of pH control

The second factor which could potentially have limited the yield of lovastatin was the drop in pH on the third day of the fermentation. In order to control this pH reduction, addition of three different buffers was tried. These were 2-(N-morpholino)-ethanesulfonic acid or MES, phosphate and 3-(N-morpholino)propanesulfonic acid or MOPS, which were used at 10 g/l. As Table 4 shows, without buffer addition lovastatin production of 70 U/l was obtained, which was substantially improved by the addition of any of the three buffers. These observations confirmed the above suggestion and indicated that the control of pH will be important in the scale-up of the process.

Effect of alternate carbon sources

Another approach to moderate the pH reduction was a partial or a complete substitution of glucose as a carbon source. A number of carbon sources were used to substitute for 50% of the initial amount of glucose in the medium. Control flasks gave a yield of 104 U/l (Table 5). When the glucose concentration was reduced to 50 g/l, the production was lowered by 50%. Proflo oil and soy bean oil supplementation did not increase the production above that seen with 50 g of glucose/l. Yields up to 90% of control were obtained with modified starch and lactose. Glycerol and methyl oleate were as good as glucose. These results, too, support the sug-

Table 3

Effect of concentration of sugar in the shots

Concentration of cerelose in shots (g/l)	Lovastatin (U/l)
None (control)	139
30	170
50	178
60	177

The initial concentration of cerelose in the medium was 100 g/l. The sugar shots were added on the fifth day.

Table 4

Effect of buffers

Buffer	Lovastatin (U/l)
None	70
0.05 M MES	121
0.07 M phosphate	135
0.05 M MOPS	138

Table 5

Effectiveness of various carbon sources as partial substitutes for cerelose

Conc. of cerelose (g/l)	Name and conc. of other C-source	Lovastatin (U/l)
100 (control)	None	104
50	None	57
50	50 g lactose/l	94
50	50 g modified starch/l	88
50	45 g Proflo oil/l	69
50	45 g soy bean oil/l	62
50	50 g glycerol/l	125
50	45 g methyl oleate/l	111

gestion that the pH control is important in this fermentation. Glycerol was further studied as a total replacement for glucose and was found to give 30% higher production than that with glucose.

Kinetics of fermentation of reisolate 46-7

Glycerol-containing medium was used in this experiment. As shown in Fig. 3, the dry cell weight increased throughout the fermentation. However, the rate was lower after the fourth day. Glycerol was used at a slower rate, 0.7 g/l·h, as compared with that of 1.1 g/l·h for glucose. The pH did not drop to 4.5 as was observed with glucose as a carbon source. Lovastatin was produced at a rate of 1.1 U/l·h from the second to the sixth day, which is about 40% higher than that with glucose. However, as with glucose, the rate of synthesis reduced after the sixth day. In this case it must have been due to the exhaustion of the energy source as pH did not go below 5.8.

Effect of shot addition to the glycerol medium

To verify that carbon source was limiting the production, either glucose or glycerol was added on the sixth day. Table 6 shows that without shot 131 U of lovastatin/l were produced and the addition of either increased the yield; however, glucose was more effective. It is possible that glucose is taken up and/or used up very rapidly and, therefore, is more efficient in averting the adverse effects of energy source depletion.

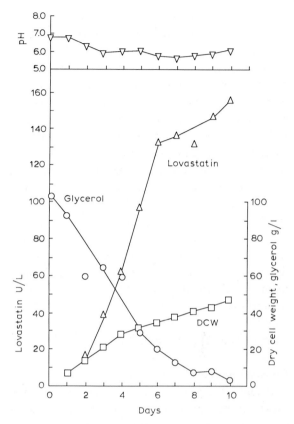

Fig. 3. Kinetics of fermentation of isolate 46-7 in glycerol medium. Dry cell weight —□—, pH —▽—, lovastatin —▽—, glycerol —○—.

Effect of buffers in glycerol medium

We also tested the effect of addition of buffers to glycerol medium and, as expected, no improvement in the production was seen (data not shown).

Scale-up studies

Scale-up of fungal mycelial fermentation poses some unique challenges. Oxygen transfer, as in other fermentation, is a critical variable. However,

Table 6

Effect of C-source addition to the glycerol medium

Initial C-source	C-source shot	Lovastatin (U/l)
Glycerol	None	131
Glycerol	20 g cerelose/l	192
Glycerol	20 g glycerol/l	154

in many fungal fermentations it is more difficult to obtain good oxygen transfer due to the non-Newtonian nature of the fermentation broths. One of the approaches used to obtain good oxygen transfer is to use a more efficient impeller design as shown in Fig. 4. This impeller is a hydrofoil axial flow impeller from Prochem (Prochem Mixing Equipment Ltd., Brampton, Ontario, Canada). The design consists of four or five hydrofoil blades set at a critical angle on a central hub. They act like the wing of an aircraft. During rotation the impeller creates high upward hydrodynamic thrust which increases the downward pumping capacity of the blades. Additionally the design minimizes the drag forces associated with the motion of the blades and thus reduces the energy losses. The hydrofoil blades tend to move the liquid in a mild top-to-bottom flow pattern. In contrast, the Rushton turbines throw liquid radially outwards from the impeller in a more turbulent agitation pattern [11].

Cascade control strategy

Table 7 illustrates this strategy. The first column shows the automatic mode of control. The set point is the value at which the variable is to be controlled. Process variable is the instantaneous value of the variable. Output is the signal sent to the device to be controlled, e.g. a cooling water valve. K, T1 and T2 are PID loop constants. In automatic mode, e.g. for temperature control, when the instantaneous value of the variable deviates from the set point, the output is sent to the device to be controlled. In cascade control, shown in the second column, the output obtained is used to reset the set point in a second loop. For example, in control of agitation,

Table 7

Cascade control strategy

	% Dissolved oxygen	Agitator speed (rpm)
Set point	10	143.9
Process variable	9.97	143.4
Output	58.6	56.2
Mode	automatic	cascade
K	1	
T_1	3	
T_2	0.035	

when the dissolved oxygen concentration deviates from the set point, the output obtained resets the set point in the agitator loop. This causes a deviation in that loop and the resultant output sends a signal to the motor controller and the rate of agitation is adjusted. During the period of low oxygen demand this type of control strategy can result in very low agitation rates, which would lead to poor mixing. To avoid this, a minimum agitation rate is set and the control system cannot reduce the agitation rate below this value.

Effectiveness of Prochem impellers

In this experiment, two 800-liter fermentors were run in parallel, one with Rushton radial flow impeller and the other with Prochem. The dissolved oxygen was controlled at 75% of air saturation with cascade control of agitation. The oxygen transfer coefficient (K_La) profiles obtained with these two types of impellers were similar (Fig. 5). The maximum K_La observed with the Rushton turbine was slightly higher than that with the Prochem impeller. Secondly, the peak was reached slightly earlier with the former. A significant difference was found when the power draw was considered. As shown in Fig. 6, the maximum power requirement with the Prochem impellers was about 66% of that with the Rushton turbines. There was no adverse impact of the Prochem impellers on the yield. Thus, these results clearly demonstrate the effectiveness of the Prochem impellers.

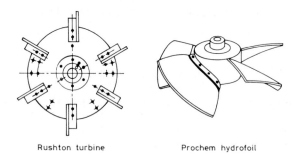

Rushton turbine   Prochem hydrofoil

Fig. 4. Types of agitator tested in the fermentors.

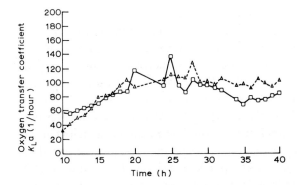

Fig. 5. Profile of oxygen transfer coefficient during the period of high oxygen demand. Prochem agitator —△—, Rushton agitator —□—.

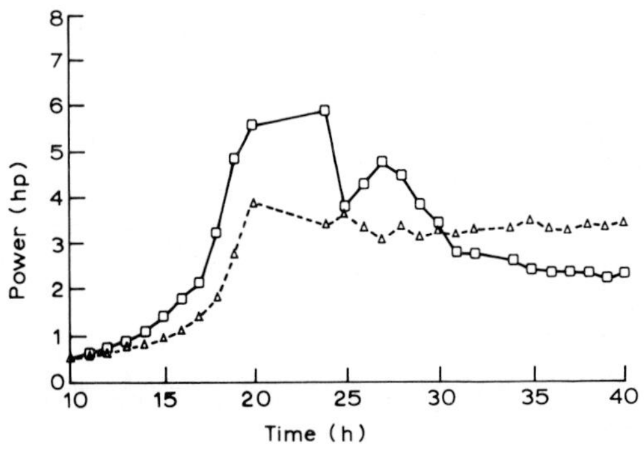

Fig. 6. Power requirements during the period of high oxygen demand. Prochem agitator —△—, Rushton agitator —□—.

Kinetics of fermentation in fermentors

The size of the fermentors used in this experiment was 800 liters. The dissolved oxygen concentration was maintained at 50% of air saturation or above by cascade control of agitator speed. Typical batch profiles are shown in Figs. 7, 8 and 9. Oxygen uptake rate and the carbon dioxide evolution rates were calculated on-line from inlet and outlet gas analysis done with mass spectrometry. There was rapid growth in the first 18 h as seen from the in-

crease in the oxygen uptake and the carbon dioxide evolution rates (Fig. 7). The reduction and subsequent leveling off of these rates indicated that the growth was complete in about 40 h. At this time the lovastatin production began. It continued linearly to 140 h. As in the shake flasks, the pH first decreased to 5.2 and then increased as the carbon source was exhausted (Fig. 8). The rate of aeration was held constant (Fig. 9). The brief deviation from the set value was due to an operator error. It oc-

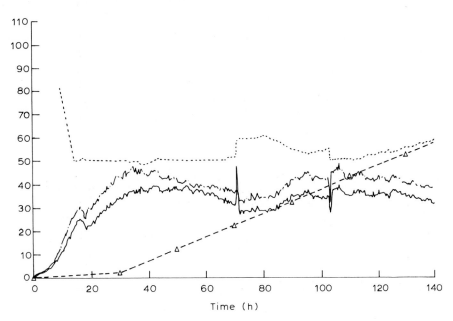

Fig. 7. Kinetics of fermentation in 800 liter fermentor. Carbon dioxide evolution rate (mmol·l^{-1}·h^{-1}) ——, oxygen uptake rate (mmol·l^{-1}·h^{-1}) —·—, dissolved oxygen (% air saturation) ..., lovastatin (U/l) △—△.

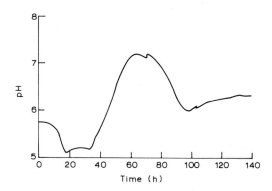

Fig. 8. pH profile during fermentation in 800 liter fermentor.

Biosynthesis of lovastatin

Information on the biosynthesis of lovastatin was obtained by studying the incorporation of ^{13}C-, ^{2}H- and ^{18}O-labeled precursors [6, 10]. Chan *et al.* [6] used ^{13}C-, ^{2}H- and ^{18}O-labeled acetate and methionine as precursors. *A. terreus* ATCC 20542 was the organism studied. NMR spectroscopy was used to analyze the results. The resulting assignments are shown in Fig. 10. The main portion of lovastatin consists of a polyketide chain of nine intact acetate units with a methionine-derived methyl group at C-6. The β-methylbutyryl side chain is constructed from two intact acetate units with a methyl group at C-2′ donated by methionine. Endo and his co-workers confirmed these results with *Penicillium citrinum* NRRL 8082 and *Monoascus ruber* M-4681 [10]. They studied the incorporation of label from [^{13}C]acetate, [^{13}C]propionate and [^{13}C]methionine. They found that the label from [^{13}C]propionate was not incorporated into either compactin or lovastatin. Their results with the ^{13}C-labeled acetate and methionine were similar to those reported by Chan *et al.* [6]. They suggested from the data of the preliminary studies with [^{14}C]acetate that the hydroxylation and subsequent methyl butyration at C-8 takes place after the cyclization. Furthermore, the

curred at the time of low oxygen demand and hence had no detrimental effect on the fermentation. Between 20 and 50 h the agitation rate was increased through cascade control as the oxygen demand increased, after which the demand decreased and the agitation rate was decreased. This approach is very energy-efficient and it minimizes any potential shear damage to the culture.

The information gained during the scale-up studies along with that obtained with shake flasks led to the successful scale-up of the process to the factory equipment.

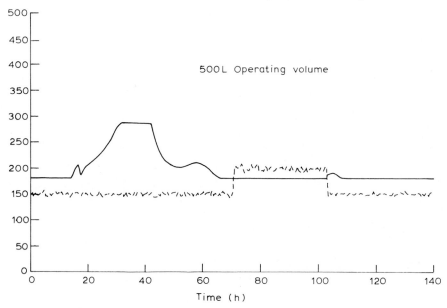

Fig. 9. Agitation and aeration during fermentation in 800 liter fermentor. Air flow (l·min^{-1}) ———, agitator speed (rpm) —. Deviation in air flow during 70–100 h was due to an operator error.

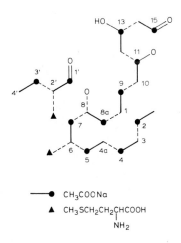

—● CH_3COONa

▲ $CH_3SCH_2CH_2\underset{\underset{\displaystyle NH_2}{|}}{C}HCOOH$

Fig. 10. Proposed precursor incorporation during the biosynthesis of lovastatin.

observation that *P. citrinum* does not produce any compounds which contain the methyl group at C-6, such as monocolin L and monocolin J, led them to propose that the methyl group at C-6 is incorporated into the linear intermediate before cyclization. At this time, none of the enzymes involved in the biosynthesis have been isolated or studied. Further work on these enzymes and understanding of their regulation will greatly facilitate future yield improvement.

In summary, lovastatin is a very efficacious drug for the therapy of hypercholesterolemia. Its production was increased 5-fold by culture reisolation and medium optimization. Process scale-up required careful monitoring of carbon utilization rate, oxygen uptake rate and pH. Lovastatin is synthesized from 11 acetate units via the polyketide pathway. Methionine is the precursor of two methyl groups. Improved knowledge of biosynthesis and of regulation of the enzymes involved will greatly facilitate future production improvements.

REFERENCES

1 Alberts, A.W., J. Chen, G. Kuron, V. Hunt, J. Huff, C. Hoffman, J. Rothrock, M. Lopez, H. Joshua, E. Harris, A. Patchett, R. Monaghan, S. Currie, E. Stapley, G. Albers-Schonberg, O. Hensens, J. Hirshfield, K. Hoogsteen, J. Liesch and J. Springer. 1980. Mevinolin: a highly potent competitive inhibitor of hydroxymethylglutaryl-coenzyme A reductase and a cholesterol-lowering agent. Proc. Natl. Acad. Sci. 77: 3957–3961.

2 Brix, T., S.W. Drew and B.C. Buckland. 1988. Fermentation process development within a computer controlled pilot plant. Computers in Fermentation Technology: Progress in Industrial Microbiology Vol. 25 (Bushnell, M.E., ed.), pp. 151–194, Elsevier Science Publishers, Amsterdam.

3 Brown, M.S., J.R. Faust, J.L. Goldstein, I. Kaneko and A. Endo. 1978. Induction of 3-hydroxy-3-methylglutaryl coenzyme A reductase activity in human fibroblasts incubated with compactin (ML-236B), a competitive inhibitor of the reductase. J. Biol. Chem. 253: 1121–1128.

4 Buckland, B.C. 1984. The translation of scale in fermentation processes: the impact of computer process control. Bio/Technology 2: 875–893.

5 Buckland, B.C., T. Brix, H. Fastert, K. Gbewonyo, G. Hunt and D. Jain. 1985. Fermentation exhaust gas analysis using mass spectrometry. Bio/Technology 3: 982–988.

6 Chan, J.K., R.N. Moore, T.T. Nakashima and J.C. Vederas. 1983. Biosynthesis of mevinolin. Spectral assignment by double-quantum coherence NMR after high carbon-13 incorporation. J. Am. Chem. Soc. 105: 3334–3336.

7 Endo, A. 1979. Monocolin K, a new hypocholesterolemic agent produced by a *Monoascus* species. J. Antibiot. 32: 852–854.

8 Endo, A., M. Kuroda and K. Tanazawa. 1976. Competitive inhibition of 3-hydroxy-3-methylglutaryl coenzyme A reductase by ML-236A and ML-236B fungal metabolites having hypocholesterolemic activity. FEBS Lett. 72: 323–326.

9 Endo, A., M. Kuroda and Y. Tsujita. 1976. ML-236A, ML-236B and ML-236C, new inhibitors of cholesterogenesis produced by *Penicillium citrinum*. J. Antibiot. 29: 1346–1348.

10 Endo, A., Y. Negishi, T. Iwashita, K. Mizukawa and M. Hirama. 1985. Biosynthesis of ML-236B (compactin) and monocolin K. J. Antibiot. 38: 444–448.

11 Gbewonyo, K., D. DiMasi and B.C. Buckland. 1986. The use of hydrofoil impellers to improve oxygen transfer efficiency in viscous mycelial fermentations. Proceedings of International Conference on BioReactor Fluid Dynamics, 1986, pp. 281–299, B.H.R. Cranfield, Cambridge, U.K.

12 Tanazawa, K. and A. Endo. 1979. Kinetic analysis of the reaction catalysed by rat-liver 3-hydroxy-3-methylglutaryl coenzyme A reductase using two specific inhibitors. Eur. J. Biochem. 98: 195–201.

13 Tobert, J.A. 1987. New developments in lipid-lowering therapy: the role of inhibitors of hydroxymethylglutaryl coenzyme A reductase. Circulation 76: 534–538.

Novel Microbial Products for Medicine and Agriculture
Editors: A.L. Demain, G.A. Somkuti, J.C. Hunter-Cevera and H.W. Rossmoore

171

CHAPTER 20

Triacsins, acyl-CoA synthetase inhibitors and F-244, a hydroxymethylglutaryl-CoA synthase inhibitor

Hiroshi Tomoda and Satoshi Ōmura[*]

The Kitasato Institute, Tokyo, Japan

SUMMARY

Triacsins isolated from *Streptomyces* sp. are potent inhibitors of acyl-CoA synthetase (EC 6.2.1.3). Inhibition of triacsin A is noncompetitive with respect to the two substrates ATP and coenzyme A, but is competitive with respect to long chain fatty acids. Growth inhibition of Raji cells caused by triacsins appears to be due to inhibition of acyl-CoA synthetase. The common N-hydroxytriazene moiety of triacsins is essential for inhibitory activity against acyl-CoA synthetase. A β-lactone termed F-244 isolated from *Scopulariopsis* sp. shows potent inhibition of cholesterogenesis. Studies on the inhibition site of F-244 revealed that the drug specifically inhibits hydroxymethylglutaryl (HMG)-CoA synthase. The hydroxymethyl-β-lactone moiety is responsible for inhibitory activity against HMG-CoA synthase.

INTRODUCTION

Lipid metabolism normally keeps an elegant balance between synthesis and degradation. When the balance is lost, hypercholesterolemia and a number of kinds of hyperlipidemia may develop. This in turn can cause, at a high rate, a variety of serious diseases, such as arteriosclerosis, atherosclerosis, hypertension, obesity, diabetes, functional depression of some organs and so on. We have been interested in drugs of microbial sources for the control of abnormal lipid metabolism.

Our efforts in this field began with the discovery of cerulenin in 1963. Cerulenin is a potent inhibitor of fatty acid synthetase [4]. It inhibits all known types of fatty acid synthetases, both the multifunc-

tional enzyme complex (Type I) and the nonaggregated enzyme system (Type II). The only exception is the fatty acid synthetase purified from a cerulenin-producing fungus, *Cephalosporium caerulens* [2, 11, 12]. The antibiotic blocks the condensing enzyme irreversibly. Unfortunately, cerulenin did not evolve into an effective chemotherapeutic because of its side effect. However, it has been widely used as a biochemical tool in the field of lipid research [3]. In 1983 we discovered thiotetromycin, an inhibitor of Type II fatty acid synthetase [5]. Recently, we have discovered two kinds of interesting inhibitors, triacsins and F-244. Triacsins are acyl-CoA synthetase inhibitors, and F-244 is an inhibitor of 3-hydroxy-3-methylglutaryl coenzyme A (HMG-CoA) synthase. Merck Sharp and Dohme Research Laboratories discovered F-244 (L-659,699) independently and almost at the same time [6]. In this

---
[*]To whom correspondence should be addressed.

symposium, we would like to describe these two inhibitors.

RESULTS AND DISCUSSION

Triacsins

During the course of our search for inhibitors of fatty acid metabolism of microbial origin, *Streptomyces* sp. SK-1894 was found to produce acyl-CoA synthetase inhibitors. Triacsins A, B, C and D (Fig. 1) were isolated from the cultured broth of this strain [7]. Triacsins C and D were identical to WS-1228 A and B, respectively, previously reported as hypotensive vasodilators [9]. They have an eleven-carbon chain and a common *N*-hydroxytriazene moiety at its terminus. Inhibition of acyl-CoA synthetase by triacsins was studied [10] and the mechanism of inhibition of animal cell growth by triacsins was also studied.

Assay of acyl-CoA synthetase

Acyl-CoA synthetase (EC 6.2.1.3) catalyzes the conversion of free long chain fatty acids to acyl-CoAs. We have developed a new assay method, using HPLC, to determine the reaction product acyl-CoA. Fig. 2 shows a typical chromatogram of the reaction mixture. Oleoyl-CoA was detectable at a picomolar level with a retention time of 15.8 min. This technique facilitated our studies considerably, and will be of wide application.

Inhibition of acyl-CoA synthetase by triacsins

The concentration of triacsins required for 50% inhibition (IC_{50} values) of acyl-CoA synthetase activity are summarized in Table 1. Acyl-CoA synthetase purified from *Pseudomonas aeruginosa* (Toyobo Co., Tokyo), microsomal fraction of rat liver and membrane fraction of Raji cells (an established cell line from human Burkett's lymphoma) were used as enzyme sources. Triacsins inhibited acyl-CoA synthetase activity from all the sources tested. Triacsin C is the most potent with IC_{50} values of 3.2–8.7 μM, followed by triacsin A with IC_{50} values of 5.3–18 μM. Triacsins B and D are much less po-

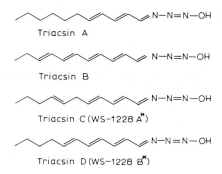

Fig. 1. Structures of triacsins.* From Ref. 9.

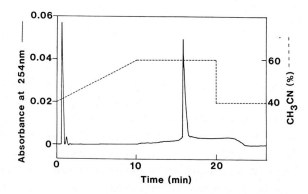

Fig. 2. HPLC of the reaction mixture of acyl-CoA synthetase from *P. aeruginosa*. Oleoyl-CoA (3.7 nmol, retention time 15.8 min) was detected. Column YMC-Pack A-302 ODS (4.6 × 150 mm); solvent, a 10-min linear gradient from 40 to 60% acetonitrile in 25 mM KH_2PO_4 then a 10-min isocratic run with 60% acetonitrile in 25 mM KH_2PO_4; flow rate, 1.0 ml/min; detection, UV at 254 nm.

tent than triacsins A and C. At higher concentrations triacsins B and D inhibited the enzymes by 40–45%. Neither (2*E*)-2,4-undecadienal nor (3*E*)-2,4,7-undecatrienal (hydrolytic products of triacsins A and C, respectively) showed inhibitory activity against acyl-CoA synthetase. This result indicates that the common *N*-hydroxytriazene moiety is essential for inhibitory activity. Furthermore, triacsins A and C have a common structural feature of a conjugated dienylidine *N*-hydroxytriazene moiety, while triacsins B and D have a longer conjugated polyene in their structure. This suggests that the common structural feature of triacsins A and C is responsible for potent inhibitory activity against acyl-CoA synthetase. On the other hand,

Table 1

Effects of triacsins on acyl-CoA synthetases and acetyl-CoA synthetase

Enzyme	IC$_{50}$ (μM)				
	triacsin A	triacsin B	triacsin C	triacsin D	(3E)-2,4,7-undeca-trienal
Acyl-CoA synthetase					
Pseudomonas sp.	17	> 200	3.6	> 200	–
Rat liver	18	> 200	8.7	> 200	–
Raji cells	5.3	> 100	3.2	> 100	–
Acetyl-CoA synthetase					
Saccharomyces cerevisiae	–	n.d.	–	n.d.	n.d.

– = no inhibition at 200 μM.
n.d. = not determined.
> 100 = inhibited by 40–45% at 100 μM of triacsins.
> 200 = inhibited by 40–45% at 200 μM of triacsins.

acetyl-CoA synthetase from *Saccharomyces cerevisiae* (short chain acyl-CoA synthetase) is not inhibited by triacsins. It is suggested that triacsins inhibit long chain acyl-CoA synthetase specifically.

Steady-state kinetics of the inhibition of acyl-CoA synthetase by triacsins

Triacsin A inhibited acyl-CoA synthetase from *P. aeruginosa* noncompetitively with respect to the two substrates ATP (K_m 0.41 mM) and CoA (K_m 1.93 mM). Triacsin A behaved in a competitive manner with respect to oleic acid. The K_m value for oleic acid was determined to be 101 μM and the apparent K_i of triacsin A was 8.97 μM.

Inhibition of Raji cell growth by triacsins

The growth of Raji cells was inhibited by triacsins in a dose-dependent fashion as shown in Fig. 3. The inhibition by triacsins A and C was clearly observed at day 2. The inhibition by triacsins B and D was not evident at this time, but after day 2 severe growth inhibition emerged. The IC$_{50}$ values (from day 2 to day 5) of triacsins for Raji cell growth were estimated from the data of Fig. 3 and are summarized in Table 2. Triacsins A and C inhibited the growth strongly, regardless of culture periods. Curiously, IC$_{50}$ values of triacsins B and D

decreased steeply after day 3. It is assumed that this is due to a secondary effect of triacsins B and D, or that their metabolites have an inhibitory effect on Raji cell growth. The order of their inhibitory potency against Raji cell growth coincides well with that against acyl-CoA synthetase from Raji cells.

The effect of triacsins on the incorporation of [^{14}C]palmitate into lipid fractions in Raji cells was studied. The incorporation was inhibited by triacsins. Triacsins A (IC$_{50}$ 14.4 μM) and C (IC$_{50}$ 6.3 μM) are much more potent than triacsins B and D (IC$_{50}$ 70 μM for both).

The hierarchies of the inhibitory potency of triacsins against the three activities, namely Raji cell growth, palmitate incorporation into lipid fraction of Raji cells, and acyl-CoA synthetase from Raji cells, are very similar. It is postulated that the inhibition of acyl-CoA synthetase by triacsins leads to the inhibition of lipid synthesis and consequently to the inhibition of Raji cell growth.

Proposed mechanism of selective toxicity of triacsins to animal cells

One of the interesting biological characteristics of triacsins is that triacsins show no antimicrobial activity but exhibit potent growth inhibition against animal cells such as Vero, HeLa and Raji cells. Triacsins appear to inhibit acyl-CoA synthetase from widely different sources. The question is why the growth of microorganisms is not inhibited by triacsins in spite of the inhibition of microbial

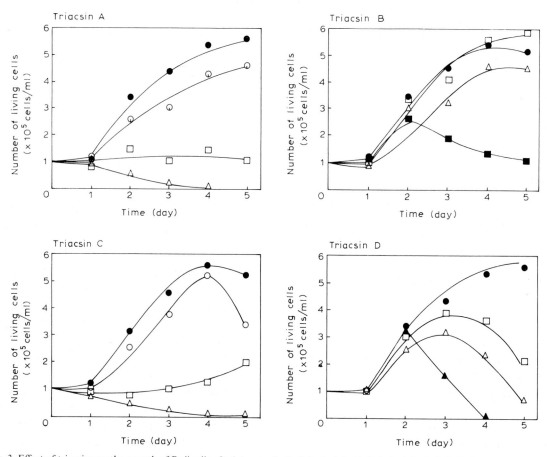

Fig. 3. Effect of triacsins on the growth of Raji cells. ●, 0 (control); ○, 0.1; ◉, 0.2; □, 0.5; △, 1.0; ▲, 2.5; ■, 3.0 μg/ml of triacsins.

Table 2

Effect of triacsins on growth of Raji cells

Day	IC$_{50}$ (μM)			
	triacsin A	triacsin B	triacsin C	triacsin D
2	1.8	> 50	1.0	> 50
3	1.4	11.2	1.3	6.1
4	1.5	10.5	1.2	4.4
5	1.5	9.3	0.9	1.8

acyl-CoA synthetase. Our speculation is as follows. Acyl-CoA, an activated form of fatty acid, is essential for both microorganisms and animal systems. It plays an important role as a metabolic intermediate in lipid biosynthesis and β-oxidation of fatty acids. Acyl-CoA also serves as a regulator in other meta-

bolic pathways [8]. In animal tissues and cells, free fatty acids are produced by fatty acid synthetase [16], and then have to be converted to acyl-CoAs by the reaction of acyl-CoA synthetase. This is the main route supplying acyl-CoA, so the inhibition of acyl-CoA synthetase by triacsins has a lethal effect on animal systems. On the other hand, acyl-CoAs are synthesized by two pathways in microorganisms. Even when triacsins block acyl-CoA synthetase, acyl-CoA is supplied *via* another route using fatty acid synthetase [16]. Therefore, triacsin action cannot be lethal to microorganisms.

F-244

In order to find new inhibitors of cholesterogenesis, our attention was directed toward mevalonate biosynthesis. A fungal β-lactone termed F-244 (Fig. 4) isolated from *Scopulariopsis* sp. [13] was found to inhibit mevalonate biosynthesis. F-244 was identical to 1233 A reported as an antibiotic by Aldridge *et al.* [1]. F-244 was found to be a potent and specific inhibitor of HMG-CoA synthase (EC 4.1.3.5). Studies on F-244 derivatives suggested that the hydroxylmethyl-β-lactone moiety is responsible for potent inhibitory activity against HMG-CoA synthase [14].

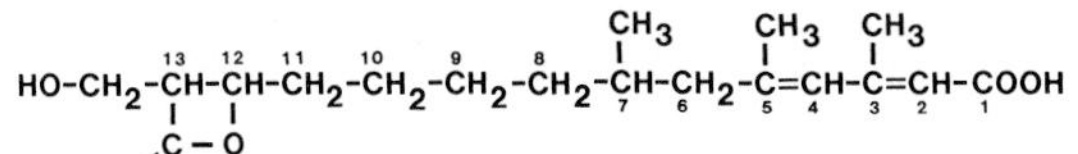

HO-CH$_2$-CH-CH-CH$_2$-CH$_2$-CH$_2$-CH$_2$-CH-CH$_2$-C=CH-C=CH-COOH

CH$_3$ CH$_3$ CH$_3$

C–O

Fig. 4. Structure of F-244 (identified as 1233A by Aldridge *et al.* [1]).

Effect of F-244 on Vero cell growth

Animal cells appear much more sensitive to inhibitors of mevalonate biosynthesis than microorganisms. Morphological changes and growth inhibition of Vero cells (an established cell line from kidney cells of African green monkey) was observed at 10 μM of F-244. However, when 1 mM mevalonate was added to the culture medium, both morphological changes and growth inhibition were overcome and the cells grew normally. Addition of 5 mM sodium acetate had no effect. The results indicated that F-244 inhibits mevalonate biosynthesis in these cultured cells.

Effect of F-244 on the incorporation of ^{14}C-labeled precursors into digitonin-precipitable sterols in a rat liver enzyme system

Degrees of inhibition of [^{14}C]acetate incorporation were similar to those of [^{14}C]acetyl-CoA incorporation at various concentrations of F-244. The IC$_{50}$ values were 1.8 μM. No inhibition of [^{14}C]-mevalonate incorporation was observed even at 300 μM of F-244.

Inhibition of HMG-CoA synthase by F-244

The results described above indicated that the inhibition site of F-244 lies within the steps between acetyl-CoA and mevalonate where the three enzymes acetoacetyl-CoA thiolase, HMG-CoA synthase and HMG-CoA reductase are involved. In order to determine the inhibition site of F-244, the effect of F-244 on the three enzymes was studied. F-244 inhibited the reaction of HMG-CoA synthase and the sequential reaction of acetoacetyl-CoA thiolase and HMG-CoA synthase (Fig. 5). However, neither acetoacetyl-CoA thiolase nor HMG-CoA reductase was inhibited at 150 μM of F-244. F-244 is a very effective inhibitor of HMG-CoA synthase with an IC$_{50}$ value of 0.2 μM. The inhibition (IC$_{50}$ 0.68 μM) of the sequential reaction of acetoacetyl-CoA thiolase and HMG-CoA synthase supported the F-244 inhibition of HMG-CoA synthase.

Effects of F-244 and its derivatives on HMG-CoA synthase and Vero cell growth

Five derivatives of F-244 were prepared chemically and their inhibitory activities against HMG-CoA synthase and Vero cell growth were compared (Table 3).

Among them F-244 was the most potent inhibitor of HMG-CoA synthase. The methyl ester derivative (6) had almost the same activity as F-244. The saturated derivative (4) was about half as active as F-244. The acetylated one (5) showed much less activity. Cleavage of β-lactone (2, 3) resulted in entire

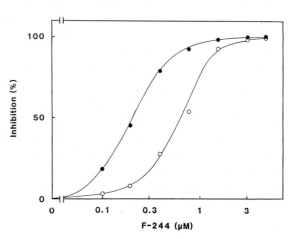

Fig. 5. Inhibition of HMG-CoA synthase ($\bullet$) and the sequential reaction of acetoacetyl-CoA thiolase and HMG-CoA synthase ($\bigcirc$) by F-244.

Table 3

Effects of F-244 and analogs on HMG-CoA synthase and the growth of Vero cells

		HMG-CoA synthase IC$_{50}$ (μM)	Vero cells MIC (μM)
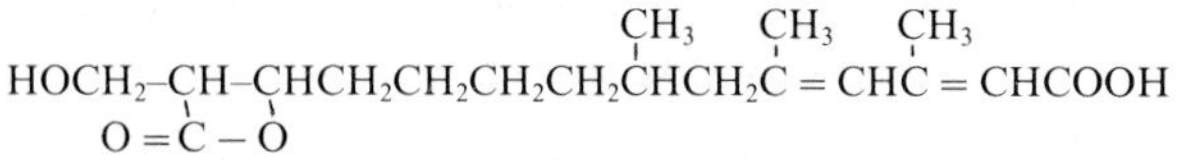 $\underset{O=C-O}{HOCH_2-CH-CHCH_2CH_2CH_2CH_2\overset{CH_3}{CHCH_2}\overset{CH_3}{C}=CH\overset{CH_3}{C}=CHCOOH}$	1	0.20	20
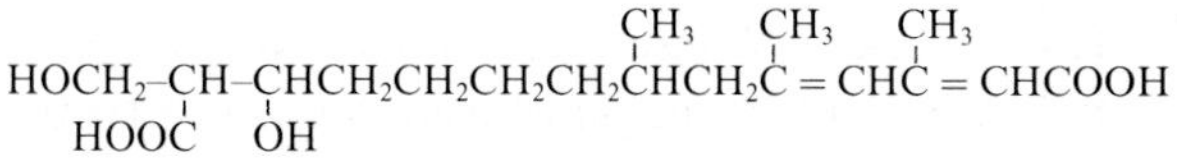 $\underset{HOOC\quad OH}{HOCH_2-CH-CHCH_2CH_2CH_2CH_2\overset{CH_3}{CHCH_2}\overset{CH_3}{C}=CH\overset{CH_3}{C}=CHCOOH}$	2	> 150	> 300
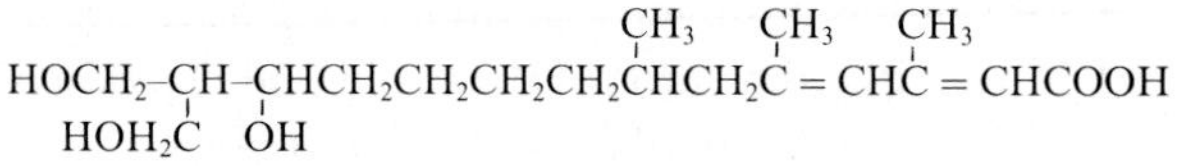 $\underset{HOH_2C\quad OH}{HOCH_2-CH-CHCH_2CH_2CH_2CH_2\overset{CH_3}{CHCH_2}\overset{CH_3}{C}=CH\overset{CH_3}{C}=CHCOOH}$	3	> 150	> 300
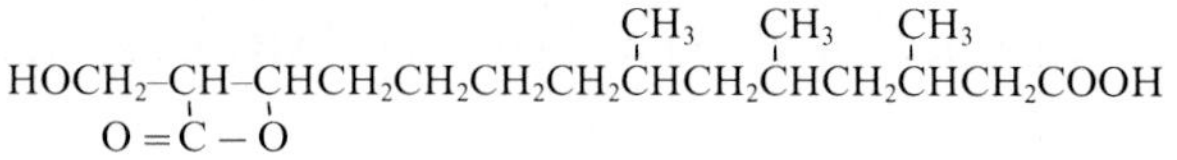 $\underset{O=C-O}{HOCH_2-CH-CHCH_2CH_2CH_2CH_2\overset{CH_3}{CHCH_2}\overset{CH_3}{CHCH_2}\overset{CH_3}{CHCH_2COOH}}$	4	0.43	5
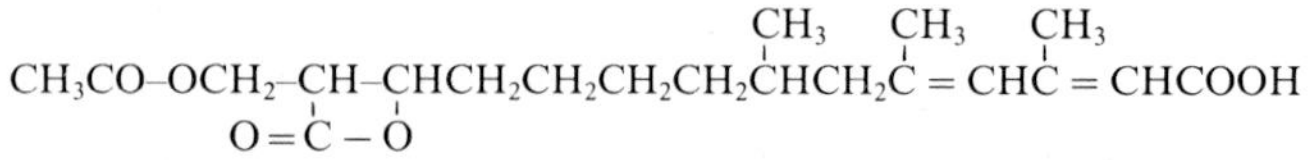 $\underset{O=C-O}{CH_3CO-OCH_2-CH-CHCH_2CH_2CH_2CH_2\overset{CH_3}{CHCH_2}\overset{CH_3}{C}=CH\overset{CH_3}{C}=CHCOOH}$	5	32% at 4.3	135
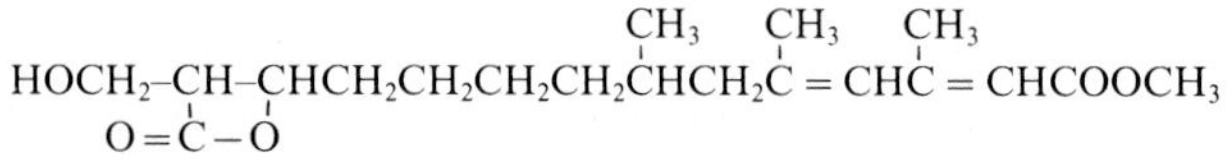 $\underset{O=C-O}{HOCH_2-CH-CHCH_2CH_2CH_2CH_2\overset{CH_3}{CHCH_2}\overset{CH_3}{C}=CH\overset{CH_3}{C}=CHCOOCH_3}$	6	0.27	75
$\underset{O=C-O}{R-CH-CHCHCH_2\overset{CH_3}{C}=CHCHC\overset{CH_3}{C}\overset{O}{C}\overset{CH_3}{CH}\overset{CH_3}{CH}CH_2CH_3}$		> 150	300

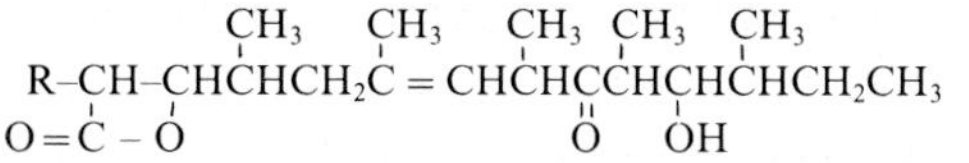

Ebelactone A: R = CH$_3$–

Ebelactone B: R = CH$_3$CH$_2$–

MIC = minimum inhibitory concentration.

loss of the inhibitory activity. Interestingly, ebelactones, which are esterase inhibitors with a β-lactone [15], had no effect on HMG-CoA synthase. These findings indicate that not only the β-lactone but also the hydroxymethyl moiety are responsible for inhibitory activity against HMG-CoA synthase.

On the other hand, the saturated derivative (4) showed the most potent inhibitory activity against Vero cell growth, followed by F-244, the methyl ester derivative (6) and the acetylated one (5). The difference in potency against the two activities (enzyme activity and Vero cell growth) might arise from different membrane permeabilities of the drugs.

ACKNOWLEDGEMENTS

The authors are grateful to Dr. T. Aoyagi, Institute of Microbial Chemistry, Tokyo, Japan, for his generous gift of ebelactones. They are also indebted to Mr. H. Kumagai and Mr. K. Igarashi for their excellent technical assistance.

REFERENCES

1 Aldridge, D.C., D. Gil and W.B. Turner. 1971. Antibiotic 1233A: a fungal β-lactone. J. Chem. Soc. (C) 3888–3891.
2 Kawaguchi, A., H. Tomoda, J. Awaya, S. Omura and S. Okuda. 1979. Cerulenin resistance in a cerulenin-producing fungus. Isolation of cerulenin resistant fatty acid synthetase. Arch. Biochem. Biophys. 197: 30–35.

3 Ōmura, S. 1976. The antibiotic cerulenin, a novel tool for biochemistry as an inhibitor of fatty acid synthesis. Bacteriol. Rev. 40: 681–697.

4 Ōmura, S. 1981. Cerulenin. Methods Enzymol. 72: 520–532.

5 Ōmura, S., Y. Iwai, A. Nakagawa, R. Iwata, Y. Takahashi, H. Shimizu and H. Tanaka. 1983. Thiotetromycin, a new antibiotic. Taxonomy, production, isolation, and physicochemical and biological properties. J. Antibiot. 36: 109–114.

6 Ōmura, S., H. Tomoda, H. Kumagai, M.D. Greenspan, J.B. Yodkovitz, J.C. Chen, A.W. Alberts, I. Martin, S. Mochals, R.L. Monaghan, J.C. Chabala, R.E. Schwartz and A.A. Patchett. 1987. Potent inhibitory effect of antibiotic 1233A on cholesterol biosynthesis which specifically blocks 3-hydroxy-3-methylglutaryl coenzyme A synthase. J. Antibiot. 40: 1356–1357.

7 Ōmura, S., H. Tomoda, Q.-M. Xu, Y. Takahashi and Y. Iwai. 1986. Traicsins, new inhibitors of acyl-CoA synthetase produced by Streptomyces sp. J. Antibiot. 39: 1211–1218.

8 Powell, G.L., P.S. Tippett, T.C. Kiorpes, J. McMillin-Wood, K.E. Coll, H. Schultz, K. Tanaka, E.S. Kang and E. Shrage. 1985. Fatty acyl-CoA as an effector molecule in metabolism. Fed. Proc. 44: 81–84.

9 Tanaka, H., K. Yoshida, Y. Itoh and H. Imanaka. 1982. Studies on new vasodilators, WS-1228A and B. I. Discovery, taxonomy, isolation and characterization. J. Antibiot. 35: 157–163.

10 Tomoda, H., K. Igarashi and S. Ōmura. 1987. Inhibition of acyl-CoA synthetase by triacsins. Biochim. Biophys. Acta 921: 595–598.

11 Tomoda, H., A. Kawaguchi, S. Ōmura and S. Okuda. 1984. Cerulenin resistance in a cerulenin-producing fungus. II. J. Biochem. 95: 1705–1712.

12 Tomoda, H., A. Kawaguchi, T. Yasuhara, T. Nakajima, S. Ōmura and S. Okuda. 1984. Cerulenin resistance in a cerulenin-producing fungus. III. J. Biochem. 95: 1712–1723.

13 Tomoda, H., H. Kumagai, Y. Takahashi, Y. Iwai, Y. Tanaka and S. Ōmura. 1988. F-244 (1233A), a specific inhibitor of 3-hydroxy-3-methylglutaryl coenzyme A synthase. Taxonomy of producing strain, fermentation, isolation and biological properties. J. Antibiot. 41: 247–249.

14 Tomoda, H., H. Kumagai, H. Tanaka and S. Ōmura. 1987. F-244 specifically inhibits 3-hydroxy-3-methylglutaryl coenzyme A synthase. Biochim. Biophys. Acta 922: 351–356.

15 Umezawa, H., T. Aoyagai, K. Uotani, K. Hamada, T. Takeuchi and S. Takahashi. 1980. Ebelactone, an inhibitor of esterase, produced by actinomycetes. J. Antibiot. 33: 1594–1595.

16 Wakil, S.J. and J.K. Stoops. 1983. Structure and mechanism of fatty acid synthetase. In: The Enzymes (Boyer, P.D., ed.), pp. 3–61, Academic Press, New York.

Novel Microbial Products for Medicine and Agriculture
Editors: A.L. Demain, G.A. Somkuti, J.C. Hunter-Cevera and H.W. Rossmoore
179

CHAPTER 21

Amicoumacin and SF-2370, pharmacologically active agents of microbial origin

Shigeharu Inouye and Shinichi Kondo

Central Research Laboratories, Meiji Seika Kaisha, Ltd., Yokohama, Japan

SUMMARY

Amicoumacins A, B and C were found in the culture broth of *Bacillus pumilus* BN-103 as new antibiotics. A similar series of metabolites, AI-77s, were isolated from *Bacillus pumilus* AI-77 as antiulcer agents. Amicoumacins A and B showed antiinflammatory activity against carrageenin-induced rat paw edema by oral administration. In addition, amicoumacin A showed antiulcer activity against water-immersion-induced gastric ulcer in rats. In experiments to elucidate the mechanism of action, amicoumacin A showed no significant influence against the enzymes involving the arachidonic acid cascade and antigen-induced histamine release from mast cells. However, it weakly suppressed the release of superoxide anion and strongly inhibited the proliferation of thymocyte cells induced by interleukin 1. An antibiotic, SF-2370, was found in the culture of *Actinomadura* sp. The same metabolite, K-252a, was isolated from *Nocardiopsis* sp. as an inhibitor of protein kinase C. SF-2370 and in particular its alkylamino derivatives, NA0344, NA0345 and NA0346, showed potent hypotensive and diuretic actions against spontaneously hypertensive and normotensive rats. In isolated vascular smooth muscles contracted by high K^+, the relaxing actions of the NA derivatives were slow in onset but gradually increased and were well sustained even after the drugs were thoroughly washed out.

AMICOUMACIN A, A POTENT ANTIINFLAMMATORY AND ANTIULCER AGENT

Introduction

An interest in screening microbial products for antiinflammatory agents dates back to as early as the 1960s, when antiinflammatory proteinases were introduced in the clinic in Japan. In addition to proteinases, a large number of microbial metabolites including amylases, polysaccharides and low molecular weight compounds have been claimed as antiinflammatory agents [24]. A systematic search for antiulcer agents of microbial origin was started in the 1970s, and polysaccharides, glycoproteins and many low molecular weight compounds were reported. Professor Hamao Umezawa made a great contribution in this field, isolating various antiinflammatory proteinases [26] and enzyme inhibitors [47].

Isolation of amicoumacins

In the course of our screening program for new antibiotics, amicoumacins were detected in the culture broth of *Bacillus pumilus* BN-103 using *Staphylococcus aureus* as a test organism in 1981. Isolation of amicoumacins was effected through

Amberlite IRC-50, active carbon and Diaion HP-20 columns to give a crude powder. Further purification by the use of a Sephadex G-10 column resulted in the separation of amicoumacins A, B and C [13, 14].

The structures of amicoumacins were determined by chemical degradation coupled to spectroscopic analysis, and especially chemical transformation of three amicoumacins shown in Fig. 1 established the structural relation of the amicoumacins. Hydrolysis of amicoumacin A by mild alkaline treatment yielded amicoumacin B, which could be converted to amicoumacin C by lactonization on treatment with trifluoroacetic acid. Opening of a lactone ring of amicoumacin C with ammonia gave amicoumacin A with an amide bond. X-ray crystallographic analysis of amicoumacin B revealed the stereochemical profile, showing a scissor-like structure consisting of an isobutyryl group and a hydroxyamino acid side chain which was ejected from the isocoumarin nucleus (Fig. 2) [12].

Amicoumacin A showed potent antibacterial activity against mainly gram-positive bacteria. The activities of amicoumacins B and C were greatly re-

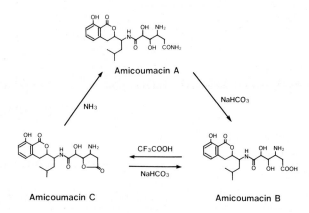

Fig. 1. Chemical transformation of amicoumacins A, B and C.

duced, weakly active against these strains (Table 1). In addition, amicoumacin A was mitocidal, especially against the two-spotted spider mite. Acute toxicity (LD_{50}) of amicoumacin A was 132 mg/kg by oral administration [14].

A search of the literature revealed that microbial metabolites containing the isocoumarin nucleus were less numerous than the coumarin derivatives. The isocoumarin derivatives [7, 9, 23, 31, 35] related

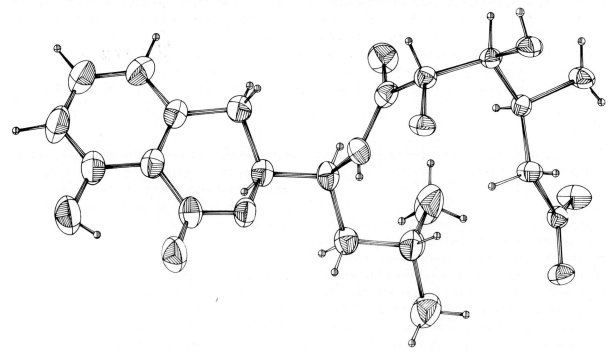

Fig. 2. A molecular profile of amicoumacin B.

Table 1

Antibacterial activity of amicoumacins A, B and C

Compound	MIC (μg/ml)[a]			
	Staphylococcus aureus 209P JC-1	Bacillus anthracis No. 119	Escherichia coli NIHJ JC-2	Salmonella enteritidis No. 11
Amicoumacin A	0.39	3.13	100	1.56
Amicoumacin B	25	>100	>100	50
Amicoumacin C	25	>100	>100	50

[a] Minimum inhibitory concentrations (MICs) were determined by the two-fold agar dilution method using heart infusion broth and an inoculum of 10^6 cfu.

to amicoumacins are shown in Fig. 3. Amicoumacins resembled most closely baciphelacin [31] and especially xenocoumacins [7] in structure and bioactivity. Xenocoumacins 1 and 2 were isolated from the culture broth of Xenorhabdus nematophilus and X. luminescens, which are symbiotic microbes present in the pathogenic nematode that is an insect parasite. They showed antiulcer activity against rat stress ulcer as well as antiinflammatory and antimicrobial activities.

Antiinflammatory and antiulcer activity of amicoumacin A

Table 2 shows the antiinflammatory activity of

amicoumacins A and B compared to phenylbutazone used as a reference drug. Amicoumacin A was effective in a dose-dependent manner against rat paw edema induced by carrageenin, and its activity was comparable to that of phenylbutazone at an oral dosage of 50 mg/kg. Amicoumacin B was only slightly active by oral administration [14].

Antiulcer activity of amicoumacin A against stress-induced gastric ulcer in rats is shown in Table 3. An oral dose of 10 mg/kg of amicoumacin A was comparable to a dose of 30 mg/kg of sulpiride in the prevention of gastric ulcer, and a higher dose (25 mg/kg) gave superior activity to that of sulpiride [14].

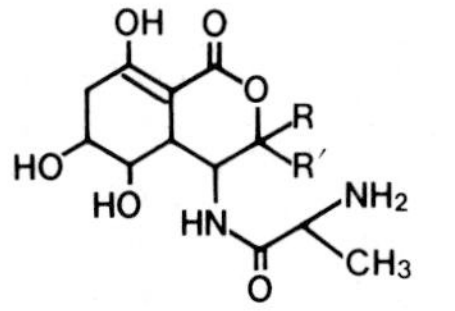

Actinobolin (1959) (R=H, R'=CH₃)
Bactobolin (1979) (R=CH₃, R'=CHCl₂)
anti-tumor activity

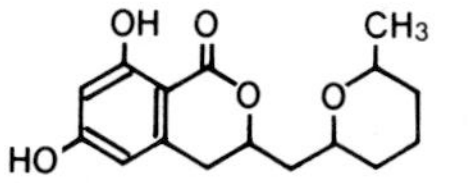

Cladosporin (1971)
antifungal activity

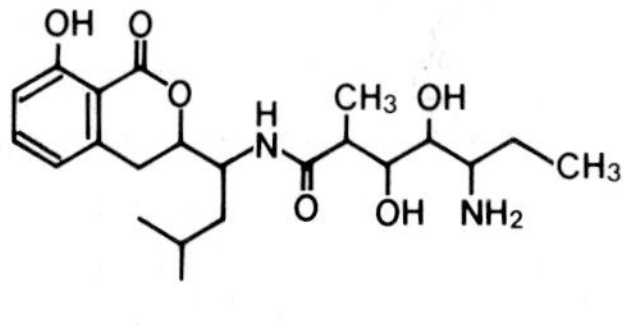

Baciphelacin (1975)
antimicrobial activity

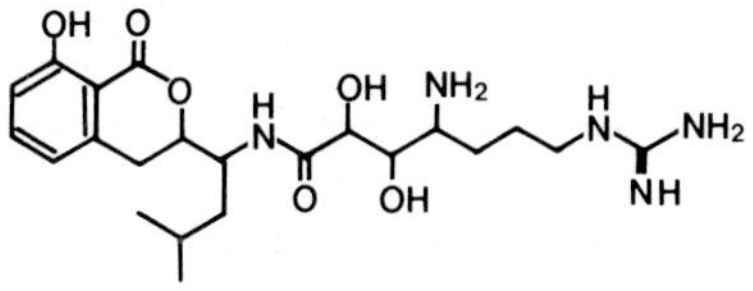

Xenocoumacin 1 (1986)
anti-ulcer activity

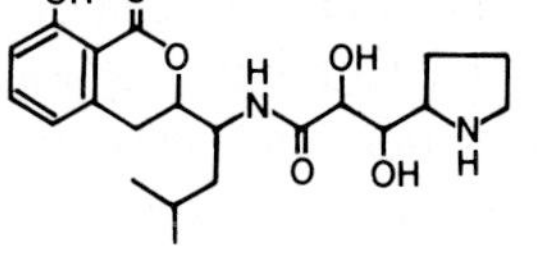

Xenocoumacin 2 (1986)
anti-ulcer activity

Fig. 3. Chemical structures of microbial metabolites related to amicoumacins.

Table 2

Antiinflammatory activity of amicoumacins A and B and phenylbutazone against rat paw edema induced by carrageenin[a]

Compound	Oral dose (mg/kg)	Swelling[b] (%)	Inhibition (%)
Amicoumacin A	10	66.9 ± 3.4	8.0
Amicoumacin A	25	61.0 ± 4.1	16.1
Amicoumacin A	50	$49.4 \pm 5.2*$	32.0
Amicoumacin B	25	62.0 ± 5.8	14.7
Amicoumacin B	50	$58.2 \pm 3.4*$	19.9
Phenylbutazone	50	$50.9 \pm 4.7*$	30.0
Vehicle	—	72.7 ± 4.7	0

[a] A drug suspended in 0.5% gum arabic was administered orally to male Wistar rats ($n = 5$), and 1.0% carrageenin solution was injected 1 h later. The size of paw edema was measured 3 h after injection.
[b] Mean $\pm$ S.E.
$*P < 0.05$.

Table 3

Antiulcer activity of amicoumacin A and sulpiride against gastric ulcer in rats induced by water-immersion[a]

Compound	Oral dose (mg/kg)	Ulcer index[b]	Prevention (%)
Amicoumacin A	10	$2.80 \pm 0.58*$	34.1
Amicoumacin A	25	$1.20 \pm 0.20**$	71.8
Sulpiride	30	$2.80 \pm 0.55*$	34.1
Saline	—	4.25 ± 0.48	–

[a] Male Sprague-Dawley rats ($n = 5$) were fixed in a rocket type cage and drugs were administered orally 30 min before immersion into water at $23 \pm 1°C$ up to the xiphoid. The rats were sacrificed after 6 h stress, and the size of ulcer inside the stomach was measured and graded into five degrees.
[b] Mean $\pm$ S.E.
$*P < 0.05$; $**P < 0.01$.

In relation to the mechanism of action, we have investigated the effect of amicoumacins on some enzymes and chemical mediators that appeared to be involved in inflammation and ulceration. Since many nonsteroidal antiinflammatory agents inhibit the key enzymes in the biosynthesis of prostaglandins [6, 42], the inhibitory activities against cyclooxygenase from sheep vesicular gland and 5-lipoxygenase from rat basophilic leukemia cells were examined. However, no inhibition was shown against cyclooxygenase at 50 μg/ml, and against 5-lipoxygenase at 25 μg/ml. Only slight inhibition was observed against phospholipase A_2 from porcine pancreas (40% inhibition at 200 μg/ml), which is related to the release of arachidonic acid from membrane. Therefore, amicoumacin has no significant influence on enzymes involving the arachidonic acid cascade, and is different from typical nonsteroidal antiinflammatory agents in its mechanism of action.

Amicoumacins A and B showed a weak inhibitory effect on histamine release from rat peritoneal exudate cells induced by DNP-ascaris as the antigen. However, as shown in Table 4, the inhibitory

Table 4

Effects of amicoumacins A and B and tranilast on the histamine release from rat peritoneal exudate cells with DNP-ascaris[a]

Compound	Concentration (μg/ml)	Histamine release[b] (ng/40 μl)	Suppression (%)
Amicoumacin A	0.1	29.4 ± 0.5	22.7
	1.0	29.9 ± 2.6	20.7
	10.0	29.3 ± 1.4	23.1
	100.0	32.0 ± 1.2	12.0
Amicoumacin B	0.1	29.6 ± 1.2	21.9
	1.0	$28.4 \pm 1.3*$	26.9
	10.0	30.1 ± 1.8	19.8
	100.0	$28.6 \pm 1.4*$	26.0
Tranilast	0.1	33.9 ± 2.8	4.1
	1.0	30.5 ± 1.2	18.2
	10.0	$21.5 \pm 0.5**$	55.4
	100.0	$18.6 \pm 0.5**$	67.4
Non-treatment control	—	34.9 ± 1.7	0.0
Spontaneous release	—	10.7 ± 1.8	—

[a] Peritoneal exudate cells collected from male Wistar rats weighing about 300 g ($n = 4$) were sensitized by incubation with rat antiserum against DNP-ascaris at 37°C for 2 h. A suspension of the mast cells in Hanks' solution was prewarmed at 37°C for 5 h, and incubated for 20 min after addition of the test sample and then the antigen (DNP-ascaris). The amount of histamine released was assayed fluorometrically with o-phthalaldehyde.
[b] Mean $\pm$ S.E.
$*P < 0.05$; $**P < 0.01$.

effect was not dose-dependent in the concentration range of 0.1–100 $\mu g/ml$, while tranilast used as a reference drug inhibited in a dose-dependent manner. These results suggested that the membrane-stabilizing effect may not be a major cause of the antiinflammatory action of amicoumacin.

Active oxygen species are known to be implicated in inflammation [10]. The effects of amicoumacins A and B on the generation of superoxide anion in rat polymorphonuclear leukocytes are shown in Table 5. Leukocytes were activated by exposure to opsonized zymosan to enhance their O_2 uptake leading to generation of superoxide anion. The inhibitory effect of amicoumacin A was dose-dependent, but its effect at 300 $\mu g/ml$ was one tenth of that of diclofenac used as a reference drug.

Table 6 shows the effect of amicoumacins A and B on the proliferation of thymocytes stimulated by interleukin 1. Amicoumacin A significantly inhibited the uptake of [3H]thymidine at 1 $\mu g/ml$, being ten times more potent than amicoumacin B, in parallel to the order of antiinflammatory activity. The inhibition of cell proliferation was not due to cytotoxicity, since most of the cells remained viable. The high inhibitory activity of amicoumacin A against the interleukin 1-stimulated reaction is worth investigating in more detail, since interleukin 1 is believed to be involved in various inflammatory pro-

Table 5

Inhibitory effects of amicoumacins A and B and diclofenac on the generation of superoxide anion in rat polymorphonuclear leukocytes induced by opsonized zymosan[a]

Compound	Suppression (%)[b]		
	30 $\mu g/ml$	100 $\mu g/ml$	300 $\mu g/ml$
Amicoumacin A	-1.12 ± 1.42	$4.72 \pm 0.73*$	$13.59 \pm 1.07**$
Amicoumacin B	-1.26 ± 1.11	-0.22 ± 0.61	$3.98 \pm 0.24**$
Diclofenac	$12.35 \pm 0.28**$	$30.08 \pm 0.36**$	$46.48 \pm 0.32**$

[a] Leukocytes (1×10^7), the test sample and ferricytochrome c (0.1 mM) were incubated in the presence of opsonized zymosan for 30 min at 37°C. The generation of O_2^- was determined by the reduction of ferricytochrome c at 550 nm.
[b] Mean $\pm$ S.E.
$*P<0.05$; $**P<0.01$.

Table 6

Inhibitory effects of amicoumacins A and B on the proliferation of thymocytes responding to interleukin 1[a]

Compound	IL 1 (U/ml)	Uptake of [3H]thymidine (uptake of vehicle = 100)			
		0.01 $\mu g/ml$	0.1 $\mu g/ml$	1 $\mu g/ml$	10 $\mu g/ml$
Amicoumacin A	0.5	128.4	77.9	22.1*	29.2*
	1.0	75.1	24.0*	2.2**	13.4*
Amicoumacin B	0.5	125.4	160.4	148.2	20.6*
	1.0	49.1	64.5	64.0	11.9*

[a] A mixture of the thymocyte suspension (5×10^6 cells/100 μl/ well) of C3H/He male mice, interleukin 1 (50 μl) and sample (50 μl) in RPMI 1140 medium containing phytohemagglutinin (1 $\mu g/ml$) was cultured for 48 h in a CO_2 incubator, and further cultured for 16 h after addition of [3H]thymidine (0.5 $\mu Ci/20$ ml/well) for pulse labeling. The uptake of [3H]thymidine (cpm) was assayed with a liquid scintillation counter.
$*P<0.05$; $**P<0.01$.

cesses [29].

Regarding the mechanism of antiulcer action, we have examined the anticholinergic property of amicoumacin A, but at 1–100 $\mu g/ml$ it showed no effect on the contraction of isolated ileum of guinea pig and rabbit with acetylcholine (10^{-6} M). The activity against H^+/K^+-ATPase from porcine gastric membrane, which is related to gastric secretion [5], was also negligible (10% inhibition at 200 $\mu g/ml$).

Amicoumacin A could be classified in the category of basic antiinflammatory drugs, but has a unique chemical and pharmacological profile. It is less active than acidic antiinflammatory drugs such as indomethacin and diclofenac, but practically equal to phenylbutazone. The most characteristic feature of amicoumacin A is that the compound has antiulcer activity, in addition to antiinflammatory activity. This is in sharp contrast to many of the nonsteroidal antiinflammatory agents that induce ulcerogenicity arising from the inhibition of prostaglandin biosynthesis. The mechanism of action of amicoumacin A is probably different from those of common antiinflammatory agents. It will be of interest to investigate in the future whether or not the same mechanism of action is operative in the antiinflammatory and antiulcer activities.

Isolation and evaluation of AI-77s

Shimojima *et al.* [38] reported in 1982 the isolation of a series of AI-77s from the culture broth of *Bacillus pumilus* AI-77 in a screening program searching for new antiulcer agents of microbial origin. They are AI-77-A, B, C, D, E, F and G, of which AI-77-B is identical to amicoumacin B, and AI-77-A is very close to amicoumacin A, probably identical [39, 40].

The structure-antiulcer activity relationships of AI-77s were extensively investigated by Shimojima *et al.* [37], and Fig. 4 illustrates a part of their work. Among nine compounds compared, the activity against the stress ulcer induced by water-immersion in rats was most potent in AI-77-B. Lactonization of AI-77-B (amicoumacin C) resulted in a slight decrease of the activity. *N*-Acylation (AI-77-C, D, diacetyl-AI-77-C), deamination (AI-77-F) or ring opening of the isocoumarin moiety (AI-77-G) led to inactivation, while *O*-methylation (*O*-methyl-AI-77-B) retained the activity. Interestingly, *N*-alkylation (AI-77-C2) did not reduce the activity, but in-

creased the activity by oral administration.

Fig. 5 shows the *in vivo* metabolic relation of AI-77s in rats. According to Shimojima *et al.* [37, 41], there were two active forms *in vivo*: one was the amide of AI-77-B (amicoumacin A) and the other, AI-77-B (amicoumacin B). About 20% of the amide was converted to AI-77-B *in vivo*. γ-Lactones of AI-77-B (amicoumacin C) and AI-77-C2 (*N*-ethylamicoumacin C) were prodrugs for oral dosing and were converted to AI-77-B *in vivo*.

AI-77-C2 showed a broad antiulcer spectrum. When given orally against a variety of rat ulceration models [48], AI-77-C2 prevented the development of stress ulcer induced by water-immersion and pylorus-ligated ulceration. More interestingly, AI-77-C2 prevented the gastric ulcer induced by indomethacin and aspirin. In addition to the antiulcer activity, AI-77-C2 showed a broad antiinflammatory spectrum [41]. It was active against bradykinin and dextran-induced paw edema, ultraviolet erythema and adjuvant arthritis, but not active against carrageenin-induced paw edema.

In connection with the mechanism of antiulcer action, Urushidani *et al.* [48] reported that, when AI-77-C2 was given intraduodenally, it exhibited

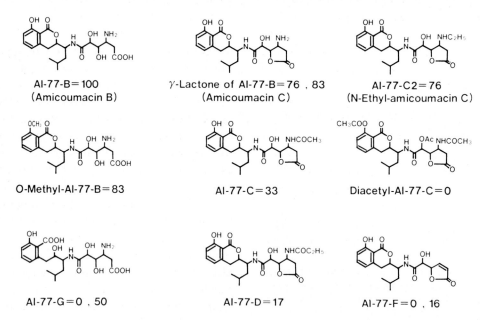

Fig. 4. Structure-antiulcer activity relationships of AI-77s. Protective values (%) at a dose of 25 mg/kg i.p. in rats are shown. Values above 60% are significantly effective. Data are cited and rearranged from Refs. 37, 38 and 41.

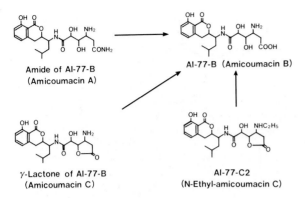

Amide of AI-77-B
(Amicoumacin A)

AI-77-B (Amicoumacin B)

γ-Lactone of AI-77-B
(Amicoumacin C)

AI-77-C2
(N-Ethyl-amicoumacin C)

Fig. 5. *In vivo* metabolism of AI-77s in rats. Data are cited and rearranged from Refs. 37 and 41.

an inhibitory activity against gastric secretion in a dose-dependent manner. Four hours after pylorus ligation, the gastric juice volume was markedly reduced at 50 mg/kg and even at 8 mg/kg. A slight reduction in acid concentration was observed, and acid output was markedly inhibited. In contrast, peptic activity largely increased, while pepsin output reduced slightly, reflecting the reduction in volume of gastric juice. These results indicated that AI-77-C2 had no effect on the secretion of pepsin and that the main action of AI-77-C2 was a marked inhibition of gastric juice secretion. In this connection, Kitagawa *et al.* [21] reported that a significant increase in gastric secretion was probably involved in the pathogenicity of stress ulcer.

Acid secretion by the parieted cells is regulated by histaminic, muscarinic and gastrinic receptors [4]. Furthermore, E-type prostaglandins modulate gastric secretion [2]. In this respect, Shimojima *et al.* [41] reported that AI-77s were not antihistaminic, anticholinergic and central suppressive. The anti-ulcer activity of AI-77-C2 was significantly enhanced by coadministration of indomethacin (5 mg/kg, s.c.), suggesting that endogenous prostaglandins were not involved in the mechanism of protection.

When injected intravenously, AI-77-C2 showed a suppression of gastric motility. It has been proposed that gastric hypermotility plays a major role in the development of gastric necrosis, especially in the stress ulcer [15], and an inhibition of such a re-

sponse may lead to protection of the gastric mucosa.

SF-2370 AND ITS DERIVATIVES, POTENT HYPOTENSIVE AGENTS

Introduction

A systemic approach to the search for microbial metabolites with hypotensive activity has been pioneered by Professor Hamao Umezawa and his group. Screening for enzyme inhibitors involved in catecholamine biosynthesis led to the discovery of a series of hypotensive agents [47].

Current interest in this field has concentrated on the screening of enzyme inhibitors from the culture broth against the renin-angiotensin system, and more than 18 metabolites have been claimed as acetylcholinesterase and renin inhibitors of microbial origin [28].

Another approach to the discovery of hypotensive agents in culture broths was to utilize the direct relaxant action on vascular smooth muscle or direct measurement of decrease in blood pressure. Along this line, various vasodilatory agents of microbial origin have been reported [45].

Isolation of SF-2370

An antibiotic, SF-2370, was discovered in 1985 in the course of our screening program using an anticoccidium assay. A culture broth of *Actinomadura* sp. SF-2370 was extracted with ethyl acetate followed by precipitation with *n*-hexane to give a crude powder. Further purification over a silica gel column and TLC gave pure SF-2370 as crystals [36].

The structure of SF-2370 (Fig. 6) was determined by chemical and physico-chemical properties, and confirmed by X-ray diffraction analysis [18]. The molecular profile of SF-2370 revealed an extremely condensed gathering in the indolocarbazole moiety, and some aromatic C=C bond lengths were unusually short. Moreover, the two terminal benzene rings made an angle of 7.4° with each other, probably due to steric hindrance.

SF-2370 is active against only a limited number

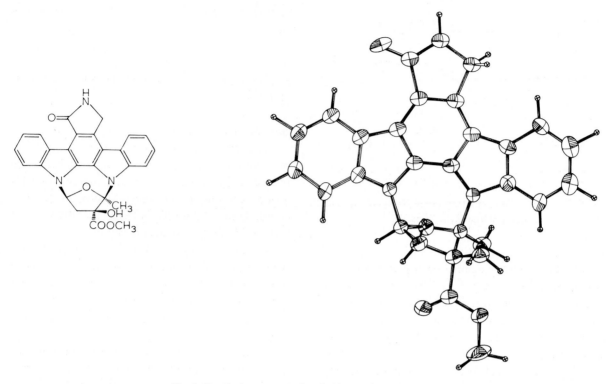

Fig. 6. Chemical structure and molecular profile of SF-2370.

of bacteria and yeasts (Table 7). Acute toxicity (LD_{50}) by intraperitoneal administration to mice was more than 300 mg/kg [36].

SF-2370 belongs to a unique class of antibiotics that have the indolocarbazole moiety in common. Among this group, staurosporine was the first to be isolated in 1977 by Professor Omura [32], followed by more than six other members [3, 11, 17, 27, 36, 43, 44] including SF-2370. K-252a, which was identical to SF-2370, was found in 1986 by Kase *et al.* [17] in the culture broth of *Nocardiopsis* sp. in a screening program aiming at inhibitors of the Ca^{2+} messenger system. As shown in Table 8, metabolites belonging to this group were produced by a variety of organisms and exhibited a variety of pharmacological activities including hypotensive action, platelet aggregation inhibition, protein kinase inhibition, and antitumor action. Especially with regard to K-252a, potent inhibitory activity against secretion and aggregation in rabbit platelet [49], secretion in rat mast cells and neutrophils [34]

and various protein kinases including protein kinase C [16] was reported.

Table 7

Antimicrobial activity and acute toxicity of SF-2370

Test organism	MIC[a] (μg/ml)
Staphylococcus aureus JC-1	>200
Bacillus subtilis ATCC 6633	>200
Escherichia coli JC-2	>200
Micrococcus luteus	6.25
Corynebacterium bovis 1810	6.25
Candida albicans C-A-24	6.25
Aspergillus fumigatis	>100
Trichophyton mentagrophytes	>100
LD_{50} (mg/kg) i.p. (mice)	>300

[a] Minimum inhibitory concentration (MIC) was determined by the agar dilution method, using a modified Mueller-Hinton medium for bacteria and a Sabouraud medium for fungi and yeast with an inoculum of 10^6 cfu.

Table 8

Producing microorganisms and screening assay methods for staurosporine and related metabolites possessing the indolocarbazole moiety

Compound	Producer	Screening assay	Ref.
Staurosporine	*Streptomyces staurosporeus*	alkaloid	32
Staurosporine	*Streptomyces actuosus*	differentiation-inducing activity	25
Staurosporine	*Streptomyces* sp.	inhibition of platelet aggregation	30
Staurosporine	*Streptomyces* sp.	inhibition of protein kinase C	46
Arcyriaflavins	*Arcyria denudata*	fungal pigment	43
SF-2370	*Actinomadura* sp.	anticoccidium activity	36
K-252a	*Nocardiopsis* sp.	inhibition of Ca^{2+} messenger system	17, 27
Rebeccamycin	*Saccharothrix aerocolonigenes*	antitumor activity	3
UCN-01	*Streptomyces* sp.	inhibition of protein kinase C	44
AT-2433	*Actinomadura melliaura*	antitumor activity	11

In the following paragraphs, the discussion is limited to the hypotensive action of SF-2370 and its chemical derivatives, NA0344, 0345, 0346 and 0339 (Fig. 7). These derivatives were prepared from SF-2370 by reduction of the methoxycarbonyl group followed by a ring opening of the intermediate epoxy function with appropriate alkylamines, and by bromination followed by hydrolysis of the methyl ester group.

So far, three microbial hypotensive agents containing the indole moiety have been reported (Fig. 8). Staurosporine [32] is most closely related to SF-2370 and in particular to NA0345 that contains an *N*-methyl group. Amauromine [45], which is a vasodilator, has some similarity to SF-2370. Rugulovasine [1] is rather similar to dihydroergotoxins which are used in the clinic for hypertensive patients.

Hypotensive activity of SF-2370 and NA derivatives [8]

In the early stage of evaluation of SF-2370, it was found that it possessed potent diuretic action

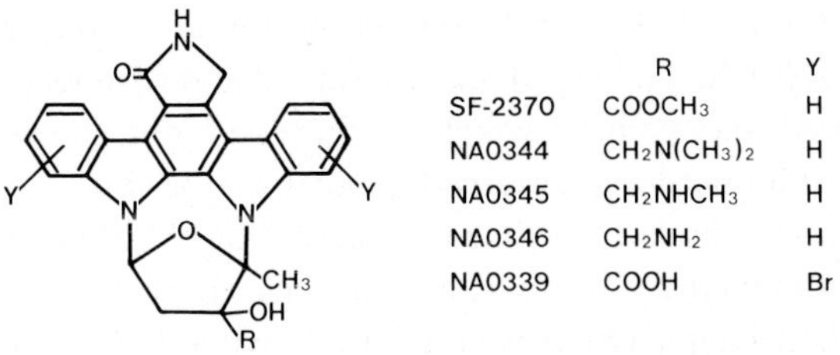

Fig. 7. Chemical structures of NA derivatives of SF-2370.

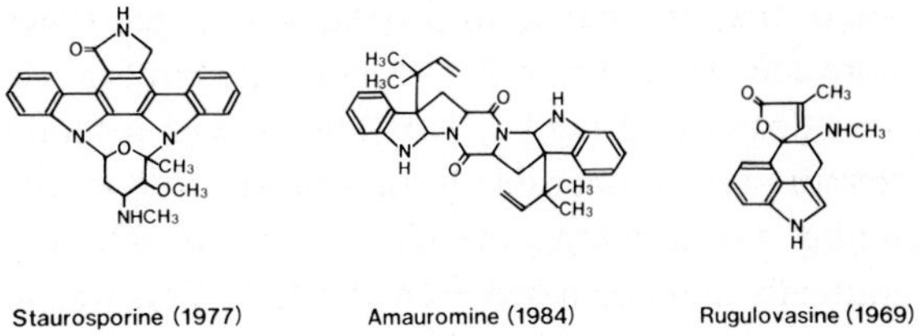

	R	Y
SF-2370	COOCH₃	H
NA0344	CH₂N(CH₃)₂	H
NA0345	CH₂NHCH₃	H
NA0346	CH₂NH₂	H
NA0339	COOH	Br

Staurosporine (1977) Amauromine (1984) Rugulovasine (1969)

Fig. 8. Chemical structures of microbial hypotensive agents possessing the indole moiety.

upon oral administration to rats (Table 9). Thus, at a dose of 10 or 30 mg/kg, SF-2370 produced an increase in urine volume and urine sodium in a dose-

Table 9

Diuretic effects of SF-2370 and hydroflumethiazide on saline-loaded rats[a]

Compound	Oral dose (mg/kg)	Urine volume (ml/100 g /5 h)	Urine sodium (μEq./100 g /5 h)
SF-2370	10	1.9±0.1*	466±46*
SF-2370	30	2.3±0.1*	519±29*
Hydroflumethiazide	30	1.9±0.1*	438±38
Vehicle	—	1.4±0.2	271±32

[a] Male Sprague-Dawley rats weighing 220–250 g were loaded with 5 ml saline 30 min after the oral administration of drug. Urine was collected for 5 h in a urine-collecting cage. The sodium ion concentration was determined with an ion-meter.
*$P < 0.05$.

dependent manner. The diuretic action of SF-2370 was more potent than that of hydroflumethiazide used as a reference drug at 30 mg/kg. Since the diuretic action is closely related to the hypotensive action [22], the vascular activity of SF-2370 was examined using DOCA/salt hypertensive rats, and spontaneously hypertensive (SH) rats. SF-2370 showed a hypotensive effect in these two models.

Fig. 9 shows the antihypertensive effect of SF-2370 on SH rats. It was orally active, and exhibited a long-lasting hypotensive action over 5 h at a dose of 100 mg/kg. The maximal depression of blood pressure was 18% at 1 h after dosing.

At an advanced stage of evaluation, it was found that alkylamino derivatives of SF-2370 were more potent than the parent antibiotic, almost ten times more active in SH rats. This is illustrated in Fig. 10. At a dose of 10 mg/kg, NA0344 showed a blood pressure fall comparable to that of SF-2370 at 100 mg/kg. Furthermore, the blood pressure fell very gradually and decreased even after 5 h. This was in contrast to the action of nicardipine, which was used as a reference drug. The blood pressure in rats treated with nicardipine decreased rapidly, reaching a minimum at 2 h, and recovered thereafter. In addition to a long duration of antihypertensive effect, NA0344 caused little change of the heart rate,

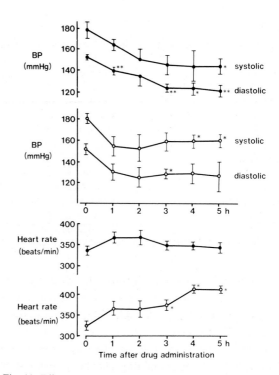

Fig. 10. Effects of orally administered NA0344 and nicardipine on the blood pressure and the heart rate of conscious SH rats ($n = 3$). Dose, 10 mg/kg. The experimental conditions were the same as in Fig. 9. The heart rate was recorded with a tachometer. ●, NA0344; ○, nicardipine. *$P < 0.05$; **$P < 0.01$.

whereas nicardipine caused a rise of heart rate, which lasted at least 5 h. It is known that nicardipine, a specific calcium channel blocker, cause an increase in the heart rate due to baroreflex [20] arising from the stimulation of reflective sympathetic response resulting from the peripheral dilation.

Table 10 compares the antihypertensive effects of three NA derivatives, nicardipine and indapamide for 24 h at an oral dose of 10 mg/kg. NA0344 showed a long-lasting action, with a maximal effect at around 12 h, NA0345 around 8 h and NA0346 around 5 h. Under the same conditions, nicardipine exhibited a maximal decrease at 2 h and then recovered. Indapamide, which is a diuretic agent, showed a mild but long-sustained hypotensive action.

The mode of hypotensive action of NA0344 was examined by intravenous administration to anesthetized normotensive rats. As shown in Fig. 11, the blood pressure gradually decreased and plateaued

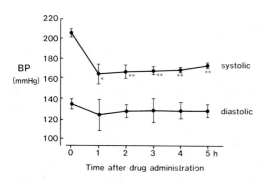

Fig. 9. Effect of orally administered SF-2370 on the blood pressure of conscious SH rats ($n = 3$). Dose, 100 mg/kg. Male SH rats weighing about 300 g were anesthetized with ethyl ether, and a polyethylene catheter was surgically implanted into the occygeal artery to directly monitor the blood pressure. The systolic and diastolic blood pressures were measured under conscious conditions with a pressure transducer coupled to a carrier amplifier and recorded on a polygraph. Vertical bars show the mean ±S.E. *$P < 0.05$ and **$P < 0.01$.

Table 10

Effects of NA derivatives, nicardipine and indapamide on blood pressure in conscious SH rats at an oral dose of 10 mg/kg ($n=4$)[a]

Compound		Before	Time after administration (h)				
			2	5	8	12	24
NA0344	blood pressure[b]	187.4 ± 1.2	176.4 ± 1.9**	163.0 ± 6.2*	163.5 ± 3.4**	157.4 ± 4.5**	168.3 ± 6.5*
	change (%)		−5.9	−13.0	−12.8	−16.0	−10.2
NA0345	blood pressure	190.9 ± 3.3	177.2 ± 5.8	165.3 ± 5.5**	157.1 ± 3.0**	157.6 ± 4.8**	168.4 ± 2.2**
	change (%)		−7.2	−13.4	−17.7	−17.4	−11.8
NA0346	blood pressure	192.7 ± 2.5	179.0 ± 3.8*	175.2 ± 3.0**	173.7 ± 3.9**	181.7 ± 5.6	183.3 ± 3.5
	change (%)		−7.1	−9.1	−9.9	−5.7	−4.9
Nicardipine	blood pressure	194.1 ± 2.9	165.0 ± 7.0**	178.2 ± 0.8*	174.7 ± 3.3**	188.1 ± 5.4	190.9 ± 5.9
	change (%)		−15.0	−8.2	−10.0	−3.1	−1.6
Indapamide	blood pressure	182.5 ± 3.3	178.9 ± 3.5	170.2 ± 3.0*	167.9 ± 4.8*	170.1 ± 4.8	170.3 ± 4.3
	change (%)		−2.0	−6.8	−8.0	−6.8	−7.2
Vehicle	blood pressure	187.5 ± 2.7	188.2 ± 1.3	187.2 ± 2.5	186.3 ± 2.9	186.3 ± 1.7	192.2 ± 3.4
	change (%)		+0.4	−0.2	−0.6	−0.6	+2.5

[a] SH rats weighing about 300 g were prewarmed in a chamber at 37°C for 5 min, and blood pressure was measured at the tail using a plethysmographic pulse pickup.

[b] Mean of systolic blood pressure (mmHg) ± S.E.

*$P < 0.05$; **$P < 0.01$.

at a minimum 2–3 min after injection of NA0344, but nicardipine sharply lowered the blood pressure after injection. Fig. 12 compares the effect of NA0344 and nicardipine on blood pressure and heart rate upon intravenous administration to normotensive rats. Nicardipine showed a hypotensive

action ten times more potent than that of NA0344, but caused an increase of the heart rate, similar to the phenomenon observed upon oral dosing. The heart rate was almost unchanged by NA0344.

Effects of SF-2370 and NA derivatives on aortic contraction [8]

With the purpose of elucidating the mechanism

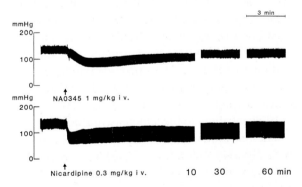

Fig. 11. Typical tracings of the blood pressure of anesthetized Sprague-Dawley rats treated with NA0344 (A, 1 mg/kg, i.v.) and nicardipine (B, 0.3 mg/kg, i.v.). Male Sprague-Dawley rats weighing 400–450 g were anesthetized with sodium pentobarbital, and blood pressure was measured from the cervical artery via an inserted polyethylene tube. A drug was injected into the femoral vein through a polyethylene cannula. Other experimental conditions were the same as in Fig. 9.

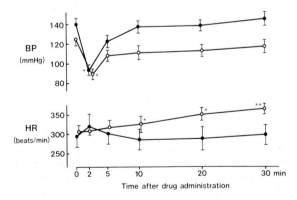

Fig. 12. Effects of intravenously administered NA0344 and nicardipine on the blood pressure and the heart rate of anesthetized normotensive rats ($n=4$). Dose: NA0344, 1 mg/kg; nicardipine, 0.1 mg/kg. The experimental conditions were the same as in Fig. 11. ●, NA0344; ○, nicardipine. *$P < 0.05$; **$P < 0.01$.

of hypotensive action, we have examined the effects of SF-2370 and NA derivatives on the contractile response of isolated thoracic aorta of guinea pigs. In the isolated guinea pig aorta precontracted by norepinephrine (10^{-7} M), SF-2370 and NA derivatives attenuated the contraction in a concentration-dependent manner, as shown in Fig. 13. Among the three compounds compared, NA0344 was the most potent followed by NA0345 and SF-2370. This order was parallel to that of the hypotensive activity.

The inhibitory effects of NA derivatives were further examined on contraction of guinea pig aorta in high-K^+ physiological solution that caused depolarization of the smooth muscle cell membrane. The results are shown in Fig. 14. NA0344 exhibited the most potent inhibition, followed by NA0346. NA0339, which showed a transient hypotensive action in rats by intravenous administration, did not cause any inhibition.

It was noted that the relaxation caused by NA0344 and especially NA0346 did not reach a steady level even after treatment for 120 min. Such

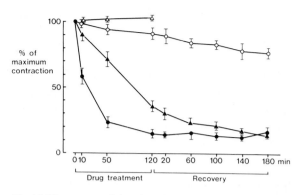

Fig. 14. Time-course of the relaxation with NA derivatives of the high-K^+ (45 mM) induced contraction in guinea pig aorta during treatment and recovery after washing out the drugs. Drug concentration, 10^{-6} M (NA0344, NA0346) or 3×10^{-6} M (NA 0339) ($n = 4$). The experimental conditions were essentially the same as in Fig. 13. The aortic strips were depolarized by raising the external KCl concentration to 45 mM. △, NA0339; ○, vehicle (0.005% dimethyl sulfoxide); ▲, NA0346; ●, NA0344.

a slow response was not common since the relaxation effect usually reached a maximum within half an hour. When the drug was removed from the bathing solution, the contractile response was not immediately recovered, and duration of the relaxation potency was observed for at least 180 min after washing out the drug.

Table 11 compares the hypotensive effect, diuretic action, relaxation of aorta and inhibition of protein kinase C of the NA derivatives. When the magnitude of blood pressure fall was compared, NA0344 was most potent, NA0345 almost equal to NA0344, and NA0346 weakest upon oral administration to SH rats. The order of diuretic activity was almost parallel to that of the hypotensive activity, and suggested that the diuretic action might partly contribute to the hypotensive effect.

The relaxation effect on aorta was most potent with NA0344 followed by NA0346, in parallel to the hypotensive effect. The relaxation by NA0339 was almost negligible. However, all of the compounds, including NA0339, showed high and comparable inhibitory activity against protein kinase C. Therefore, there was an inconsistency between the relaxation activity and the inhibitory activity. It has been reported that protein kinase C is involved in the contraction of vascular smooth muscle [33]. It

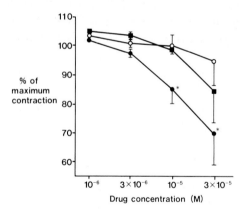

Fig. 13. Dose-response curves of SF-2370 and NA derivatives on the relaxation of guinea pig aortic strips precontracted by norepinephrine ($n = 3$). Spiral strips (2×50 mm) made from thoracic aorta of guinea pigs were suspended in aerated Tyrode solution. The tissues were equilibrated for 30 min, and contracted with 10^{-7} M norepinephrine. Cumulative dose-response curves were obtained by a stepwise increase in the concentration of a drug that was added to the bathing solution. After 20 min, the change of tension was recorded isometrically on a minipolygraph using an FD-pickup. The force of contraction induced with norepinephrine (10^{-7} M) was taken as 100%. ○, SF-2370; ■, NA-0345; ●, NA0344. *$P < 0.05$.

Table 11

A comparison of the NA derivatives in hypotensive and diuretic activities and inhibition of high-K^+-induced aortic contraction and protein kinase C

Compound	Maximum change of BP (mmHg)[a]	Urine volume[b] (ml/100 g/5 h)	Urine sodium[b] (μEq./100 g/5 h)	IC_{50} (μg/ml)	
				aortic contraction[c]	protein kinase C
NA0344	-39.2 ± 2.2	2.6 ± 0.3*	478 ± 19*	0.10	0.053
NA0345	-35.0 ± 5.2	1.9 ± 0.1*	471 ± 53*		0.031
NA0346	-14.2 ± 8.7	1.4 ± 0.1	291 ± 19	0.50	0.027
NA0339				$>> 1.5$	0.050

[a] Systolic blood pressure was determined by the tail-cuff method using male SH rats ($n=4$) by oral administration of 10 mg/kg.

[b] To male Sprague-Dawley rats ($n=5$), saline (2.5 ml/100 g) was loaded 30 min after oral administration of 10 mg/kg. Urine was collected for 5 h.

[c] Inhibitory concentration of a drug causing 50% relaxation of the contractile force induced by high K^+ (45 mM) in guinea pig thoracic aorta. For detailed experimental conditions, see legend to Fig. 13.

[d] The concentration of a drug inhibiting by 50% the activity of protein kinase C from mouse brain was determined according to Kikkawa et al. [19] in the presence of 12-O-tetradecanoylphorbol-13-acetate.

*$P < 0.05$.

is not clear so far why the kinase inhibitory activity was not correlated with the relaxant activity on vascular smooth muscle. An antagonistic action against Ca^{2+} was improbable, since the NA derivatives did not inhibit atrial muscle contraction (data not shown). Other mechanisms are currently under investigation.

In conclusion, SF-2370 and in particular NA derivatives possess a unique pharmacological profile showing a long-lasting hypotensive action, potent diuretic action and slow relaxation and sustained effect even after the drugs are thoroughly washed out.

ACKNOWLEDGEMENTS

We thank J. Itoh, M. Koyama and M. Sezaki for the isolation and preparation of amicoumacins, SF-2370 and its chemical derivatives, Y. Yuda for the antiinflammatory and antiulcer evaluations, M. Hachisu for the hypotensive evaluation, and H. Ikeda for the literature search.

REFERENCES

1 Abe, M., S. Ohmomo, T. Ohashi and T. Tabuchi. 1969. Isolation of chanoclavine-(1) and two new interconvertible alkaloids, rugulovasine A and B, from the culture of *Penicillium concavorugulosum*. Agric. Biol. Chem. 33: 469–471.

2 Banerjee, A.K., A.J. Christmas and C.E. Hall. 1979. A comparative study of the effects of prostaglandins and H_2-receptor antagonists on gastric acid secretion, mucosal blood flow and ulcer formation. Arzneim.-Forsch./Drug Res. 29: 634–639.

3 Bush, J.A., B.H. Long, J.J. Catino and W.T. Bradner. 1987. Production and biological activity of rebeccamycin, a novel antitumor agent. J. Antibiot. 40: 668–678.

4 Debas, H.T. 1977. Regulation of gastric acid secretion. Fed. Proc. 36: 1933–1941.

5 Fellenius, E., T. Berglindh, G. Sachs, L. Olbe, B. Elander, S.-E. Sjostrand and B. Wallmark. 1981. Substituted benzimidazoles inhibit gastric acid secretion by blocking (H^+/K^+)ATPase. Nature 290: 159–161.

6 Garcia-Rafanell, J. and J. Forn. 1979. Correlation between antiinflammatory activity and inhibition of prostaglandin biosynthesis induced by various non-steroidal antiinflammatory agents. Arzneim.-Forsch./Drug Res. 29: 630–633.

7 Gregson, R.P. and B.V. McInerney. 1986. Xenocoumacins, PCT Patent WO 8601509.

8 Hachisu, M., T. Hiranuma, S. Sagawa, M. Koyama and M. Nishio. 1987. Antihypertensive activity of SF-2370 derivatives, a potent protein kinase C inhibitor. Jpn. J. Pharmacol. 43: 295P.

9 Haskell, T.H. and Q.R. Bartz. 1959. Actinobolin, a new broad-spectrum antibiotic. Isolation and characterization. Antibiot. Ann. 1958–1959: 505–509.

10 Hirschelmann, R. and H. Bekemeier. 1981. Effects of catalase, peroxidase, superoxide dismutase and 10 scavengers of oxygen radicals in carrageenin edema and in adjuvant arthritis of rats. Experientia 37: 1313–1314.

11 Horan, A.C., J. Golik, J.A. Matson and M.G. Patel. 1986. Novel antibiotics, process for their preparation and pharmaceutical compositions containing them. Jap Kokai Pat. 61: 106592.

12 Itoh, J., S. Omoto, N. Nishizawa, Y. Kodama and S. Inouye. 1982. Chemical structures of amicoumacins produced by *Bacillus pumilus*. Agric. Biol. Chem. 46: 2659–2665.

13 Itoh, J., S. Omoto, T. Shomura, N. Nishizawa, S. Miyado, Y. Yuda, U. Shibata and S. Inouye. 1981. Amicoumacin-A, a new antibiotic with strong antiinflammatory and antiulcer activity. J. Antibiot. 34: 611–613.

14 Itoh, J., T. Shomura, S. Omoto, S. Miyado, Y. Yuda, U. Shibata and S. Inouye. 1982. Isolation, physicochemical properties and biological activities of amicoumacins produced by *Bacillus pumilus*. Agric. Biol. Chem. 46: 1255–1259.

15 Kagoshima, M. and N. Suguro. 1982. Gastric movement of the rat in reserpine-induced ulcer. Folia Pharmacol. Japon. 80: 231–238.

16 Kase, H., K. Iwahashi, M. Kaneko, C. Murakata, Y. Matsuda, S. Nakanishi, K. Yamada, M. Takahashi and A. Sato. 1987. K-252 compounds, potent inhibitors of protein kinase C and cyclic nucleotide-dependent protein kinases. Jpn. J. Pharmacol. 43 (Suppl.): 202P.

17 Kase, H., K. Iwahashi and Y. Matsuda. 1986. K-252a, a potent inhibitor of protein kinase C from microbial origin. J. Antibiot. 39: 1059–1065.

18 Kasuya, A., A. Itai, Y. Iitaka, Y. Takeuchi, Y. Kodama, K. Kawamura, T. Sasaki, M. Koyama and M. Sezaki. 1986. X-Ray crystal structure of a new indolocarbazole antibiotic, SF-2370. Ann. Rep. Meiji Seika Kaisha 25: 64–69.

19 Kikkawa, U., Y. Takai, R. Minakuchi, S. Inohara and Y. Nishizuka. 1982. Calcium-activated, phospholipid-dependent protein kinase from rat brain. J. Biol. Chem. 257: 13341–13348.

20 Kirchheim, H.R. 1976. Systemic arterial baroceptor reflexes. Physiol. Rev. 56: 100–176.

21 Kitagawa, H., M. Fujiwara and Y. Osumui. 1979. Effect of water-immersion stress on gastric secretion and mucosal blood flow in rats. Gastroenterology 77: 298–302.

22 Koeda, T., M. Hachisu, T. Niizato and Y. Sekizawa. 1979. Influence on blood pressure and some laboratory findings of spontaneously hypertensive rats (SHR) after continuous administration of a combination of hydroflumethiazide and mebutamate or hydroflumethiazide. Pharmacometrics 17: 569–573.

23 Kondo, S., Y. Horiuchi, M. Hamada, T. Takeuchi and H. Umezawa. 1979. A new antitumor antibiotic, bactobolin produced by *Pseudomonas*. J. Antibiot. 32: 1069–1071.

24 Matthews, H.W. and B.F. Wade. 1977. Pharmacologically active compounds from microbial origin. Adv. Appl. Microb. 21: 269–288.

25 Morioka, H., M. Ishihara, H. Shibai and T. Suzuki. 1985. Staurosporine-induced differentiation in a human neuroblastoma cell line, NB-1. Agric. Biol. Chem. 49: 1959–1963.

26 Nakamura, S., M. Hamada, M. Ishizuka and H. Umezawa. 1970. Anti-inflammatory neutral proteinases, retikinonase I and II obtained from *Streptomyces verticillatus* var. *zynogenes*. Chem. Pharm. Bull. 18: 2112–2118.

27 Nakanishi, S., Y. Matsuda, K. Iwahashi and H. Kase. 1986. K-252b, c and d, potent inhibitors of protein kinase C from microbial origin. J. Antibiot. 39: 1066–1071.

28 Nisbet, L.J. and J.W. Westley. 1986. Developments in microbial products screening. Ann. Rep. Med. Chem. 21: 149–157.

29 Nouri, A.M.E., G.S. Panayi and S.M. Goodman. 1984. Cytokines and the chronic inflammation of rheumatic disease. I. The presence of interleukin-1 in synovial fluids. Clin. Exp. Immunol. 55: 295–302.

30 Oka, S., M. Kodama, H. Takeda, N. Tomizuka and H. Suzuki. 1986. Staurosporine, a potent platelet aggregation inhibitor from a *Streptomyces* species. Agric. Biol. Chem. 50: 2723–2727.

31 Okazaki, H., T. Kishi, T. Beppu and K. Arima. 1975. A new antibiotic, baciphelacin. J. Antibiot. 28: 717–719.

32 Ōmura, S., Y. Iwai, A. Hirano, A. Nakagawa, J. Awaya, H. Tsuchiya, Y. Takahashi and R. Masuma. 1977. A new alkaloid AM-2282 of *Streptomyces* origin. Taxonomy, fermentation, isolation and preliminary characterization. J. Antibiot. 30: 275–282.

33 Rasmussen, H., Y. Takuwa and S. Park. 1987. Protein kinase C in the regulation of smooth muscle contraction. FASEB J. 1: 177–185.

34 Satoh, H., K. Ohmori, H. Manabe, K. Yamada, K. Iwahashi and H. Kase. 1987. Effect of K-252a, a new microbial metabolite, on the secretory responses in isolated rat mast cells and neutrophils. Jpn. J. Pharmacol. 43 (Suppl.): 202P.

35 Scott, P.M., W. van Walbeek and W.M. MacLean. 1971. Cladosporin, a new antifungal metabolite from *Cladosporium cladosporioides*. J. Antibiot. 24: 747–755.

36 Sezaki, M., T. Sasaki, T. Nakazawa, U. Takeda, M. Iwata, T. Watanabe, M. Koyama, F. Kai, T. Shomura and M. Kojima. 1985. A new antibiotic SF-2370 produced by *Actinomadura*. J. Antibiot. 38: 1437–1439.

37 Shimojima, Y. and H. Hayashi. 1983. 1H-2-Benzopyran-1-one derivatives, microbial products with pharmacological activity. Relationship between structure and activity in 6-((1(S),-(3(S), 4-dihydro-8-hydroxy-1-oxo-1H-2-benzopyran-3-yl)-3-methylbutyl)-amino)-4(S), 5 (S)-dihydroxy-6-oxo-3(S)-ammoniohexanoate. J. Med. Chem. 26: 1370–1374.

38 Shimojima, Y., H. Hayashi, T. Ooka and M. Shibukawa. 1982. Production, isolation and pharmacological studies of AI-77s. Agric. Biol. Chem. 46: 1823–1829.

39 Shimojima, Y., H. Hayashi, T. Ooka, M. Shibukawa and Y. Iitaka. 1982. Studies on AI-77s, microbial products with

pharmacological activity. Structures and the chemical nature of AI-77s. Tetrahedron Lett. 23: 5435–5438.

40 Shimojima, Y., H. Hayashi, T. Ooka, M. Shibukawa and Y. Iitaka. 1984. Studies on AI-77s, microbial products with gastroprotective activity. Structures and the chemical nature of AI-77s. Tetrahedron 40: 2519–2527.

41 Shimojima, Y., T. Shirai, T. Baba and H. Hayashi. 1985. 1H-2-Benzopyran-1-one derivatives, microbial products with pharmacological activity. Conversion into orally active derivatives with antiinflammatory and antiulcer activities. J. Med. Chem. 28: 3–9.

42 Siegel, M.I., R.T. McConnell, N.A. Portes and P. Cuatrecasas. 1980. Arachidonate metabolism via lipoxygenase and 12L-hydroperoxy-5,8,10,14-icosatetraenoic acid peroxidase sensitive to anti-inflammatory drugs. Proc. Natl. Acad. Sci. USA 77: 308–312.

43 Steglich, W., B. Steffan, L. Lopanski and G. Eckhardt. 1980. Indole pigments from the fruiting bodies of the slime mold *Arcyria denudata*. Angew. Chem. Intern. Ed. 19: 459–460.

44 Takahashi, I., E. Kobayashi, K. Asano, M. Yoshida and H. Nakano. 1987. UCN-01, a selective inhibitor of protein kinase C from *Streptomyces*. J. Antibiot. 40: 1782–1784.

45 Takase, S., M. Iwami, T. Ando, M. Okamoto, K. Yoshida, H. Horiai, M. Kohsaka, H. Aoki and H. Imanaka. 1984. Amauromine, a new vasodilator. Taxonomy, isolation and characterization. J. Antibiot. 37: 1320–1323.

46 Tamaoki, T., H. Nomoto, I. Takahashi, Y. Kato, M. Morimoto and F. Tomita. 1986. Staurosporine, a potent inhibitor of phospholipid/Ca^{++} dependent protein kinase. Biochem. Biophys. Res. Commun. 135: 397–402.

47 Umezawa, H. 1972. Enzyme Inhibitors of Microbial Origin, University of Tokyo Press, Tokyo.

48 Urushidani, T., Y. Kasuya and S. Yano. 1986. Ulcerogenic and antiulcerogenic effects of a new antiinflammatory drug, the r-lactone-N-ethyl derivatives of 6-(1S-(3S, 4-dihydro-8-hydroxy-1H-2-benzo-pyran-1-one-3-yl) -3-methylbutylamino)-4S,5S-dihydroxy-6-oxo-3S-ammoniohexanoate, on gastrointestinal tract in rats. Arzneim.-Forsch./Drug Res. 36: 1383–1390.

49 Yamada, K., H. Kase and K. Kubo. 1986. Effect of a new microbial metabolite, K-252, on secretion and aggregation in rabbit platelets. Jpn. J. Pharmacol. 42 (Suppl.): 265P.

Novel Microbial Products for Medicine and Agriculture

Editors: A.L. Demain, G.A. Somkuti, J.C. Hunter-Cevera and H.W. Rossmoore

195

CHAPTER 22

Screening of microbial products affecting plant metabolism

Takao Kida

Central Research Laboratories, Ajinomoto Co., Inc., Kawasaki, Japan

SUMMARY

A simple and sensitive assay system was developed in the search for new herbicidal substances by using blue-green algae and excised leaf segments of barnyard millet. We isolated a new compound, pereniporin A, which inhibited the root elongation of lettuce at 100 ppm, from the culture broth of *Perenniporia medullaepanis* Aj 8345 by using a routine antimetabolite assay. A weak antibacterial substance, 7-deoxy-D-glycero-D-gluco-heptose, was isolated again as an inhibitor of the greening of dark-grown *Scenedesmus obliquus* C-2A' from the culture broth of *Streptomyces*. We also isolated streptothricin-like antibiotics, Nos. 6241-A and -B, as active substances that inhibited *de novo* starch synthesis in excised leaf segments of barnyard millet. No. 6241-B, identified as SF-701, showed remarkable herbicidal activity against barnyard millet with slight phyto-toxicity to rice plant at concentrations above 500 ppm.

INTRODUCTION

Microbial metabolites, in addition to synthetic chemicals, are possible sources of new herbicides. Recently, bialaphos [11] was developed as the first practical herbicide of microbial origin.

A desired herbicidal compound should control weeds with as little toxicity to other organisms as possible. A herbicide that inhibits photosynthesis has a remarkable selective toxicity between plants and animals. Plants and animals also differ in their ability to synthesize amino acids and vitamins.

It is important to develop a sensitive and simple bioassay system for the detection of photosynthesis inhibitors and amino acid synthesis inhibitors in microbial culture broths. An assay method to discover amino acid synthesis inhibitors has already been applied by many researchers. Ōmura et al. [10] found phosalacine in 1984 by using this assay method. Assay methods usually employed to detect photosynthesis inhibitors, however, are unsuitable for screening thousands of culture broths. Therefore, we attempted to develop a new assay system to detect the inhibition of photosynthesis to screen a large number of microbial culture broths. It consisted of detecting *de novo* starch synthesis in excised leaf segments and greening of dark-grown *Scenedesmus obliquus* C-2A'.

During the screening for herbicidal substances by using this assay system, we isolated pereniporin A, 7-deoxy-D-glycero-D-glucoheptose, laidlomycin and streptothricin-like antibiotics, Nos. 6241-A and -B. This paper describes the assay system, isolation of active compounds, as well as their structures and biological activities.

MATERIALS AND METHODS

Microbial strains

Microbial strains used in this experiment are listed in Table 1.

Culture media

The fermentation medium for the production of pereniporins A and B contained soluble starch 10 g, glucose 20 g, $(NH_4)_2SO_4$ 5 g, KH_2PO_4 0.5 g, $MgSO_4 \cdot 7H_2O$ 0.5 g, NaCl 0.5 g, potato extract 20 g, 1 ml of a trace salt mixture which was composed of $CuSO_4 \cdot 7H_2O$ 0.6 g, $FeSO_4 \cdot 7H_2O$ 0.11 g, $MnCl_2 \cdot 4H_2O$ 0.79 g and $ZnSO_4 \cdot 7H_2O$ 0.15 g per 100 ml, in 1 liter of distilled water. The medium for *Streptomyces* and *Penicillium* contained soluble starch 20 g, glucose 10 g, KH_2PO_4 1 g, $MgSO_4 \cdot 7H_2O$ 1 g, yeast extract 2 g, and Bacto-soytone (Difco) 7 g in 1 liter of distilled water. The basal medium for blue-green algae contained KNO_3 0.808 g, NaCl 0.46 g, $Na_2HPO_4 \cdot 12H_2O$ 0.358 g, $NaH_2PO_4 \cdot 2H_2O$ 0.468 g, $CaCl_2 \cdot 2H_2O$ 0.015 g, $MgSO_4 \cdot 7H_2O$ 0.246 g, and 1 ml of Arnon's microelement solution in 1 liter of distilled water.

Plants

Plants used in this experiment are listed in Table 2.

Antimicrobial assay

The minimum inhibitory concentration (MIC) was determined by the two-fold agar dilution method using the test microorganisms shown in Table 1.

Table 1

Microbial strains

Perenniporia medullaepanis Aj 8345
Streptomyces purpeofuscus No. 381
Streptomyces No. 317
Streptomyces No. 701
Streptomyces No. 6241
Penicillium No. 467
Bacillus subtilis Aj 1316
Scenedesmus obliquus C-2A′
Scenedesmus obliquus
Euglena gracilis ATCC30581

Table 2

List of plants

Italian ryegrass (*Lolium multiflorum* LAM.)
Rice plant (*Oryza sativa* L. cv Nihonbare)
Barnyard millet (*Panicum crus-galli*)
Lettuce (*Lactuca sativa* L.)

The assay media were Bouillon agar for bacteria and potato dextrose agar for yeast and fungi. In the case of the antimetabolite assay, a culture filtrate which inhibits the growth of *Bacillus subtilis* Aj 1316 in Davis minimum medium, but not with casamino acid, was selected.

Detection of the greening of dark-grown S. obliquus C-2A′ [5]

The dark-grown algal cells were suspended in the basal medium for blue-green algae, poured into a plastic petri dish containing the test solution, and then illuminated at an intensity of 14 kilolux for 14 h at 27°C. The newly synthesized pigments were extracted from algal cells with hot methanol, and chlorophyll was measured spectrophotometrically at 665 nm.

Detection of de novo starch synthesis [7]

The effect of the test compounds on *de novo* starch synthesis was examined by using the excised leaf segments of barnyard millet (*Panicum crus-galli*), which had been incubated in a dark chamber for 12 h. After the leaf segments which were floating on the surface of the test solution in a petri dish had been illuminated for 16 h at 25°C, *de novo* synthesized starch was determined by staining them with iodine.

Detection of oxygen evolution of the algal cells [7]

The effect of test compounds on oxygen evolution of *S. obliquus* under illumination was observed with a membrane-coated oxygen electrode. To determine their inhibitory activity, the rate of oxygen evolution was measured before and after adding the sample solution.

Assay of herbicidal activity [2]

Germinated rice plant seeds and barnyard millet seeds were sown in plastic pots (60 mm in diameter) filled with paddy soil, were watered and were allowed to grow in a growth chamber illuminated to an intensity of 14 kilolux at 25°C. On the 6th day after seeding, each test solution was applied for foliar treatment. On the 4th day after application, the degree of herbicidal effect was observed.

RESULTS AND DISCUSSION

Structures and biological activity of new antibiotics, pereniporins A and B [6]

The six candidates were selected by the amino acid antimetabolite assay from about 340 strains of basidiomycetes which are the type cultures of our laboratories. Among them, the ethyl acetate extract of the culture filtrate of *Perenniporia medullaepanis* Aj 8345 inhibited the growth of lettuce after germination. This active compound was purified by the following procedure. From 6 liters of culture filtrate, ethyl acetate extraction, silica gel column chromatography, gel filtration on Sephadex LH-20 and further purification by HPLC gave two pure samples of new antibiotics, named pereniporins A and B, in an overall yield of 19 mg and 6 mg, respectively.

The physico-chemical properties of pereniporins A (1) and B (2) are shown in Table 3. In 2 there are 2 less hydrogen atoms than 1. The IR spectra of these compounds showed characteristic bands ranging from 3400 to 3440 cm^{-1} attributable to hydroxyl groups. The UV absorption at 225 nm and the IR absorption at 1750 cm^{-1} of 2 suggested the presence of an α,β-unsaturated γ-lactone. The ^{1}H- and ^{13}C-NMR spectra of 1 and 2 taken in CD$_3$OD are shown in Table 4. The assignments of functional groups were made with the aid of INEPT and two-dimensional C-H correlation spectra of 1 and 2. Their spectra were very similar, particularly the ^{1}H and ^{13}C data; the exception being the UV and IR data mentioned above. In the case of 1, analysis of the ^{13}C-NMR spectrum accounted for 21 protons directly attached to carbons. The remaining 3 pro-

Table 3

Physico-chemical properties of pereniporins A and B

	Pereniporin A	Pereniporin B
Appearance	white powder	white powder
m.p. (°C)	164–166	181–183
$[\alpha]_D^{24}$ (MeOH)	$-181°$ (c 0.25)	$-208°$ (c 0.05)
FD-MS m/z (M$^+$)	268	266
Molecular formula	C$_{15}$H$_{24}$O$_4$	C$_{15}$H$_{22}$O$_4$
IR ν_{max}^{KBr} cm^{-1}	3400, 1050, 1030	3440, 1750, 1040
UV λ_{max}^{MeOH} nm	end absorption	225
Color reaction		
positive	KMnO$_4$	KMnO$_4$
negative	ninhydrin	ninhydrin
Silica gel TLC^a R_f	0.73	0.86

^{a} Using a solvent system of MeOH/EtOAc (5:95).

Table 4

Assignments of the chemical shifts in ^{1}H-NMR and ^{13}C-NMR spectra of pereniporins A and B

	Pereniporin A	Pereniporin B
-CH$_3$	19.4 (1.14)	20.3 (1.12)
	25.1 (1.34)	24.9 (1.35)
	33.4 (1.08)	33.4 (1.12)
-CH$_2$-	19.3 (1.46, 1.70)	19.2 (1.51, 1.72)
	33.3 (1.27, 1.92)	33.3 (1.19, 2.05)
	45.9 (1.27, 1.34)	45.7 (1.32, 1.36)
-CH$_2$O-	67.8 (4.17, 4.53)	76.5 (4.17, 4.47)
>CH-	47.8 (1.83)	47.3 (1.87)
>CHO-	66.0 (4.45)	65.6 (4.60)
-CH<$^{O-}_{O-}$	99.3 (5.31)	
=CH-	124.8 (5.64)	140.8 (6.77)
≥C-	35.0	35.0
	39.3	39.9
≥CO-	78.5	78.2
=C<	140.1	130.8
>C=O		172.1

The chemical shifts of protons are given in parentheses.

exchangeable protons are assumed to exist as hydroxyl groups from the IR spectrum and ^{13}C-NMR spectral data.

The structural elucidation of 1 was mainly performed with the aid of its long-range C-H shift correlated spectra shown in Fig. 1. In this figure, many cross-peaks were observed between ^{13}C and ^{1}H sig-

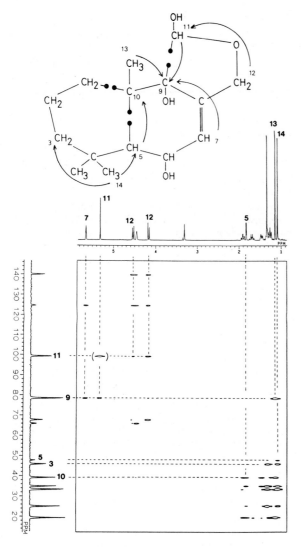

Fig. 1. Long-range C-H shift correlated spectrum of pereniporin A.

Pereniporin A   Pereniporin B

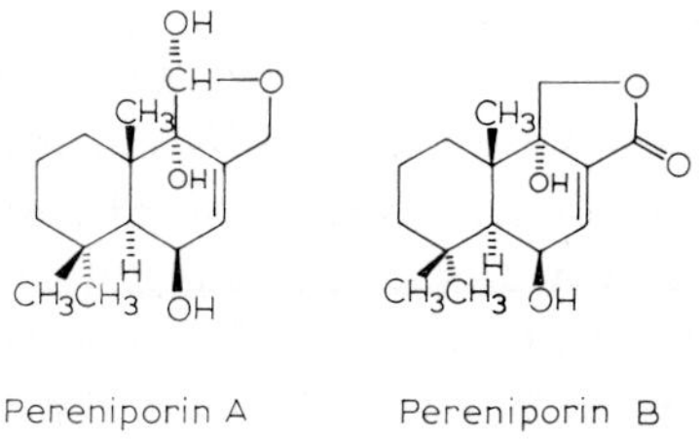

Fig. 2. Structures of pereniporins A and B.

alkaline treatment.

Antimicrobial activity was shown by 1 against *B. subtilis* Aj 1316 in Davis minimum medium (MIC 6.25 μg/ml) but was inactive against gram-negative bacteria. The root elongation of lettuce was inhibited by 1 at 100 ppm (Table 5).

7-Deoxy-D-glycero-D-glucoheptose, as an inhibitor of the greening of dark-grown S. oliquus C-2A' [5]

The culture filtrate of *Strep. purpeofuscus* No. 381 was selected as a candidate for further purification studies, from about 4000 different microbial culture filtrates. This culture filtrate inhibited the greening but did not show antimicrobial activity against heterotrophically dark-grown algae. From 20 liters of culture filtrate, an active compound, No. 381, was obtained with a yield of 640 mg by *n*-butanol extraction, partition chromatography, and silica gel column chromatography.

Based on physico-chemical and ^{1}H-NMR spectral data, this active compound (No. 381) was iden-

nals. They are the cross-peaks between H-7 and C-9, H-14 and C-3, H-14 and C-5, H-13 and C-9, H-5 and C-10, and H-12 and C-11. Consequently the planar structure of 1 was determined as shown in Fig. 2. This is a new compound. The structural elucidation of 2 was performed by comparing its ^{13}C-NMR signals with those of 1. From these NMR spectral data and the evidence of the existence of an α,β-unsaturated γ-lactone moiety, 2 was identified as 6β,-9α-dihydroxydrimenine [9], which was chemically derived from mukaadial by

Table 5

Plant growth inhibitory activity of pereniporin A

Concentration (μg/ml)	Relative length (% of control)		
	lettuce:	barnyard millet	
	root	root	shoot
500	0	18	0
250	0	57	26
100	39	76	108
50	108	79	93
10	96	89	115

tified as SF-666 A (7-deoxy-D-glycero-D-glucoheptose) (Fig. 3) which was previously isolated as a weak antimicrobial substance in 1970 [1].

This No. 381 (SF-666 A) inhibited the greening of dark-grown *S. obliquus* C-2A′ at a concentration of 12.5 µg/ml (Table 6). Its effects on photosynthetic oxygen evolution and the Hill reaction were examined. Oxygen evolution was not affected by this compound when illumination was begun immediately after its addition at a concentration of 100 µg/ml to the reaction mixture. However, when the algal cells were first incubated at 27°C for 40 min in the presence of this compound at concentrations of 1–100 µg/ml before illumination, dose-dependent inhibition occurred (Table 7). It did not inhibit the Hill reaction of spinach chloroplasts (Table 7). We believe that No. 381 (SF-666 A) inhibits the carbon dioxide fixation system and thus inhibits greening.

A new assay method to detect photosynthesis inhibitors by examining de novo starch synthesis [7]

We attempted to detect inhibitory activity against starch synthesis in excised leaf segments. In leaf segments cut off the whole plant which were grown under light, we might expect to detect starch

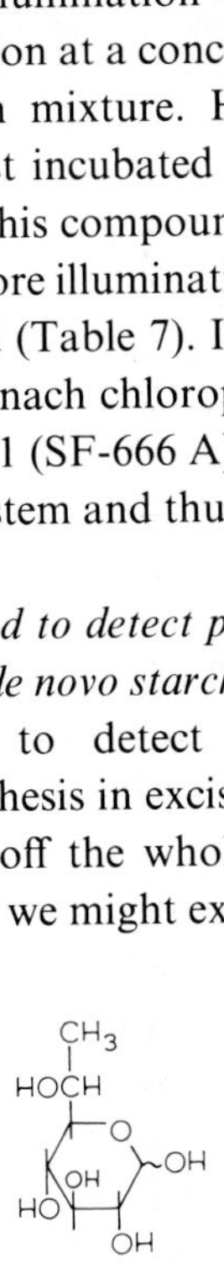

Fig. 3. Structure of No. 381 (SF-666 A).

Table 6

Effect of compound No. 381 (SF-666 A) on greening

Concentration (µg/ml)	Greening[a]
12.5	0
6.25	4.1
3.12	16
1.56	24
0.78	50
0.39	77
0	100

[a] % of control (control: 11.8 µg chlorophyll/mg cell).

Table 7

Effects of No. 381 on photosynthesis

Compound	Concentration (µg/ml)	Oxygen evolution[a] (% of control[b])	Hill reaction (% of control[c])
No. 381	100	16	100
	10	29	100
	1.0	97	100
Diuron	1.0	0	13
	0	100	100

[a] Oxygen evolution was measured after the algal cells were incubated with different concentrations of No. 381 solution for 40 min at 27°C.
[b] Control: 180–200 nmol O_2/mg cell/h.
[c] Control: ferricyanide reduction, 100 µmol/mg chlorophyll/h.

by iodine staining. However, we might not detect starch in leaf segments cut off the whole plant if that plant had been transferred to a dark chamber and kept for 12 h at 25°C. If these segments which were negative for starch with iodine staining were illuminated at an intensity of 14 kilolux for 16 h at 25°C, we might detect starch in these segments again by iodine staining. Italian ryegrass (*Lolium multiflorum* LAM., C_3) and barnyard millet (*Panicum crus-galli*, C_4) were selected as plants suitable for detecting *de novo* starch synthesis from several kinds of C_3 and C_4 plants.

A variety of biologically active compounds were examined for inhibition of *de novo* starch synthesis in the excised leaf segments of barnyard millet (Table 8). The most potent inhibitors of *de novo* starch synthesis were the photosynthesis inhibitors, diuron, propanil, and linuron. They inhibited starch synthesis at a concentration of 0.1 ppm. Other compounds without photosynthesis inhibitory activity also inhibited starch synthesis. These compounds included paraquat, which reportedly generates superoxide, sodium azide and 2,4-dinitrophenol, which are respiratory inhibitors, and protein synthesis inhibitors such as cyclohexamide, gentamicin, or streptomycin.

To distinguish between photosynthetic electron transport inhibitors and the others, another assay method is necessary. *De novo* starch synthesis is

Table 8

Effects of several types of biologically active compounds on *de novo* starch synthesis in leaf segments of barnyard millet

Chemicals	Inhibitory activity[a]				
μg/ml:	0	0.1	1.0	10	100
Photosynthesis inhibitors					
diuron	−	+ +	+ +	+ +	+ +
propanil	−	+	+ +	+ +	+ +
swep	−	−	+	+ +	+ +
linuron	−	+	+ +	+ +	+ +
Non-photosynthesis inhibitors					
paraquat	−	−	+	+ +	+ +
nitrofen	−	−	−	−	
methoxyphenone	−	−	−	−	−
amitrole	−	−	−	−	−
glyphosate	−	−	−	−	−
2,4-D	−	−	−	−	−
phenazine	−	−	−	−	−
isoprothiolane	−	−	−	−	−
2,4-dinitrophenol	−	−	−	+	+
sodium azide	−	−	+	+	+ +
antimycin A	−	−	−	−	−
olygomycin	−	−	−	−	−
cycloheximide	−	−	+ +	+ +	+ +
gentamicin	−	−	−	−	+
streptomycin	−	−	−	−	+
kasugamycin	−	−	−	−	−
chloramphenicol	−	−	−	−	−
actinomycin C	−	−	−	−	−
rifamycin	−	−	−	−	−
bleomycin	−	−	−	−	−

[a] Inhibitory activity was expressed as follows: −, no effect (staining with iodine); +, active (partial staining); + +, active (not staining).

closely associated with oxygen evolution in excised leaf photosynthesis. Therefore, several kinds of potent inhibitors as detected by the starch synthesis system were examined for their effects on algal photosynthetic oxygen evolution by a membrane-coated oxygen electrode (Table 9). Photosynthesis inhibitors tested (diuron, propanil, swep and linuron) inhibited photosynthetic oxygen evolution at 1.0 ppm. On the other hand, non-photosynthesis inhibitors such as paraquat, sodium azide, 2,4-dinitrophenol, or cyclohexamide did not affect the oxy-

Table 9

Effects of herbicides and other chemicals on oxygen evolution

Chemicals	Oxygen evolution (% of control)				
μg/ml:	0	0.1	1.0	10	100
Photosynthesis inhibitors					
diuron	100	35	0	0	0
propanil	100	100	33	0	0
swep	100	100	69	13	0
linuron	100	6	0	0	0
Non-photosynthesis inhibitors					
paraquat	100	−[a]	−	−	100
2,4-dinitrophenol	100	−	−	−	100
sodium azide	100	−	−	−	100
cycloheximide	100	−	−	−	100

[a] −, not examined.

gen evolution at all. Thus, we can distinguish between photosynthetic electron transport inhibitors and the others by using these two assay methods.

Active compounds as inhibitors of de novo starch synthesis in excised leaf segments of barnyard millet [2–4]

Approximately 6500 kinds of microbial culture filtrates were tested in this assay system. Only four culture filtrates were obtained as candidates for further purification studies (Table 10). Among them *Streptomyces* sp. No. 701 inhibited both starch synthesis and photosynthetic oxygen evolution. These

Table 10

Results of screening of culture filtrates

Culture No.	Assay methods	
	starch synthesis	O₂ evolution
Streptomyces No. 317	+	−
Streptomyces No. 701	+	+
Streptomyces No. 6241	+	−
Penicillium No. 467	+	−

active compounds were isolated and their structures were determined. They are hadacidin, duazomycin A, streptothricin-like antibiotics (Nos. 6241-A and -B) and laidlomycin. No. 6241-A was a new compound and No. 6241-B was identified as SF-701 [12] which was isolated as an antimicrobial substance (Fig. 4).

Laidlomycin, which was isolated as an antimycoplasmal antibiotic in 1974 [8], inhibited starch synthesis at a concentration of 1.0 μg/ml and also inhibited oxygen evolution (Table 11). It inhibited photophosphorylation at a concentration of 1.0 μg/ml but promoted the Hill reaction (electron acceptor, ferricyanide) at this concentration (Table 11). These data indicate that laidlomycin may be an uncoupler of photophosphorylation. We believe that laidlomycin inhibits *de novo* starch synthesis by inhibiting photophosphorylation. In a pot test, it was not strongly herbicidal in foliar treatment even at a concentration of 2000 ppm.

Streptothricin-like antibiotics, Nos. 6241-A and -B, inhibited *de novo* starch synthesis in excised leaf segments at concentrations ranging from 1.0 to 10 μg/ml (Table 12). The activity of No. 6241-A was approximately one tenth that of No. 6241-B. On the other hand, neither compound inhibited the photosynthetic oxygen evolution of *S. obliquus* at a concentration as high as 100 μg/ml. Streptothricin-

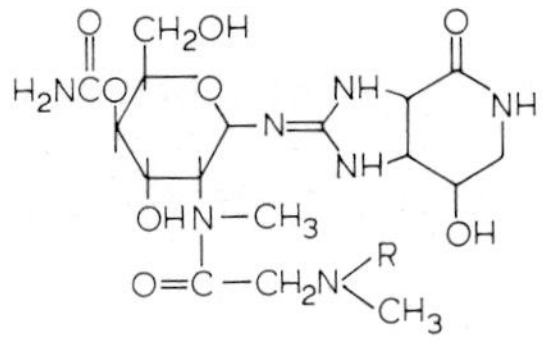

R = CH$_3$, No. 6241 – A
R = H,   No. 6241 – B (SF – 701)

Fig. 4. Structures of Nos. 6241-A and -B.

group antibiotics are known as protein synthesis inhibitors. Thus, we think that Nos. 6241-A and -B inhibited *de novo* starch synthesis as a result of effects such as the inhibition of protein synthesis. These compounds, especially No. 6241-B, showed remarkable herbicidal activity against barnyard millet with little phytotoxicity to rice plants at a concentration above 500 μg/ml (Fig. 5). However, this selective toxicity may not be due to a difference between C$_4$ and C$_3$ plants because these antibiotics inhibited *de novo* starch synthesis in the leaf segments of C$_3$ and C$_4$ plants. The selectivity observed in this study may be due to the difference in drug permeability between barnyard millet and rice plants.

Table 11

Effects of laidlomycin on photosynthesis

Compound	Concentration (μg/ml)	Inhibition of starch synthesis[a]	CO$_2$-dependent O$_2$ evolution[b]	Hill reaction[c]	Photophosphorylation[c]
Laidlomycin	100	+ +	39.5	233	
	10	+	100	260	
	1.0	+	100	200	0
	0.1	−		128	
DCMU	1.0	+ +	0	13.0	
CCCP	0.4				0
	0	−	100	100	100

[a] Using excised leaf segments of barnyard millet: −, no effect (staining with iodine); +, active (partial staining); + +, active (not staining).
[b] Using *S. obliquus*: % of control.
[c] Using spinach chloroplasts: % of control.
DCMU = 3-(3,4-dichlorophenyl)-1,1-dimethylurea; CCCP = carbonylcyanide *m*-chlorophenylhydrazone.

Table 12

Effects of Nos. 6241-A and -B on photosynthesis

Compound	Concentration (μg/ml)	Inhibitory activity	
		starch synthesis[a]	O_2 evolution[b]
No. 6241-A	100	+ +	100
	10	+	
	1.0	−	
	0.1	−	
No. 6241-B	100	+ +	100
	10	+ +	
	1.0	+ +	
	0.1	−	
	0	−	100

[a] −, no effect; +, active (partial staining); + +, active (no staining).

[b] % of control.

Barnyard millet   Rice plant

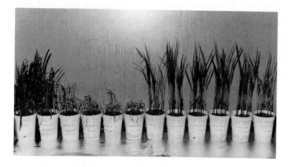

0 250 500 750 1000 2000

0 250 500 750 1000 2000

Fig. 5. Herbicidal activity of No. 6241-B against barnyard millet. Concentrations are given in μg/ml.

ACKNOWLEDGEMENTS

The author is grateful to Dr. T. Oh-hama of the University of Tokyo for providing a strain of *S. obliquus*. He also thanks Professor H. Seto for his measurement of the NMR and helpful suggestions.

REFERENCES

1 Ito, T., N. Ezaki, T. Tsuruoka and T. Niida. 1971. Structure of SF-666 A and SF-666 B, new monosaccharides. Carbohydr. Res. 17: 375–382.

2 Kida, T., T. Ishikawa and H. Shibai. 1985. Isolation of two streptothricin-like antibiotics, Nos. 6241-A and B, as inhibitors of de novo starch synthesis and their herbicidal activity. Agric. Biol. Chem. 49: 1839–1844.

3 Kida, T. and H. Shibai. 1985. Inhibition by hadacidin, duazomycin A, and other amino acid derivatives of de novo starch synthesis. Agric. Biol. Chem. 49: 3231–3237.

4 Kida, T. and H. Shibai. 1986. Inhibition of de novo starch synthesis and photosynthesis by laidlomycin. Agric. Biol. Chem. 50: 485–486.

5 Kida, T. and H. Shibai. 1986. Screening for inhibitors of the greening of dark-grown *Scenedesmus obliquus* C-2A′, and isolation and biological activity of an active compound, No. 381. Agric. Biol. Chem. 50: 483–484.

6 Kida, T., H. Shibai and H. Seto. 1986. Structure of new antibiotics, pereniporins A and B, from a basidiomycete. J. Antibiot. 39: 613–615.

7 Kida, T., S. Takano, T. Ishikawa and H. Shibai. 1985. A simple bioassay for herbicidal substances of microbial origin by determining de novo starch synthesis in leaf segments. Agric. Biol. Chem. 49: 1299–1303.

8 Kitame, F., K. Utsushikawa, T. Kohama, T. Saito, M. Kikuchi and N. Ishida. 1974. Laidlomycin, a new antimycoplasmal polyether antibiotic. J. Antibiot. 27: 884–888.

9 Kubo, I., T. Matsumoto, A.B. Kakooko and N.K. Mubiru. 1983. Structure of mukaadial, a molluscicide from Warburgia plants. Chem. Lett. 979–980.

10 Ōmura, S., M. Murata, H. Hanaki, K. Hinotozawa, R. Oiwa and H. Tanaka. 1984. Phosalacine, a new herbicidal antibiotic containing phosphinothricin. Fermentation, isolation, biological activity and mechanism of action. J. Antibiot. 37: 829–835.

11 Tachibana, K., T. Watanabe, Y. Sekizawa, M. Konnai and T. Takematsu. 1982. Finding of the herbicidal activity and the mode of action of bialaphos, L-2-amino-4-[(hydroxy)-(methyl)phosphinoyl]butyrylalanylalanine. In: Abstracts of Papers, 5th International Congress of Pesticide Chemistry, Kyoto, Japan, IVa-19.

12 Tsuruoka, T., T. Shoumura, N. Ezaki, T. Niwa and T. Niida. 1968. SF-701, a new streptothricin-like antibiotic. J. Antibiot. 21: 237–238.

Novel Microbial Products for Medicine and Agriculture
Editors: A.L. Demain, G.A. Somkuti, J.C. Hunter-Cevera and H.W. Rossmoore
© 1989, Society for Industrial Microbiology

CHAPTER 23

Novel second-generation avermectin insecticides and miticides for crop protection

Richard A. Dybas[1,*], Nancy J. Hilton[2], J.R. Babu[1], Franz A. Preiser[2], and Gary J. Dolce[3]

Merck Sharp & Dohme Research Laboratories, [1]Three Bridges, NJ, and [2]Rahway, NJ, and [3]Boyce Thompson Institute for Plant Research, Ithaca, NY, U.S.A.

SUMMARY

The avermectin family of macrocyclic lactone natural products, produced by fermentation of the soil microorganism *Streptomyces avermitilis*, were discovered in the mid-1970's. The major component avermectin B_1 (abamectin) displayed the best activity against arthropods and is currently under development for control of a number of phytophagous mites and insects on horticultural and agronomic crops worldwide. Improvement in the activity of avermectins against economically important lepidopteran larvae and increased stability on plant foliage was recently achieved through chemical modifications of avermectin B_1. It was found that a series of $4''$-substituted amino-$4''$-deoxyavermectin B_1 derivatives were highly effective against a broad spectrum of Lepidoptera. $4''$-*epi*-Methylamino-$4''$-deoxyavermectin B_1 (EMA) was the most active derivative with over 1500 times greater potency against armyworm species compared to abamectin. Modification of the reactive avermectin pentadiene chromophore led to novel compounds with improved persistence on foliage. One derivative, avermectin B_1 8,9-oxide, was found to have 2–4 times greater potency than abamectin against spider mites in foliar residual bioassays. These improvements should allow a new second generation of avermectins to come forward into development in future years to expand the importance of this class of natural products in crop protection.

INTRODUCTION

Avermectins are a family of 16-membered lactone natural products produced by the soil microorganism, *Streptomyces avermitilis*. They were discovered in the mid-1970's as a direct result of a screening effort for natural products with anthelmintic properties [5]. Avermectin B_1 (1, AVM B_1, MK-936), the

major component of the fermentation, is a mixture of homologous avermectins, containing a minimum of 80% AVM B_1a and a maximum of 20% AVM B_1b. It was subsequently shown to have high potency against arthropods of importance in crop protection [9]. AVM B_1, under the generic name abamectin, is currently under development in agriculture for control of economically important mite and insect pests of agronomic and horticultural crops worldwide [11]. Ivermectin, the 22,23-di-

---

*To whom correspondence should be addressed.

4″-EPI-METHYLAMINO-4″-
DEOXYAVERMECTIN B1 (EMA)

ABAMECTIN
8,9-OXIDE

a-Component R = $C_2H_5 \geq 80\%$
b-Component R = $CH_3 \leq 20\%$

**AVERMECTIN B1
ABAMECTIN**

hydro derivative of AVM B_1, is a chemically modified derivative of abamectin that has found use as a systemic antiparasitic agent against endo- and ecto-parasites of animals [4,6]. Ivermectin, in addition, is now used for the prevention of onchocerciasis (river blindness) in man caused by the filarial worm *Onchocerca volvulus* [2,8,27].

The avermectins are believed to exert their toxic effects by interference with nerve transmission via opening of chloride ion channels [17,20,28]. As a result, a flaccid paralysis is initially observed in many invertebrates exposed to lethal avermectin concentrations. Some of the effects observed with the avermectins can be reversed by picrotoxin, known to close chloride ion channels, and to a lesser degree by bicuculline, a GABA (γ-aminobutyric acid) receptor antagonist [29]. This mode of action of the avermectins is unique and not shared by other chemical classes of compounds. Cross-resistance with existing conventional insecticides and miticides has not been observed [13, 23].

Under both laboratory conditions and in the environment, abamectin is rapidly degraded by ultraviolet light and has only a short half-life, less than 1 day, following spray application to crops [15,16]. Effective practical control of mites and insects on plants occurs as a result of the ability of abamectin

to penetrate the cuticle of fruit and foliage (translaminar movement) to provide a pesticidally active residue which is protected from further degradation by sunlight [3]. Significant differences in penetration of abamectin into various foliage types have been reported [30]. Consequently, abamectin's utility in some crops for mite control has been limited, in particular on apple, where rapid photodegradation and poor cuticular transport of abamectin has resulted in inadequate residual control of mite populations in field trials [14].

Abamectin has shown potent broad-spectrum activity against phytophagous mites with LC_{90}'s of 0.02 ppm for the eriophyid citrus rust mite, *Phyllocoptruta oleivora* (Ashmead) and the tetranychid twospotted spider mite, *Tetranychus urticae* Koch [5].

However, abamectin is much less toxic to insects, especially lepidopteran larvae such as cabbage looper, *Trichoplusia ni* (Huebner), cotton bollworm, *Heliothis zea* (Boddie), and southern armyworm, *Spodoptera eridania* (Cramer), where abamectin doses of 1.0, 1.5 and 6.0 ppm, respectively, were required to achieve an LC_{90} level [5,21]. Therefore, by comparison with the most sensitive mite and insect species, abamectin is shown to be 300 times less toxic to southern armyworm larvae. Toxicity to other lepidopteran larvae, and especially armyworm species, varies enough to preclude economic control of these worms in commercial agricultural practice [7,22].

An extensive effort at chemical modification of the avermectins was carried out in recent years in an attempt to extend the potential applications of the avermectins and to fill some of the deficiencies of this novel class of compounds in crop protection [12]. The chemical and biological studies have focused mainly on two areas: (i) to discover new avermectin derivatives with increased potency and spectrum of activity against armyworm species and other economically important lepidopteran larval pests of vegetables, corn, cotton, and soybeans; and (ii) to find avermectin compounds with increased miticidal activity, cuticular penetration, and stability (persistence) on foliage for potential application on apple, among other crops.

During the effort at chemical modification, it was discovered that the introduction of an amino substituent at the 4″-position in the terminal disaccharide unit of abamectin dramatically increased activity against lepidopteran larvae, especially armyworms [19]. Likewise, it was found that catalytic reduction and/or the addition of oxygen to the pentadiene system of AVM B_1 resulted in avermectin derivatives with potent miticidal activity, increased persistence on foliage, and apparent improved stability to ultraviolet light [18]. The results of bioassays of these novel second-generation avermectin derivatives against insects and mites are presented and discussed in this paper.

MATERIALS AND METHODS

Avermectin formulations

Laboratory formulations of technical grade avermectin derivatives were used in all of the following bioassays. For all foliar bioassays, each derivative was dissolved in a 1000 ppm solution of the surfactant Triton X-155 (Rohm & Haas) in acetone. The compounds in solution were further diluted with water in the ratio of 1:9 to yield a stock solution of the avermectin derivative in 10% acetone, 100 ppm

surfactant and water. All subsequent dilutions with the stock solution were made with a diluent of 10% acetone, 100 ppm surfactant and water. For the insect contact activity bioassay, the avermectin derivatives were dissolved in acetone.

Insecticide formulations

Formulated thiodicarb (Larvin 3.2 F (flowable), Union Carbide) and methomyl (Lannate 1.8 L (soluble liquid), DuPont) were diluted with distilled water for use in the foliar ingestion bioassays. For the same bioassay, technical grade cypermethrin (95% ai, Shell) and fenvalerate (93.5% ai, Shell) were formulated following the same procedure as outlined above for the avermectin derivatives.

For the topical bioassay, the technical grade cypermethrin and fenvalerate were each dissolved in acetone.

Insect bioassays

The southern armyworm larvae (*S. eridania*) used in the following bioassays were from a laboratory colony maintained at the Boyce Thompson Institute for Plant Research at Cornell University, Ithaca, NY. Tobacco budworm eggs (*H. virescens* (F.)) were received on a regular basis from the USDA – Cotton Research Laboratories, Stoneville, MS. Cotton bollworm eggs (*H. zea*) were received as weekly shipments from the Department of Entomology, University of North Carolina at Raleigh.

For the foliar ingestion and the foliar residual bioassays, sieva bean plants (*Phaseolus lunatus* L.) were used for the southern armyworm, *S. eridania*, while chick-pea plants (*Cicer arietinum* L.) were used for the tobacco budworm, *H. virescens*, and the cotton bollworm, *H. zea*. The foliage was sprayed with the formulated avermectin derivatives using a hand-held sprayer. All compounds were sprayed until run-off. After the residues had dried for 2 h, sections of the treated foliage were placed in plastic containers (11.5 × 4.5 cm) with water-moistened filter paper (9 cm diameter) and neonates placed onto the treated foliage. In the foliar residual bioassay, neonates were placed onto the foliage 9 days after treatment. The containers were covered with plastic lids and placed in growth chambers at

25°C with a 24-h photoperiod. Thirty larvae were evaluated per concentration for the southern armyworm (10 larvae per container), and 20 larvae evaluated per concentration for each *Heliothis* species (5 larvae per container). Mortality readings were made 96 h after the treated foliage was infested with the insects.

For the contact activity bioassay, third instar larvae were used. Each insect species was reared on artificial diet until the desired instar was reached. The *Spodoptera* larvae tested weighed in the range of 60–70 mg while the *Heliothis* species weighed in the range of 20–30 mg. Approximately. 10 ml of medium was poured into clear plastic cups (29.6 ml). One larva was placed per cup. One microliter of the prepared solution was placed on the thorax of each larva by using a Hamilton microsyringe. The cups were covered with plastic lids and held in growth chambers at 25°C for a 24-h photoperiod. For each insect species, 20 larvae were treated for each concentration tested. The percent mortality was evaluated 120 h after treatment.

Spider mite bioassays

The twospotted spider mites (*T. urticae*) used in the following bioassays were from a laboratory susceptible strain cultured at Merck & Co. Twelve-day-old bush bean plants (*Phaseolus vulgaris* L. cv. 'Tendercrop'), were used for the twospotted spider mite contact and residual activity bioassays. The first true leaves on each plant (one plant per pot) were trimmed into 2.0 cm squares. For the contact activity bioassay, 30–50 adult female twospotted spider mites were placed onto the untreated foliage and 24 h later the acaricidal treatments made. The treatments consisted of dipping each mite-infested leaf into the prepared solutions for approximately 2 s. For the residual bioassay, uninfested plants were treated with each acaricide as outlined above, then at 0 and 15 days after treatment (DAT) 30–50 adult female spider mites were introduced onto the treated foliage. Four plants (8 leaves) were treated for each concentration tested. All treatments were held in growth chambers at 22°C under a 24-h photoperiod. For both the contact and the residual bioassays, the mortality readings were made 96 h

after treatment/infestation.

For the translaminar residual spider mite bioassay, 12-day-old bush bean plants were used. The first true leaves on each plant (one plant per pot) were trimmed so that a strip 1 cm wide was remaining on each side of the mid-rib, thereby producing a 2 cm wide strip on each leaf. For the bioassay, a 2 cm^2 area was marked off. Within this marked area on the upper leaf surface, 16 1 μl droplets of avermectin solution were placed by using a Hamilton microsyringe. The droplets were allowed to air-dry. In order to confine the spider mites to the lower leaf surface, a Tanglefoot/castor oil mixture was placed around the leaf perimeter outlining the entire 2 cm^2 area. Thirty to fifty adult female spider mites were placed onto the lower leaf surface 1 day after treatment (1 DAT), 9 DAT and 12 DAT. Four plants (8 leaves) were treated for each concentration tested. All treatments were held in growth chambers at 22° C under a 24-h photoperiod. Mortality counts were made 96 h after mite infestation on the leaves.

RESULTS AND DISCUSSION

Insecticidal activities

Several bioassays were used in the evaluation and characterization of the insecticidal activities of the chemically modified avermectins in order to select compounds for further development. Previous testing had shown that the avermectins were most effective as stomach poisons, i.e., when they were ingested by insect larvae as residues on foliage [1]. The foliage spray bioassay was used as the initial screen to evaluate the direct entry of the avermectin compounds into the insect through the gut. Avermectins which showed high insecticidal activity in the foliage bioassay as stomach poisons were advanced to the foliar residual test to measure the persistence of the derivative in/on plant surfaces and the length of insect control following application. Under commercial conditions, at the time of pesticide application, mixed populations of insect larvae and egg masses are normally found on the treated foliage. Therefore, it was important that a new derivative be able to control existing larval populations but also demonstrate sufficient persistence or residual activity to kill newly hatched larvae. Avermectin derivatives were also evaluated for contact toxicity to insect larvae by topical application to the thorax to evaluate direct entry into the insect through the cuticle as would be the case by direct exposure to foliar sprays or contact with dried foliar residues.

While carrying out extensive modifications at the 4″-position, the only free hydroxy group of the disaccharide substituent, good activities were observed with several variants against Lepidoptera [10,19]. The activities of the 4″-substituted amino derivatives were initially determined against southern armyworm, *S. eridania*, and tobacco budworm, *H. virescens*. Southern armyworm and tobacco budworm larvae are rather easy to rear in the laboratory. The southern armyworm represents an excellent test model for other economically important *Spodoptera* species while tobacco budworm is a major pest of cotton and vegetables among other crops. The mortality at two concentrations, 0.1 and 0.02 ppm, was used for comparative purposes against larvae of both insects to optimize the biological activities within the series of avermectin derivatives.

From these studies, 4″-*epi*-amino and 4″-*epi*-methylamino-4″-deoxyavermectin B₁ were selected for comprehensive evaluation. The activities of the 4″-*epi*-amino (2) and 4″-*epi*-methylamino (EMA, 3) avermectin derivatives were compared by topical application to the three lepidopteran larvae included in the primary foliage bioassay tests (Table 1). EMA was the more toxic by contact action to southern armyworm, tobacco budworm, and cotton bollworm third instar larvae. At dose levels of 0.1 and 0.4 μg/g body weight for southern armyworm and tobacco budworm, respectively, 100% larval mortality was observed while 90% kill of cotton bollworm larvae was obtained at 0.4 μg/g body weight after 120 h. In contrast, 55, 30, and 70% mortality of southern armyworm, tobacco budworm, and cotton bollworm larvae, respectively, was shown with the 4″-*epi*-amino derivative at the same dose levels. The ability of an insecticide to control insect larvae by contact toxicity through

Table 1

Insecticidal activity of topically applied 4″-*epi*-amino- and 4″-*epi*-methylamino-4″-deoxyavermectin B₁ against southern armyworm (SAW), tobacco budworm (TBW) and cotton bollworm (CBW) third instar larvae

Compound	Percent mortality at 120 h		
	SAW (0.1 μg/g)[a]	TBW (0.4 μg/g)	CBW (0.4 μg/g)
2: Amino	55	30	70
3: EMA	100	100	90

[a] μg/g = μg active ingredient per g body weight of larva.

penetration of the insect cuticle represents an important attribute for optimal effectiveness in crop protection. On the basis of its spectrum of activity and greater facility for control of lepidopteran larvae by topical application, EMA was shown to have the best overall biological profile from the series of 4″-substituted amino avermectin derivatives and potential for further evaluation as an insecticide for crop protection.

Foliar ingestion and topical application bioassays were conducted in which the LC₉₀ values of EMA were determined against the three test lepidopteran larvae in comparison to abamectin and a number of standard insecticides. As shown in Table 2, it is clearly evident that EMA is highly toxic to the lepidopteran larvae by ingestion, with LC₉₀ values in the range of 0.002–0.005 ppm for the three test species. Southern armyworm, which is relatively insensitive to abamectin, was easily killed by the *epi*-methylamino derivative. EMA was found to be 1166-fold more potent than abamectin for southern armyworm, thus exhibiting a significant improvement over the parent molecule in intrinsic activity. These results are similar to those reported by Trumble *et al.* [26] who observed that in diet-incorporation assays the *epi*-methylamino analog EMA (L-656,748) was about 1500 times more active against neonate beet armyworm, *Spodoptera exigua* (Huebner), than abamectin. EMA was also more toxic to southern armyworm larvae than the standard carbamate or pyrethroid insecticides, being

Table 2

Comparative foliar ingestion toxicity of EMA, abamectin and standard insecticides against southern armyworm (SAW), tobacco budworm (TBW) and cotton bollworm (CBW) neonates

Compound	LC_{90} (ppm) at 96 h		
	SAW	TBW	CBW
3: EMA	0.005	0.003	0.002
1: Abamectin	5.83	0.128	0.21
Methomyl	8.6	10.0	8.1
Thiodicarb	4.42	5.0	6.6
Cypermethrin	—	—	0.41
Fenvalerate	1.34	1.5	—

Table 3

Foliar residual activity of EMA against southern armyworm (SAW) and tobacco budworm (TBW) neonates

Compound	LC_{90} ppm (9 DAT)[a]	
	SAW	TBW
3: EMA	0.153	0.10
Thiodicarb	34.8	40.0
Fenvalerate	7.41	5

[a] 9 DAT = 9 days after insecticidal treatment insects placed onto foliage; mortality counts made 96 h after infestation.

1720, 884 and 268 times more potent than the carbamates methomyl and thiodicarb and the pyrethroid fenvalerate, respectively.

EMA was also more toxic than abamectin to the two *Heliothis* species, being 43 and 105 times more effective than abamectin against tobacco budworm and cotton bollworm neonates. While abamectin is slightly less effective against cotton bollworm than tobacco budworm, the results in Table 2 show that EMA is essentially equitoxic for both insect species with LC_{90} values of 0.002 and 0.003 ppm. EMA was also 3300, 1666 and 500 times more effective than methomyl, thiodicarb and fenvalerate against tobacco budworm and 4050, 3300 and 205-fold more potent than methomyl, thiodicarb and the pyrethroid cypermethrin against the cotton bollworm. The results of the foliar ingestion assay indicate that EMA is two to three orders of magnitude more potent against Lepidoptera than the current insecticide standards.

EMA (3) showed long foliar residual activity for lepidopteran larvae under laboratory conditions, although toxicity to the neonates declined with time after application (Table 3). For southern armyworm and tobacco budworm larvae, LC_{90} values of 0.153 and 0.10 ppm were obtained following exposure of larvae to 9-day-old foliar residues (9 DAT). This compares to LC_{90} values of 0.005 and 0.003 ppm obtained when neonates were exposed to fresh foliar residues (0 DAT) of the *epi*-methylamino de-

rivative (Table 2). Although the toxicities of the foliar residues were observed to decline following application, EMA remained more active than the standard insecticides. For southern armyworm, EMA was about 230 times more toxic than thiodicarb and approximately 50 times more effective than the pyrethroid fenvalerate at 9 days after treatment (9 DAT). Similarly, EMA was 400-fold more toxic to tobacco budworm than the carbamate thiodicarb and over 50 times more toxic than fenvalerate in the residual assay at 9 DAT. The results of these assays indicate that the *epi*-methylamino derivative has sufficient persistence to effectively kill lepidopteran larvae which hatch onto previously treated plant foliage.

As shown in Table 4, EMA is also highly toxic

Table 4

Comparative toxicity of topically applied EMA and two pyrethroid insecticides against southern armyworm (SAW), tobacco budworm (TBW) and cotton bollworm (CBW) third instar larvae

Compound	LC_{90} (μg/g b.w.)[a] at 120 h		
	SAW	TBW	CBW
3: EMA	0.542	0.385	0.36
Fenvalerate	2.58	0.567	—
Cypermethrin	—	—	3.0

[a] μg/g b.w. = μg active ingredient per g body weight of larva.

to lepidopteran larvae by topical contact. LD_{90} values ranged from 0.36 μg/g b.w. for cotton bollworm larvae to 0.542 μg/g b.w. for third instar southern armyworm, again indicating the high susceptibility of all three lepidopteran larvae to EMA. The compound showed greater potency than the pyrethroid insecticides fenvalerate and cypermethrin. Against southern armyworm and tobacco budworm, EMA was 4.7 and 1.5 times more potent than fenvalerate, while against cotton bollworm it was 8.3-fold more toxic than cypermethrin.

The results of the topical application assays, however, indicate that insect cuticle appears to represent an effective barrier to the penetration of the avermectins, including the *epi*-methylamino derivative. For example, while EMA was found to be approximately 270 times as effective as fenvalerate against southern armyworm larvae as a stomach or ingestion poison (Table 2), it was only about 5-fold more toxic via topical application. Similarly, EMA was about 200 times more toxic than cypermethrin to cotton bollworm neonates in the foliage ingestion assay (Table 2) but was only 8-fold more potent in the contact toxicity bioassay. These data suggest that EMA has greater potential for applications on those crops on which lepidopteran larvae are primarily foliage feeders such as vegetables, corn, tobacco, and soybean and less promise on crops where the larvae have limited foliage feeding habits and where contact with pesticide residues on foliage or fruit are required to obtain a lethal dose. Crops such as cotton and apple fall into the latter category.

The spectrum of activity of EMA was determined against spider mites and against insects of several orders including Coleoptera, Homoptera, and other Lepidoptera. The LC_{90} values are presented in Table 5. The high susceptibility of lepidopteran larvae to EMA was further demonstrated in foliar bioassays with the tobacco hornworm, cabbage looper, beet armyworm, and fall armyworm where LC_{90} values of 0.003, 0.014, 0.005, and 0.01 ppm, respectively, were obtained against these four insects. The methylamino derivative also showed high toxicity for the two coleopteran in species included in the bioassay, the Colorado potato beetle

Table 5

Foliar ingestion activity of EMA against insect larvae and adult spider mites and aphids

Species (common name)	LC_{90} (ppm) at 96 h
Manduca sexta (L.) (tobacco hornworm)	0.003
Trichoplusia ni (Huebner) (cabbage looper)	0.014
Spodoptera exigua (Huebner) (beet armyworm)	0.005
Spodoptera frugiperda (J.E. Smith) (fall armyworm)	0.01
Leptinotarsa decemlineata (Say) (Colorado potato beetle)	0.032
Epilachna varivestis Mulsant (Mexican bean beetle)	0.20
Tetranychus urticae Koch (twospotted spider mite)	0.29
Aphis fabae Scopoli (bean aphid)	19.9

and Mexican bean beetle, with LC_{90}'s of 0.03 and 0.20 ppm. The foliage bioassays, in addition, showed that EMA was very toxic to the twospotted spider mite (LC_{90} 0.29 ppm); however, it was about 15 times less potent for this mite than abamectin for which an LC_{90} of 0.02 ppm was observed in the assay. The homopteran insect, the adult bean aphid, was least susceptible to EMA of the insects tested, with an LC_{90} value of 19.9 ppm.

Our studies have shown that extensive chemical modification at the terminal 4″-position of the disaccharide substituent of AVM B_1 has surprisingly led to the discovery of a series of 4″-*epi*-substituted amino-4″-deoxyavermectin B_1 derivatives which display a dramatic increase in toxicity to southern armyworm larvae and other lepidopteran larvae compared to the natural product abamectin. These derivatives were also two to three orders of magnitude more toxic to lepidopteran larvae than the current standard carbamate or pyrethroid insecticides. Following evaluation in several bioassay systems, EMA (3) proved to be the most potent derivative from this group and is currently undergoing tests in the field against major lepidopteran pests of vegetables, corn, cotton, and soybeans [10].

Miticidal activities

Studies conducted in our laboratories and elsewhere have indicated that the macrocyclic lactone ring system of abamectin (AVM B$_1$) is highly susceptible to rapid oxidative-photooxidative degradation in the presence of ultraviolet light [3,15,16]. Although this is not necessarily a disadvantage, since it assures the rapid removal of abamectin residues from the environment, the facile decomposition by sunlight has nonetheless resulted in short persistence and poor performance of the compound on certain crops [14]. Extensive chemical modification of the abamectin pentadiene system has been carried out in an attempt to stabilize the avermectins to light [18].

The activities of a number of abamectin derivatives, in which the macrocyclic diene chromophore has been modified chemically by catalytic reduction and/or the addition of oxygen (epoxidation), were determined in bioassays against the twospotted spider mite. The mortality to spider mites was evaluated initially at 0.05 ppm, a concentration of abamectin (1) which provides 100% kill of adult twospotted spider mites in the contact toxicity bioassay. In addition to abamectin, five avermectins including AVM B$_1$ 8,9-oxide (4), 10,11-dihydro-AVM B$_1$ (5), 22,23-dihydro-AVM B$_1$ (6; ivermectin), 10,11,22-23-tetrahydro-AVM B$_1$ (7) and 10-fluoro-10,11-dihydro-AVM B$_1$ (8) showed greater than 90% mortality to mites at 0.05 ppm. From this group, compound 4 represented an avermectin derivative in which the double bond of abamectin at the 8,9-position was modified by the addition of oxygen to form an epoxide, while derivatives 5, 6, and 7 reflected modifications in which the diene chromophore at the 10,11- and/or the 22,23-positions were saturated by the catalytic addition of hydrogen. In compound 8, a fluorine atom was substituted for hydrogen at the 10-position of 10,11-dihydro-AVM B$_1$ (5). It was surprising to note that whereas AVM B$_1$ 8,9-oxide (4) provided 100% kill of mites at 0.05 ppm, the 8,9-oxide of a 13-deoxyaglycone related to the milbemycins was virtually inactive at this concentration and resulted in only 20% mite mortality [24,25].

Four avermectin compounds which provided high mite mortality in the contact activity screen were advanced to the foliar residual bioassay to determine their length of residual control (persistence) against mites in comparison to abamectin (1). In this assay mites were introduced onto bean plants which had been previously treated with the various miticides and mortality was assessed 96 h after infestation. The results in Table 6 indicate that all four of the avermectin derivatives were highly toxic to spider mites immediately following introduction onto foliage (0 DAT), providing 90% or greater kill. At the 15 DAT evaluation, where mites were introduced onto treated foliage 15 days after application, only three of the derivatives, including AVM B$_1$ 8,9-oxide (4), 10,11-dihydro-AVM B$_1$ (5), and 10-fluoro-10,11-dihydro-AVM B$_1$ (8), showed good residual activity against twospotted spider mites, resulting in 60% or greater mortality. AVM B$_1$ 8,9-oxide (4) was the most effective derivative in the residual bioassay at the 0.1 ppm concentration evaluated, providing 70.7% mite mortality at 15 DAT compared to only 16.9% for abamectin.

The activity of AVM B$_1$ 8,9-oxide (4) was compared to abamectin in the plant cuticular penetration (translaminar) bioassay in which both compounds were applied to the upper leaf surface of bean leaves at 0.10 and 0.03 ppm and mites allowed to feed on the lower leaf surface (Table 7). The results indicate that abamectin 8,9-oxide has more effective cuticular penetration and/or persistence on

Table 6

Foliar residual activity of avermectin derivatives against adult female twospotted spider mites

Compound	Percent mortality at 0.1 ppm	
	0 DAT[a]	15 DAT[a]
1: AVM B$_1$	96.2	16.9
4: AVM B$_1$ 8,9-oxide	99.5	70.7
5: 10,11-dihydro-AVM B$_1$	98.0	67.0
7: 10,11,22,23-tetrahydro-AVM B$_1$	95.1	5
8: 10-fluoro-10,11-dihydro-AVM B$_1$	92.3	60.2

[a] 0 DAT and 15 DAT = 0 and 15 days after treatment spider mites placed onto foliage; mortality counts made 96 h after infestation.

Table 7

Translaminar activity of abamectin in comparison to AVM B$_1$ 8,9-oxide against adult female twospotted spider mites

Compound	Percent mortality[a]			
	Rate (ppm)	1 DAT[b]	9 DAT	12 DAT
1: AVM B$_1$	0.1	54.7	47.2	31.5
	0.03	24.0	9.3	5.0
4: AVM B$_1$ 8,9-oxide	0.1	94.2	100	72.1
	0.03	59.4	53.9	30.1

[a] Average of two bioassays.

[b] 1, 9 and 12 DAT = 1, 9 and 12 days after treatment mites placed onto foliage; mortality counts made 96 h after infestation.

bean foliage than does abamectin. At the 0.10 ppm applied concentration, AVM B$_1$ 8,9-oxide provided essentially 100% mortality to adult twospotted spider mites 9 days after treatment (9 DAT) compared to only 47.2% kill with abamectin. At 12 DAT, control had declined to 72.1% with the 8,9-oxide at 0.10 ppm concentration compared to 31.5% for abamectin. The data further show that mite mortality obtained with 0.03 ppm abamectin 8,9-oxide at 1, 9, and 12 DAT evaluations was essentially identical to that shown by abamectin at 0.1 ppm, a 3.3-fold higher concentration than that of the 8,9-oxide.

The results of dose-mortality titrations of abamectin (1) and abamectin 8,9-oxide (4) for contact toxicity to adult twospotted spider mites indicated that both compounds were equitoxic, providing LC$_{90}$ and LC$_{50}$ values of 0.04 and 0.0096 ppm, respectively, in a comparative bioassay. Therefore, the data presented in Tables 6 and 7 would appear to indicate that abamectin 8,9-oxide has greater foliar residual and translaminar activities than abamectin either due to improved cuticular penetration of bean plants or increased stability in the presence of light. Recent laboratory studies in which thin films of abamectin 8,9-oxide on petri dishes or citrus foliage were irradiated with a Kratos solar

simulator have shown that residues of the 8,9-oxide were 2–4 times more stable than abamectin in the presence of light on both substrates [16]. These results are consistent with the spider mite bioassay data and provide direct evidence that the increased miticidal activity of abamectin 8,9-oxide (4) has been accomplished through stabilization of its 8,9-diene function. Additional studies are still required to determine whether this increased stability under laboratory conditions will translate to improved activity against spider mites under practical field conditions on apple and other agronomic and horticultural crops.

REFERENCES

1 Anderson, T.E., J.R. Babu, R.A. Dybas and H. Mehta. 1986. Avermectin B$_1$ ingestion and contact toxicity against *Spodoptera eridania* and *Heliothis virescens* (Lepidoptera: Noctuidae) and potentiation by oil and piperonyl butoxide. J. Econ. Entomol. 79: 197–201.

2 Aziz, M.A. 1986. Chemotherapeutic approach to control of onchocerciasis. Rev. Infect. Dis. 8: 500–504.

3 Bull, D.L., G.W. Ivie, J.G. MacConnell, V.F. Gruber, C.C. Ku, B.H. Arison, J.M. Stevenson and W.J.A. VandenHeuvel. 1984. Fate of avermectin B$_1$a in soil and plants. J. Agric. Food Chem. 32: 94–102.

4 Campbell, W.C. 1985. Ivermectin: an update. Parasit. Today 1: 10–16.

5 Campbell, W.C., R.W. Burg, M.H. Fisher and R.A. Dybas. 1984. The discovery of ivermectin and other avermectins. In: Pesticide Synthesis Through Rational Approaches (Magee, P.S., G.K. Kohn and J.J. Menn, eds.), ACS Symposium Series No. 255, pp. 5–20, American Chemical Society, Washington, DC.

6 Campbell, W.C., M.H. Fisher, E.O. Stapley, G. Albers-Schonberg and T.A. Jacob. 1983. Ivermectin: a potent new antiparasitic agent. Science 221: 823–828.

7 Corbitt, T.S., D.J. Wright and A.St.J. Green. 1985. The toxicity of abamectin (MK-936) on cabbage to first and third larval instars of *Spodoptera littoralis* (Boisd.). Med. Fac. Landbouwwet. Rijksuniv. Gent 50: 639–642.

8 Dadzie, K.Y., A.C. Bird, K. Awadzi, H. Schulz-Key, H.M. Gilles and M.A. Aziz. 1987. Ocular findings in a double-blind study of ivermectin versus diethylcarbamazine versus placebo in the treatment of onchocerciasis. Br. J. Ophthalmol. 71: 78–85.

9 Dybas, R.A. 1983. Avermectins: their chemistry and pesticidal activities. In: Pesticide Chemistry: Human Welfare and the Environment (Miyamoto, J., ed.), pp. 83–90, Pergamon Press, New York.

10 Dybas, R.A. and J.R. Babu. 1988. 4″-Deoxy-4″-methyla-mino-4″-epiavermectin B_1 hydrochloride (MK-243): a novel avermectin insecticide for crop protection. In: 1988 British Crop Protection Conference. Pests and Diseases, pp. 57–64, British Crop Protection Council, Croydon, U.K.

11 Dybas, R.A. and A.St.J. Green. 1984. Avermectins: their chemistry and pesticidal activity. In: 1984 British Crop Protection Conference. Pests and Diseases, pp. 947–954, British Crop Protection Council, Croydon, U.K.

12 Fisher, M.H. and H. Mrozik. 1984. The avermectin family of macrolide-like antibiotics. In: Macrolide Antibiotics (Omura, S., ed.), pp. 553–606, Academic Press, New York.

13 Hoy, M.A. and J. Conley. 1987. Selection for abamectin resistance in Tetranychus urticae and T. pacificus (Acari: Tetranychidae). J. Econ. Entomol. 80: 221–225.

14 Hull, L.A. 1982. Apple, test of acaricides, 1981. Insect. Acar. Tests 7: 17.

15 Iwata, Y., J. MacConnell, J.E. Flor, I. Putter and T.M. Dinoff. 1985. Residues of the natural products acaricide avermectin B_1a on and in citrus fruits and foliage. J. Agric. Food Chem. 33: 467–471.

16 MacConnell, J.G., R.J. Demchak, F.A. Preiser and R.A. Dybas. 1989. A study of the relative stability, toxicity and penetrability of abamectin and its 8,9-oxide. J. Agric. Food Chem. in press.

17 Mellin, T.N., R.D. Busch and C.C. Wang. 1983. Postsynaptic inhibition of invertebrate neuromuscular transmission by avermectin B_1a. Neuropharmacology 22: 89–96.

18 Mrozik, H. 1985. Avermectin epoxide derivatives and method of use. U.S. Patent, 4,530,921.

19 Mrozik, H., P. Eskola, B.O. Linn, A. Lusi, T.L. Shih, M. Tishler, F.S. Waksmunski, M.J. Wyvratt, N.J. Hilton, T.E. Anderson, J.R. Babu, R.A. Dybas, F.A. Preiser and M.H. Fisher. 1989. Discovery of novel avermectins with unprecedented insecticidal activity. Experientia. In press.

20 Pong, S.S. and C.C. Wang. 1982. Avermectin B_1a modulation of gamma-aminobutyric acid receptors in rat brain membranes. J. Neurochem. 38: 375–379.

21 Putter, I., J.G. MacConnell, F.A. Preiser, A.A. Haidri, S.S. Ristich and R.A. Dybas. 1981. Avermectins: novel insecticides, acaricides and nematicides from a soil microorganism. Experientia 37: 963–964.

22 Robb, K.L. and M.P. Parrella. 1984. Efficacy of selected insecticides against beet armyworm and thrips on chrysanthemum. In: Proceedings of the Fourth Annual Industry Conference on Leafminer (Poe, S.L., ed.), pp. 33–39.

23 Roush, R.T. and J.E. Wright. 1986. Abamectin: toxicity to house flies (Diptera: Muscidae) resistant to synthetic organic insecticides. J. Econ. Entomol. 79: 562–564.

24 Takiguchi, Y., H. Mishima, M. Okuda, M. Terao, A. Aoki and R. Fukuda. 1980. Milbemycins, a new family of macrolide antibiotics: fermentation, isolation and physico-chemical properties. J. Antibiot. 33: 1120–1127.

25 Takiguchi, Y., M. Ono, S. Muramatsu, J. Ide, H. Mishima and M. Terao. 1983. Milbemycins, a new family of macrolide antibiotics. Fermentation, isolation, and physico-chemical properties of milbemycins D, E, F, G and H. J. Antibiot. 36: 502–508.

26 Trumble, J.T., W.J. Moar, J.R. Babu and R.A. Dybas. 1987. Laboratory bioassays of the acute and antifeedant effects of avermectin B_1 and a related analogue of Spodoptera exigua (Huebner). J. Agric. Entomol. 4: 21–28.

27 White, A.T., H.S. Newland, H.R. Taylor, K.D. Erttmann, E. Keyvan-Larijani, A. Nara, M.A. Aziz, S.A. D'Anna, P.N. Williams and B.M. Greene. 1987. Controlled trial and dose-finding study of ivermectin for treatment of onchocerciasis. J. Infect. Dis. 156: 463–470.

28 Wright, D.J. 1986. Biological activity and mode of action of avermectins. In: Neuropharmacology and Pesticide Action (Ford, M.G., G.G. Lunt, R.C. Deay and P.N.R. Usherwood, eds.), pp. 174–202, Ellis Horwood, Chichester.

29 Wright, D.J., A.J. Birtle and I.T.J. Roberts. 1984. Triphasic locomotor response of a plant-parasitic nematode to avermectin: inhibition by the GABA antagonists bicuculline and picrotoxin. Parasitology 8: 375–382.

30 Wright, D.J., A. Loy, A.St.J. Green and R.A. Dybas. 1985. The translaminar activity of abamectin (MK-936) against mites and aphids. Med. Fac. Landbouwwet. Rijksuniv. Gent 50: 595–601.

Novel Microbial Products for Medicine and Agriculture
Editors: A.L. Demain, G.A. Somkuti, J.C. Hunter-Cevera and H.W. Rossmoore
© 1989, Society for Industrial Microbiology

CHAPTER 24

Unique strains of *Bacillus thuringiensis* with activity against Coleoptera

Henry W. Talbot*, Michelle Burrascano, Octavio Espinosa, Robert Everich, Kathryn M. Nette, Jewel Payne and George Soares

Mycogen Corporation, San Diego, CA, U.S.A.

SUMMARY

During the past year of the screening program at Mycogen, more than 850 new, naturally occurring strains of *Bacillus thuringiensis* have been isolated from a variety of sources. Of these, 55 isolates have activity against Coleoptera, and were recovered from a diversity of locations across the continental United States. The coleopteran-active strains were found to belong to five different serotypes of *B. thuringiensis*. Electron micrographs prepared for eight isolates revealed some strains with multiple inclusions of varying morphologies. Assays of insecticidal activity against the Colorado potato beetle have shown that the new strains have a wide range of potency relative to *B. thuringiensis* var. *san diego*.

INTRODUCTION

Bacillus thuringiensis is the most widely used bacterial insect pathogen in commercial bioinsecticide preparations. At the present time, products are available for the control of lepidopteran pests (*B. thuringiensis* var. *kurstaki*) and dipteran pests (*B. thuringiensis* var. *israelensis*). Recently, the use of these *B. thuringiensis* products has increased substantially [6]. The availability of new isolates with different insecticidal activities would further expand this market; therefore, the recovery of novel *B. thuringiensis* strains has become increasingly important.

B. thuringiensis var. *san diego* (discovered at Mycogen in 1985) and *B. thuringiensis* var. *tenebrionis* are examples of strains that produce coleopteran-active insecticidal proteins which are toxic to the Colorado potato beetle (CPB) [3,5]. The CPB is the most damaging foliar pest of potatoes grown in North America and Europe. If populations are not controlled, CPB densities can reach hundreds of insects per plant. In addition, the CPB has developed resistance to many insecticides and control of this pest is difficult, especially in the northeastern United States. A *B. thuringiensis* product with efficacy for CPB control would be very useful for the potato-growing industry.

The search for additional coleopteran-active strains has been part of the *B. thuringiensis* screen-

---

*To whom correspondence should be addressed.

ing program at Mycogen. A variety of environmental samples from a wide diversity of locations within the United States have been examined during the past year, and isolated strains have been screened for insecticidal activity against various groups of insects. This paper describes the new, recently isolated coleopteran-active *B. thuringiensis* strains, including crystal morphologies, serotyping, and assays of insecticidal activity.

MATERIALS AND METHODS

Primary screen of B. thuringiensis isolates for activity against Coleoptera

Initial screening for insecticidal activity against Coleoptera was done with a diet overlay assay in which *Leptinotarsa texana* was used as a surrogate for the CPB (*L. decemlineata*). Isolates were grown in peptone glucose salts media (PGSM) for production of toxin [1,4]. Assays were repeated at least twice.

Secondary screen of B. thuringiensis isolates for activity against the CPB

Early second instar larvae of *L. decemlineata* were placed on potato leaves which were dipped in suspensions containing the *B. thuringiensis* preparations. The larvae were incubated at 25°C for 4 days, and larval mortality was recorded and analyzed using probit analysis. Potency ratios were calculated based on insect mortality with the control organism (*B. thuringiensis* var. *san diego*) as compared to that obtained with the test organism, and based on μg toxin per ml of both suspensions.

Electron micrographs

Samples were prepared for electron microscopy by Dr. Cheng-Ming Chang, Electron Microscopy Lab, Scripps Clinic and Research Foundation, La Jolla, California.

Serotyping of B. thuringiensis strains

Serotyping was carried out according to the procedure described by De Barjac [2].

RESULTS AND DISCUSSION

During the past year of the *B. thuringiensis* screening program at Mycogen, more than 850 new, naturally occurring strains were isolated. These isolates were obtained from a variety of environmental samples. Of these strains, 55 were found to have activity against Coleoptera. The data obtained for the primary screen against Coleoptera are presented for 42 strains in Table 1. This information suggested that there was a range of toxin potencies among the coleopteran-active strains. Bioassays against the CPB confirmed that this was the case (Table 2). Among the ten strains that were tested, one strain (T-4) exhibited significantly higher activity against the CPB than the control organism (*B. thuringiensis* var. *san diego*). On the other hand, other isolates such as T-8 and T-9 produced proteins that were far less toxic than those produced by the control. Clearly, there is a variety of coleopteran-active proteins produced by different strains of *B. thuringiensis*, some of which are significantly more toxic than others.

Further evidence for a number of different coleopteran-active proteins is found in the electron micrographs of several of the isolates. Fig. 1 is an electron micrograph of *B. thuringiensis* var. *san diego*. Figs. 2 through 9 show a variety of crystal types, and that some of the coleopteran-active isolates have multiple inclusions. Fig. 3 shows a spherical inclusion which is very different from others studied, and Figs. 2, 4, 6, 7, and 8 reveal various combinations of multiple inclusions. The strain shown in Fig. 6 appears to have as many as seven separate crystals. Studies are currently under way to determine which crystal type is associated with high or low toxicity to Coleoptera or other groups of insects.

Serotyping of the *B. thuringiensis* strains active against Coleoptera revealed that these isolates could be grouped into five different serotypes (Table 3). From the results of this investigation, it can be concluded that coleopteran-active *B. thuringiensis* can be isolated from numerous locations, and that there are a number of different protein toxins with varying potencies produced by these di-

215

Table 1

Primary screen for biological activity of *B. thuringiensis* strains against *L. texana*

Strain	Percent mortality	
	assay 1	assay 2
B. thuringiensis var. *kurstaki* HD-1	0	0
B. thuringiensis var. *san diego*	100	100
1	100	92
2	92	100
3	100	100
4	92	100
5	92	100
6	92	100
7	100	100
8	75	100
9	92	100
10	100	83
11	100	92
12	100	100
13	100	100
14	100	100
15	100	100
16	100	100
17	100	83
18	100	83
19	100	100
20	100	100
21	100	100
22	100	83
23	75	100
24	88	83
25	100	100
26	100	100
27	75	100
28	100	86
29	100	100
30	86	100
31	86	100
32	100	100
33	83	100
34	87	83
35	83	100
36	100	83
37	100	100
38	100	67
39	75	100
40	86	83
41	88	87

Table 2

Relative potency of *B. thuringiensis* isolates against the CPB (*L. decemlineata*)

Isolate	Potency ratio[a]
B. thuringiensis var. *san diego*	1.00
T-1	1.00
T-2	0.58
T-3	0.98
T-4	1.44
T-5	1.16
T-6	0.61
T-7	0.87
T-8	0.04
T-9	0.12
T-10	0.15

[a] Potency ratios were calculated based on insect mortality with the control organism (*B. thuringiensis* var. *san diego*) as compared to that obtained with the test organism, and based on μg toxin per ml of both suspensions.

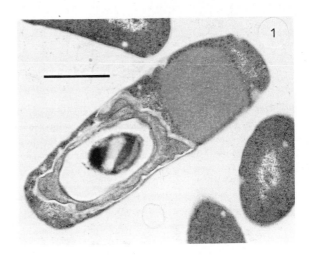

Fig. 1. Electron micrograph of *B. thuringiensis* var. *san diego*, showing refractile spore and crystalline inclusion toxic to Coleoptera. Bar = 1 μm.

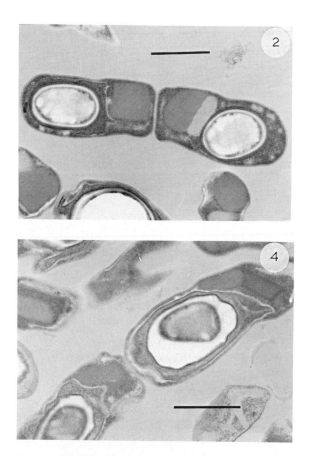

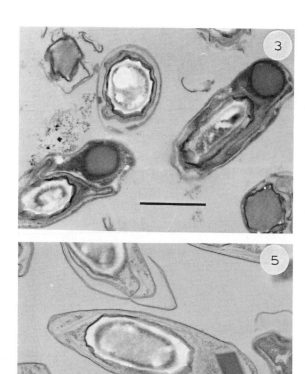

Figs. 2–5. Electron micrographs of newly isolated strains of *B. thuringiensis* with activity against Coleoptera. The strains shown in Fig. 2 and 4 appear to have multiple inclusions, and the strain shown in Fig. 3 has a spherical inclusion. Bar = 1 μm.

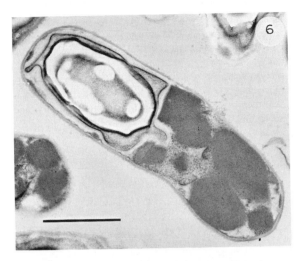

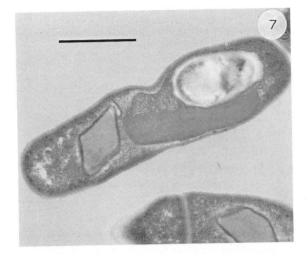

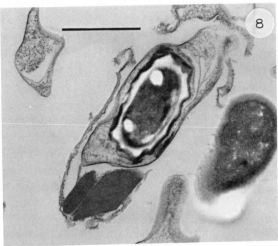

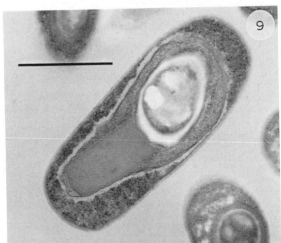

Figs. 6–9. Electron micrographs of newly isolated strains of *B. thuringiensis* with activity against Coleoptera. The strain shown in Fig. 6 has as many as seven separate inclusions. Bar = 1 μm.

Table 3

Serotypes of *B. thuringiensis* isolates active against Coleoptera

Serotype No.	Serotype name
1	*thuringiensis*
6	*entomocidus, subtoxicus*
8a 8b	*morrisoni*
9	*tolworthi*
18	*kumanotoensis*

verse strains. Further work is planned to characterize these proteins.

REFERENCES

1 Brownbridge, M. and J. Margalit. 1986. New *Bacillus thuringiensis* isolated in Israel are highly toxic to mosquito larvae. J. Invert. Pathol. 48: 216–222.
2 De Barjac, H. 1981. Identification of H-serotypes of *Bacillus thuringiensis*. In: Microbial Control of Pests and Plant Diseases 1970–1980 (Burges, H.D., ed.), p. 35, Academic Press, London.

218

3 Herrnstadt, C., G. Soares, E. Wilcox and D. Edwards. 1986. A new strain of *Bacillus thuringiensis* with activity against coleopteran insects. Bio/Technology 4: 305–308.

4 Kalfor, A.R. and H. de Barjac. 1985. Screening of the insecticidal activity of *Bacillus thuringiensis* strains against the Egyptian cotton leaf worm *Spodoptera littoralis*. Entomophaga 30: 177–186.

5 Krieg, V.A., A.M. Huger, G.A. Langenbruch and W. Schnetter. 1983. *Bacillus thuringiensis* var. *tenebrionis*, a new pathotype effective against larvae of Coleoptera. Z. Angew. Entomol. 96: 500–508.

6 Morris, O.N., J.C. Cunningham, J.R. Finney-Crawley, R.P. Jaques and G. Kinoshita. 1986. Microbial insecticides in Canada: their registration and use in agriculture, forestry, and public and animal health. Bull. Entomol. Soc. Canada 18: 1–43.

Novel Microbial Products for Medicine and Agriculture
Editors: A.L. Demain, G.A. Somkuti, J.C. Hunter-Cevera and H.W. Rossmoore
© 1989, Society for Industrial Microbiology

CHAPTER 25

Fermentation alternatives for commercial production of a mycoherbicide

Larry J. Stowell*, Kathy Nette, Brad Heath and Robert Shutter

Mycogen Corporation, San Diego, CA, U.S.A.

SUMMARY

Mycoherbicides have been used as weed control agents in commercial agriculture for nearly a decade. Until recently, mycoherbicide production has relied upon the natural ability of certain fungi to grow and sporulate in submerged fermentation. However, many plant pathogenic fungi do not sporulate under these conditions. In order to fully exploit the potential of mycoherbicides, research and development efforts should be directed towards discovery of fermentation systems which allow commercialization of fungi regardless of their sporulation habit. These systems include: fermentation of mycelia in submerged culture, induction of sporulation in liquid, and production of spores on artificial surfaces or living plant surfaces.

INTRODUCTION

Mycoherbicide candidates can be categorized into two groups based upon differences in their physiology and pathology: (i) fungi which attack plants and sporulate within the plant tissues (e.g. *Phytophthora* sp.) or sporulate under the plant epidermis in pycnidia or acervuli (e.g. *Colletotrichum* sp.), and (ii) fungi which push conidiophores through the plant surface and form conidia in the gaseous environment outside the plant (e.g. *Alternaria* sp.). Based on examples in the literature, it appears that fungi which normally sporulate within the plant readily produce spores in submerged fermentation, whereas fungi that sporulate outside the plant are reluctant to sporulate in submerged fermentation

(refer to Table 1). In order to simplify the following discussion, fungi that sporulate in liquid culture will be designated as Group 1 fungi and those which are reluctant to sporulate in liquid culture will be referred to as Group 2 fungi. Representative examples of both Group 1 and Group 2 fungi are listed in Table 1.

The ability of Group 1 fungi to sporulate in liquid culture may reflect their adaption to growth and reproduction in the aqueous environment present in plant tissues. Submerged fermentation adequately mimics the nutritional and physical environment present within the plant to stimulate sporulation. These fungi will also sporulate on agar surfaces, indicating that submerged culture is not required for sporulation. Because of their ease of production, Group 1 fungi are prime candidates for mycoherbicide development.

The first commercial mycoherbicide products were based upon Group 1 fungi. In 1981, Abbott

---

* To whom correspondence should be addressed.

Current address: PACE Consulting, San Diego, CA, U.S.A.

Table 1

Examples of plant pathogenic fungi belonging to Group 1 and Group 2

Genus	Sporulating structure	Location of *in situ* sporulation	Ref.
Group 1 – sporulate readily in liquid culture			
Ascochyta	pycnidium	under epidermis	21
Colletotri-chum	acervulus	under epidermis	4,10,27
Coniothyrium	pycnidium	under epidermis	30
Fusarium	conidiophore	vascular system	21
Phytophthora	chlamydo-spore	intercellular	24
Verticillium	conidiophore	vascular system	5
Group 2 – reluctant to sporulate in liquid culture			
Alternaria	conidiophore	through plant surface	1,31,33
Bipolaris	conidiophore	through plant surface	12
Cercospora	conidiophore	through plant surface	7
Curvularia	conidiophore	through plant surface	30
Fusarium	sporodochium	through plant surface	34

introduced Devine® for control of strangler vine in Florida citrus. The active ingredient, *Phytophthora palmivora*, is a pathogen that normally produces chlamydospores inside the plant. Devine consists of chlamydospores produced in submerged fermentation. A second product, Collego®, was introduced in 1982 by Upjohn for control of northern jointvetch in Arkansas rice and soybeans [28]. The active ingredient, *Colletotrichum gloeosporioides* f. sp. *aeschynomene* (CGA), is a pathogen that produces conidia in acervuli. Collego is also produced in submerged fermentation and is comprised of conidia, blastospores, and fission spores [6]. Manufacture of both of these products was readily adapted to the submerged fermentation facilities available at Abbott and Upjohn. At that time, industry did not seriously consider developing a mycoherbicide unless it could be produced in liquid culture. The requirement for submerged fermenta-

tion of mycoherbicides was expressed by Templeton, one of the scientists who discovered CGA, when he wrote: '... from a practical standpoint, growth and sporulation by liquid culture technology may well be an essential requirement additional to the previously described attributes of activity, specificity and viability' [29]. This requirement would prevent consideration of Group 2 fungi as mycoherbicide candidates.

The reluctance of Group 2 fungi to sporulate in liquid indicates that these fungi have a more defined requirement for sporulation than Group 1 fungi. Sporulation in Group 2 fungi requires a solid–gas interface, absence of a sporulation inhibitor (e.g. CO_2) in the gaseous phase or the presence of a sporulation stimulus outside the plant (e.g. light). Like Group 1 fungi, these pathogens sporulate readily on agar surfaces. However, Group 2 fungi do not readily sporulate in liquid or inside plant tissues.

Since the introduction of Collego and Devine, the agricultural biotechnology industry has grown, bringing with it a new interest in mycoherbicide development. Group 2 fungi are being developed despite the initial difficulties encountered in their production. In 1985, Mycogen Corporation was granted a multistate Experimental Use Permit by the Environmental Protection Agency for large-scale field evaluation of CASST™, a mycoherbicide for control of sicklepod in peanuts, soybeans, and cotton. Because this product is based on the Group 2 fungus *Alternaria cassiae*, CASST represents a new direction in mycoherbicide development. Mycoherbicide technologists are no longer restricting discovery and development efforts to organisms that readily produce spores in liquid. The arsenal now spans the entire range of plant pathogenic fungi.

The following discussion will review strategies that were developed to permit production of fungi from both Group 1 and Group 2. These include production of mycelium in submerged fermentation, spore production in submerged fermentation, spore production on artificial surfaces, and spore production on living plants.

PROPAGULE PRODUCTION USING SUBMERGED FERMENTATION

Submerged fermentation of fungi remains the most successful method of mycoherbicide production, as represented by Collego® and Devine®. However, Group 2 fungi normally require a solid–gas interface, which cannot be provided in liquid culture, to induce sporulation. Production of these fungi in liquid culture therefore requires use of an alternative propagule (e.g. mycelial fragments), or development of new processes or strains of the fungi which sporulate in liquid.

Mycelia production using submerged fermentation

Both Group 1 and Group 2 fungi produce mycelia in submerged culture. Therefore, developing a method for production and stabilization of mycelia would have broad application for both groups of fungi. In addition, a subset of the Group 2 fungi includes plant pathogens which do not sporulate during any portion of their life cycle (e.g. *Rhizoctonia* sp.) or only sporulate after formation of complex sexual fruiting structures (e.g. *Sclerotinia* sp.). In order to utilize these fungi for mycoherbicides, production and stabilization of mycelium would be essential: the need to develop mycelial production systems for these fungi is evident. Although the use of mycelial fragments has been suggested in the past, it has not gained widespread acceptance [6, 17].

The Group 2 fungus, *A. cassiae* (CASST™), has been formulated directly from submerged fermentation by harvesting mycelia, mixing with inert ingredients, and mechanically reducing the size of propagules. Similar processes have been developed and patented for fungal insect pathogens [16].

The success of a mycelial preparation can be evaluated by the ability of the final product to kill the target weed. For example, Fig. 1 illustrates the activity of CASST mycelial and spore formulations. The probit-dose response is linear in both cases. The regression equations are listed below:

Mycelia: probit = 3.0 [log(PPA)] − 22.4
             $r = 0.99$

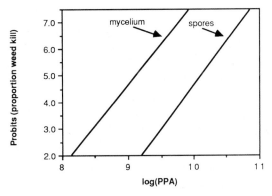

Fig. 1. Comparison between the activity of mycelium formulations and spores of *A. cassiae* (CASST™) in controlling sicklepod. Data represent the mean dose response of nine mycelium formulations and seven spore formulations expressed in Propagules Per Acre (PPA), evaluated under greenhouse conditions in 1986. All treatments were applied at 30 gallons water per acre using a precision track sprayer.

Spores: probit = 3.3 [log(PPA)] − 28.4
            $r = 0.98$

The slopes of both dose-response relationships are approximately the same (spore-dose relationship = 3.3, mycelia-dose relationship = 3.0), indicating similar specific activity and demonstrating the commercial potential of mycelial propagules.

Spore production using submerged fermentation

Spores of fungi are generally considered to be the most desirable propagule for use in mycoherbicide products because they are the natural survival and dissemination structure of many fungi. By definition, spores of Group 1 fungi are readily produced in liquid culture. However, production of spores by Group 2 fungi in submerged fermentation is under development.

The genus *Fusarium* is listed as belonging to both Group 1 and Group 2 in Table 1. The Group 1 *Fusarium* belongs to the root-infecting wilt and rot species that produce spores inside plant tissues. The Group 2 *Fusarium* produces cankers on aboveground plant parts and sporulates on sporodochia outside the plant. Walker reported that the Group 2 species, *F. lateritium*, does not produce macroconidia in liquid culture and proposed the use of surface production techniques for this fungus [34]. However, submerged fermentation research on this organism has revealed that macrospore production can be induced in liquid culture (unpublished, Mycogen Corporation). *F. lateritium* is therefore properly associated with other Group 2 fungi that are reluctant to sporulate in liquid culture.

In addition to the example above, Vezina and Singh [30] reported that the Group 2 fungus *Curvularia luminata*, produced conidia in one of the two media tested. However, the level of sporulation (spores/ml) was the lowest of the 20 different fungi evaluated. In contrast, *C. pallescens* did not produce spores in liquid culture. Like *Fusarium*, *Curvularia* is reluctant but not incapable of sporulating in liquid. These examples illustrate the potential of certain Group 2 fungi to sporulate in liquid culture. They also indicate that future research to broaden our understanding of fungal physiology is necessary to provide methods of producing many Group 2 fungi in liquid. The following example demonstrates the value of studying the physiology of spore production by Group 2 fungi.

Recent work by Cotty revealed several approaches to induction of sporulation in Group 2 fungi. He observed that CO_2 concentration is a critical factor in sporulation of *A. tagetica* [9]. High levels of CO_2 prevented sporulation on agar surfaces while removal of CO_2 induced sporulation. Cotty also selected a mutant of *A. tagetica* which was insensitive to CO_2 modulation of sporulation; this strain produced spores not only in the presence of CO_2 but also in submerged culture [8]. Research conducted at Mycogen with *A. cassiae* (CASST[TM]) has revealed a similar response to CO_2, confirming Cotty's speculation that CO_2 will modulate sporulation in other species of *Alternaria*. Induction of sporulation of Group 2 fungi in liquid will probably result from combinations of several processes including, but not limited to, strain selection and control of the gaseous environment. However, each species will have unique requirements making a general solution for all Group 2 fungi unlikely.

PROPAGULE PRODUCTION ON ARTIFICIAL SURFACES

Many plant pathogenic fungi from both Group 1 and Group 2 sporulate on agar surfaces. Therefore, the use of surface production systems may allow a broad range of fungi to be evaluated for use as mycoherbicides. For example, the alginate granule system developed by Walker has been used to produce fungi representing both Group 1 (*Colletotrichum malvarum* and *Phylosticta* sp.) and Group 2 (*F. lateritium*, *A. cassiae* and *A. macrospora*) [35]. In addition to alginate granules and agar surfaces, plant pathogenic fungal spores have been produced on the surface of mycelia in pans [12,31,35]. These techniques are similar to those used in production of spores for transformation of organic compounds and for use as insecticides [20,30].

The limiting factors for production of spores from surfaces must be identified before a production process can be optimized. As with any fermentation process, nutrition and environment play a major role. However, another important parameter, steric hindrance, must be considered during development of surface sporulation processes. Spore production will be limited if the space available for sporulation is not sufficiently large to allow spores to form normally. Steric hindrance of sporulation was found to be a limiting factor in production of *A. cassiae* (CASST) on solid surfaces. The following model of spore yield is based upon steric hindrance and allows efficiency of several experimental systems for spore production to be compared. In addition, the importance of spore size and mycelium concentration beneath the sporulation surface are discussed.

Mathematical model of sporulation from a solid surface

Group 2 mycoherbicides belonging to the dematiaceous hyphomycetes (e.g. *Alternaria*) sometimes produce single spores on erect conidiophores causing a velvet-like appearance in sporulating cultures. Fig. 2 is a stylized representation of a plant pathogenic *Alternaria* sp. sporulating on a solid surface (plant leaf, agar plate, or alginate granule). This or-

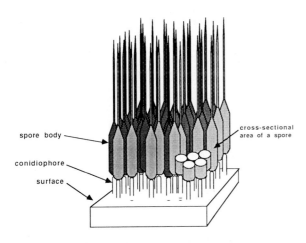

Fig. 2. Stylized representation illustrating dense-pack sporulation of plant pathogenic fungi that produce single spores on erect conidiophores from solid surfaces. The cross-sectional area of the spores provides an estimation of maximum yield per unit production area.

ganized production of conidia lends itself to the development of a simple mathematical model which describes the yield of spores based upon the cross-sectional area of a spore.

This model is a modification of that reported by Laukevics *et al.* describing steric hindrance of fungal growth on solid substrates [15]. It has been simplified from the three dimensions described by Laukevics *et al.*, to two dimensions with the radius of the spore being the single parameter determining yield of spores per unit area. We have assumed that there is no steric hindrance imposed from above the sporulating surface.

The area needed for sporulation exceeds the cross-sectional area of a spore by the wasted space between densely-packed circles. This area is illustrated in Fig. 3. The maximum packing density (Ψ) for congruent circles is equivalent to the ratio between the area of the equilateral triangle formed by connecting the center points of the circles and the area occupied by the three arcs.

$$A_t = R^2 \sqrt{3}$$
$$A_a = (1/2) R^2 \theta$$

where A_t = area of the equilateral triangle, R = cross-sectional radius of a spore, A_a = area of a single arc, and θ = angle of the arc in radians ($\pi/3$). Therefore:

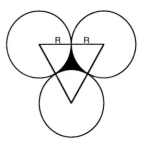

Fig. 3. Graphic representation of the unused space created by contact between three congruent circles.

$$\Psi = 3A_a/A_t = [3((1/2) R^2 \pi/3)]/[2R^2 \sqrt{3}] = 0.907$$

The general model for yield of fungi that produces spores singly on erect conidiophores is:

$$Y_E = (\Psi)/\pi R^2 = (0.907)/\pi R^2$$

where Y_E = expected yield of spores.

To evaluate the performance of a spore production system, the ratio of observed yield (Y_O) and expected yield (Y_E) can be used to estimate percent yield efficiency ($Y_\%$):

$$Y_\% = 100 \cdot Y_O/Y_E.$$

The efficiencies of several spore production systems are summarized in Table 2. The four sporulation processes evaluated include: (i) sporulation on agar in petri plates, (ii) sporulation on alginate granules, (iii) sporulation in pans from the surface of whole fermentation broth poured into the pans, and (iv) the Mycogen Sporulation Process (MSP) which is used to produce large quantities of spores for advanced product evaluations. Sporulation on petri plates and alginate granules were the least space-efficient ($Y_\% < 30$). The pan technique and the MSP both provided efficient utilization of space with $Y_\%$ greater than 80%.

The high-yield efficiency of the pan technique for *A. cassiae* production ($Y_\% = 118$) can be explained by error in the value of R listed in Table 2. Exact spore measurements were only available for the MSP system. The R values listed for other production techniques represent the mean values reported in the taxonomic literature for each fungus [11,26]. Fig. 4 illustrates the relationship between yield of spores in dense pack as a function of spore radius. A small reduction in spore radius can have a significant influence on yield. Additionally, the size of

Table 2

Alternaria spore production efficiencies on solid surfaces

Species	Ref.[a]	Surface type[b]	R (μm)[c]	Y_E[d]	Y_O[e]	$Y_{\%}$[f]
A. tagetica	9	agar	15	1.4×10^9	2.4×10^6	<1
A. macrospora	35	alginate granule	9	3.6×10^9	2.6×10^8	7
A. cassiae	35	alginate granule	17	1.1×10^9	1.8×10^8	16
A. macrospora	31	agar	9	3.6×10^9	1.0×10^9	28
A. macrospora	31	pan	9	3.6×10^9	3.6×10^9	100
A. cassiae	32	pan	17	1.1×10^9	1.3×10^9	118
A. cassiae	—	MSP	13	1.8×10^9	1.5×10^9	83

[a] Original reference in which Y_O and production techniques are described.

[b] Agar refers to production in petri plates on agar media. Pan refers to a technique of spore production in shallow pans filled with a thin layer of whole fermentation broth of the fungus. Sporulation occurs at the surface of the mycelium after treatment with light. Alginate granules are prepared by immobilizing mycelium through calcium polymerization of an alginate–mycelium suspension. Granules are dried and re-wet and treated with light to induce sporulation. The MSP surface refers to a proprietary process developed at Mycogen Corporation to produce large quantities of spores of fungi that are reluctant to sporulate in liquid culture.

[c] R is the radius of a typical spore of the fungus described in the taxonomic literature [6,18].

[d] Y_E is the expected yield per meter square based upon the dense packing model for congruent circles: $Y_E = (0.907/\pi R^2) \cdot 1.0 \times 10^{12}$.

[e] Y_O is the yield of spores per meter square projected from the production area reported in the original reference.

[f] $Y_{\%}$ is the percent efficiency of the production system: $Y_{\%} = 100 \cdot Y_O/Y_E$.

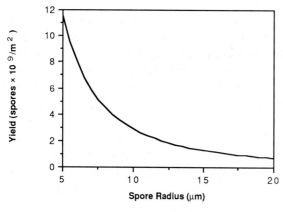

Fig. 4. Relationship between spore radius and yield per meter square using the densely packed congruent circle model.

spores can be altered by culture media [19]. The abnormally high $Y_{\%}$ for the pan technique probably results in part from production of spores with radii less than 17 μm. For example, spores of *A. cassiae* produced in high density by the MSP system are only 13 ± 3.5 μm in radius as compared to the average value of 17 μm reported for *A. cassiae* [26]. The efficiency of the MSP system using $R = 17$ μm is $Y_{\%} = 136$. This would be the highest efficiency based upon published spore radii. Despite this source of error, this model can be used to compare production efficiencies of different surface sporulation systems.

In addition to spore radius, the concentration of mycelia directly under conidiophore-bearing hyphae can influence the yield of spores per unit area. A high mycelia concentration results in the maximum number of conidiophores and conidia per unit area. Both the agar plate and the alginate granule techniques require mycelia to compete with conidiophores for space and nutrients while growing across the plate or over the surface of a granule. This competition for growing space and nutrition can be prevented by increasing the amount of mycelium directly beneath the sporulating surface while reducing the nutrients available. Conidiophores are then produced in the gaseous environment without competition from rapidly growing mycelium. For example, the pan techniques listed in Table 2 represent the highest possible concentration of mycelium (whole fermentation broth poured undiluted into a pan) and most efficient space utilization ($Y_{\%} \approx 100$). Fig. 5 illustrates the interaction of mycelia concen-

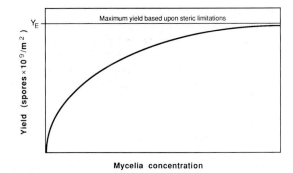

Fig. 5. Relationship between mycelia concentration in the sporulating surface and spore yield per meter square. Based upon data obtained from production of *A. cassiae* in the MSP.

tration and spore yield using the MSP. Yield increases asymptotically to the limit imposed by steric hindrance of densely packed spores. Therefore, the optimum concentration of mycelium below the spore-bearing hyphae is equal to the minimum concentration of mycelia that provides a yield (Y_O) which is not significantly less than the maximum expected yield (Y_E). Under these conditions, maximum sporulation is obtained from the production area using the smallest amount of mycelium.

SPORE PRODUCTION ON LIVING PLANT SURFACES

When spore production using artificial media fails, spore production of both Group 1 and Group 2 fungi can be carried out using infected host plants. In particular, this technique is used to produce fungi that cannot be cultured on artificial media. These fastidious pathogens belong to the Teliomycetidae (rusts) and the Albuginaceae (white rusts). Their life habit most closely resembles that of Group 1 fungi with sporulation occurring under the plant epidermis. Although these fungi are still considered obligate parasites, advances in biotechnology and fungal genetics/physiology are likely to remove existing production barriers. Until these barriers are removed, the only method of culturing rusts and white rusts for evaluation as mycoherbicides is on the living plant host.

Production of small research quantities of rust spores can be carried out under greenhouse conditions by inoculating the host with spores of the rust and providing a conducive moist environment for disease development. After pustule formation, spores can be collected with a cyclone spore trap in quantities sufficient for field evaluation [22]. Production of large quantities of rust spores has been accomplished to help study the epidemiology of wheat stem rust [14]. Specialized harvesting equipment has been developed to collect spores from rust-infected plants under field conditions (C.H. Kingsolver, personal communication). However, this technology has not reached commercial application in the mycoherbicide industry.

Commercial production of rusts might occur in fields of infected weed hosts. The spores could be harvested with specialized spore combines. Unfortunately, several problems become evident when this process is considered further. For example, weeds are known to harbor a variety of diseases of economic crops. Therefore, care would have to be taken to insure that the spores harvested are not contaminated with other organisms which might cause damage to crops, a nearly impossible task under field conditions [13]. In addition, the quality of the product might vary beyond acceptable limits when produced under constantly changing field conditions. For these reasons, the Teliomycetidae and the Albuginaceae are not likely to be developed as commercial mycoherbicides until economical production on artificial media in controlled fermentation is achieved. Fortunately, research into artificial culture of rust fungi is under way [25].

DISCUSSION

In 1980 Templeton stressed the importance of producing mycoherbicides in submerged culture, realizing the need to match mycoherbicide production technology with existing industrial fermentation capability [29]. He also suggested that only mycoherbicide candidates which sporulate in liquid would be seriously considered for development by industry. At that time, it was pharmaceutical companies [6] that produced mycoherbicides, while the

226

university system and the U.S. Department of Agriculture were almost exclusively responsible for mycoherbicide discovery and early development.

Discovery of new mycoherbicides should no longer be restricted by the lack of existing technology for production of fungi that are reluctant to sporulate in submerged culture. Rather, mycoherbicide discovery efforts should be targeted at weed pathogens addressing important and profitable market opportunities. If the most virulent and best adapted organism in the target market area does not initially produce propagules in liquid culture, alternative production systems, like the MSP, will be used to carry the product through large-scale field evaluations. At the same time, concentrated research efforts in plant pathology, fermentation, formulation and weed science will strive to optimize production economics.

Future mycoherbicide products will demonstrate the benefits provided by rapidly developing opportunities in fungal biotechnology, formulation and fermentation. Advances in formulating mycoherbicides have resulted in improved activity under an expanded range of environmental conditions [2,23] and have broadened the host range of specific fungi [3]. In addition, highly virulent, broad-spectrum pathogens have been genetically modified to limit their host range [18]. Accordingly, fermentation discoveries will be needed to meet the challenges encountered in production of an expanding range of mycoherbicides representing a broad range of natural fungal isolates, in addition to variants of these strains produced by classical genetic and recombinant DNA techniques.

REFERENCES

1 Allen, S.J. and J.F. Brown. 1983. Production of inoculum and field assessment of *Alternaria helianthi* on sunflower. Plant Dis. 67: 665–668.

2 Bannon, J.S. and H.L. Walker. 1987. Influence of non-ionic surfactants and non-phytotoxic crop oils on control of sicklepod by *Alternaria cassiae*. Proc. South. Weed Sci Soc. 40: 288.

3 Boyette, C.D. 1987. Biocontrol of hemp sesbania [*Sesbania exalta* (Raf.) Cory] by an induced host range alteration of *Alternaria crassa*. Abstr. Weed Sci. Soc. Am. 27: 129.

4 Cardina, J., R.H. Littrel and L.J. Stowell. 1987. Bioherbicide for florida beggarweed. U.S. Patent No. 4,643,756.

5 Christen, A.A. 1982. Growth and pathogenicity of alfalfa strain of *Verticillium albo-atrum*. Plant Dis. 66: 416–418.

6 Churchill, B.W. 1982. Mass production of microorganisms for biological control. In: Biological Control of Weeds With Plant Pathogens (Charudattan, R. and H.L. Walker, eds.), pp. 134–156, John Wiley & Sons, New York.

7 Conway, K.E., T.E. Freeman and R. Charudattan. 1978. Method and composition for controlling waterhyancinth. U.S. Patent No. 4,097,261.

8 Cotty, P.J. 1985. Carbon dioxide modulates the sporulation of *Alternaria* species. Phytopathology 75: 1297.

9 Cotty, P.J. 1987. Modulation of sporulation of *Alternaria tagetica* by carbon dioxide. Mycologia 79: 508–513.

10 Daniel, J.T., G.E. Templeton and J. Smith, Jr. 1974. Control of aschynomene sp. with *Colletotrichum gloeosporiodes* penz. f.sp. *aeschynomene*. U.S. Patent No. 3,849,104.

11 Ellis, M.B. 1971. Dematiaceous Hyphomycetes. Commonwealth Mycological Institute, Kew, U.K.

12 Foudin, A.S. and O.H. Calvert. 1987. A consistent method for producing gram quantities of typical *Bipolaris zeicola* and *B. maydis* conidia. Mycologia 79: 117–122.

13 Hasan, S. 1974. First introduction of a rust fungus in Australia for the biological control of skeleton weed. Phytopathology 64: 253–254.

14 Kingsolver, C.H., C.E. Peet and J.F. Underwood. 1984. Measurement of the epidemiologic potential of wheat stem rust: St. Croix, U.S. Virgin Islands 1954–1957. Bulletin 854, The Pennsylvania State University, College of Agriculture, University Park, PA.

15 Laukevics, J.J., A.F. Apsite, U.S. Viesturs and R.P. Tengerdy. 1985. Steric hindrance of growth of filamentous fungi in solid state fermentation of wheat straw. Biotechnol. Bioeng. 27: 1687–1691.

16 McCabe, D. and R.S. Soper. 1985. Preparation of an entomopathogenic fungal insect control agent. U.S. Patent No. 4,530,834.

17 Miller, T.L. and B.W. Churchill. 1986. Substrates for large scale fermentations. In: Manual of Industrial Microbiology and Biotechnology (Demain, A.L. and N.A. Solomon, eds.), pp. 122–136, American Society for Microbiology, Washington, DC.

18 Miller, R.V., E.J. Ford and D.C. Sands. 1987. Reduced host-range mutants of *Sclerotinia sclerotiorum*. Phytopathology 77: 1695.

19 Misaghi, I.J., R.G. Grogan, J.M. Duniway and K.A. Kimble. 1978. Influence of environment and culture media on spore morphology of *Alternaria alternata*. Phytopathology 68: 29–34.

20 Mudgett, R.E. 1986. Solid-state fermentations. In: Manual of Industrial Microbiology and Biotechnology (Demain, A.L. and N.A. Solomon, eds.), pp. 66–83, American Society for Microbiology, Washington, DC.

21 Nene, Y.L., M.P. Haware and M.V. Reddy. 1981. Chickpea

diseases: resistance-screening techniques. Information Bulletin No. 10. International Crops Research Institute for the Semi-Arid Tropics, Patancheru, A.P., India.

22 Phatak, S.C., D.R. Summer, H.D. Wells, D.K. Bell and N.C. Glaze. 1983. Biological control of yellow nutsedge with the indigenous rust fungus *Puccinia canaliculata*. Science 219: 1446–1447.

23 Quimby, P.C., Jr., F.E. Fulghum, C.D. Boyette and W.J. Connick, Jr. 1988. An invert emulsion replaces dew in biocontrol of sicklepod – a preliminary study. In: Pesticide Formulations and Application Systems: Vol. 8, ASTM STP 980 (Haude, D.A. and G.B. Beestam, eds.), American Society of Testing and Materials, Philadelphia, PA (in press).

24 Ribeiro, O.K. 1983. Physiology of asexual sporulation and spore germination in *Phytophthora*. In: Phytophthora, its Biology, Taxonomy, Ecology, and Pathology (Erwin, D.C., S. Bartnicki-Garcia and P.H. Tsao, eds.), pp. 55–70, American Phytopathological Society, St. Paul, MN.

25 Scott, K.J. 1976. Growth of biotrophic parasites in axenic culture. In: Encyclopedia of Plant Physiology, New Series Vol. 4 (Pirson, A. and M.H. Zimmermann, eds.), pp. 719–742, Springer-Verlag, New York.

26 Simmons, E.G. 1982. *Alternaria* themes and variation (7–10). Mycotaxon 14: 17–43.

27 Templeton, G.E. 1976. *C. malvarum* spore concentrate, formulation, and agricultural process. U.S. Patent No. 3,999,973.

28 Templeton, G.E. 1982. Biological herbicides: discovery, development, deployment. Weed Sci. 30: 430–433.

29 Templeton, G.E., R.J. Smith and W. Kolmparens. 1980. Commercialization of fungi and bacteria for biological control. Biocontrol News Inf. 1: 291–294.

30 Vezina, C. and K. Singh. 1975. Transformation of organic compounds by fungal spores. In: The Filamentous Fungi, Vol. 1: Industrial Mycology (Smith, J.E. and D.R. Berry, eds.), pp. 158–192, Edward Arnold, London.

31 Walker, H.L. 1980. *Alternaria macrospora* as a potential biocontrol agent for spurred anoda: production of spores for field studies. USDA, SEA, Advances in Technology AAT-S-12/April 1980.

32 Walker, H.L. 1982. Seedling blight of sicklepod caused by *Alternaria cassiae*. Plant Dis. 66: 426–428.

33 Walker, H.L. 1983. Control of sicklepod, showy crotalaria and coffee senna with a fungal pathogen. U.S. Patent No. 4,390,360.

34 Walker, H.L. 1983. Control of prickly sida, velvetleaf, and spurred anoda with fungal pathogens. U.S. Patent No. 4,419,120.

35 Walker, H.L. and W.J. Connick, Jr. 1983. Sodium alginate for production and formulation of mycoherbicides. Weed Sci. 31: 333–338.

Novel Microbial Products for Medicine and Agriculture
Editors: A.L. Demain, G.A. Somkuti, J.C. Hunter-Cevera and H.W. Rossmoore
© 1989, Society for Industrial Microbiology

CHAPTER 26

New anthelmintic and growth promoting agents from actinomycetes

Guy T. Carter

American Cyanamid Company, Medical Research Division, Lederle Laboratories, Pearl River, NY, U.S.A.

INTRODUCTION

Over the past decade, we at Cyanamid have been screening microorganisms for the production of compounds useful in the livestock industry. The primary goal of this work has been the discovery of novel anthelmintic, anticoccidial and growth-promoting agents. During this time, a number of new anticoccidial antibiotics were found, including the polyether maduramicin [7] from *Actinomadura yumaensis*, now the commercial product Cygro®, and the extremely potent xanthone antibiotics LL-D42067α and β from *Actinomadura madura* ssp. *simaoensis* [8]. Another organism which produced anticoccidial compounds is *Streptomyces lydicus* ssp. *tanzanius*, LL-E19020. This organism proved to be the source of extremely effective growth-promoting agents [4]. In the anthelmintic area, a group of macrocyclic lactones, the LL-F28249 series [2], was discovered. These compounds have shown very promising activity against endo- and ecto-parasites of mammals. In this report, aspects of the discovery, isolation, structure determination, biosynthesis, and bioactivity of the LL-F28249 anthelmintic agents, the anticoccidial agents Cygro®, and LL-D42067, and the growth-promotants from culture LL-E19020 will be discussed.

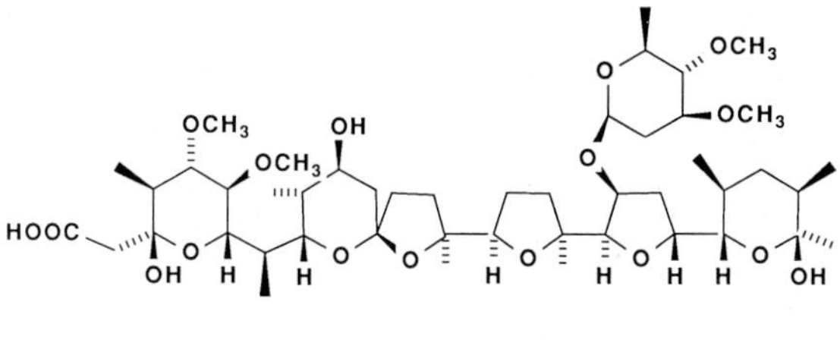

maduramicin (CYGRO)

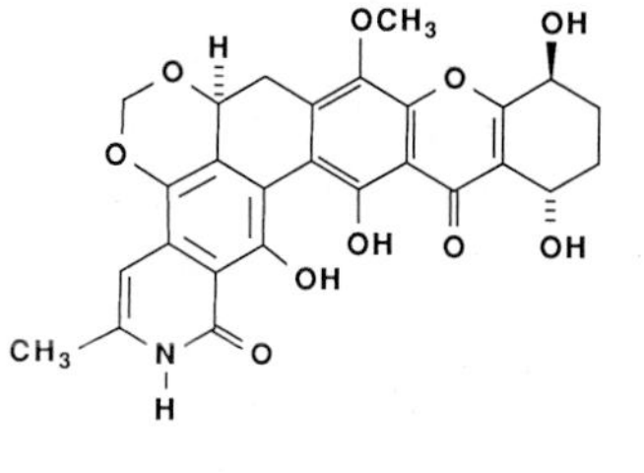

LL-D42067 ALPHA

LL-F28249 ANTHELMINTIC AGENTS

Culture LL-F28249, identified as *Streptomyces cyaneogriseus* ssp. *noncyanogenus*, was found to produce anthelmintic activity in our *Caenorhabditis elegans in vitro* prescreen. *C. elegans* is a free-living soil nematode which responds to the majority of known anthelmintic compounds. It has been incorporated into a rapid, high-capacity bioassay for the testing of fermentation broths. In liquid medium in 96-well plates, this organism is normally in constant motion. Anthelmintic activity is assessed by changes in the motility of the organism. When fermentation broth from LL-F28249 was tested in this system, complete paralysis of *C. elegans* resulted. The next stage of the evaluation process involved an *in vivo* gerbil model infected with the sheep bankrupt worm *Trichostrongylus colubriformis*.

Whole lyophilized fermentation broth from LL-F28249 demonstrated excellent activity in this model, as shown in Table 1. The effectiveness of this crude preparation prompted further investigation of the active material produced by this culture.

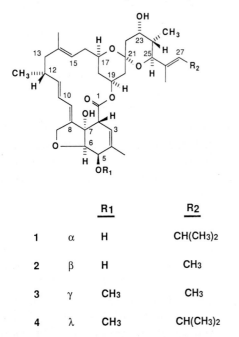

		R1	R2
1	α	H	CH(CH3)2
2	β	H	CH3
3	γ	CH3	CH3
4	λ	CH3	CH(CH3)2

The isolation and purification procedures employed to obtain the four major anthelmintic components LL-F28249α, β, γ and λ (1–4) are outlined in Fig. 1. The macrolides were recovered from the cell mass by extraction with methanol. This metha-

Table 1

Anthelmintic efficacy of lyophilized whole fermentation mash of F28249 against *Trichostrongylus colubriformis* in gerbils

	Efficacy (%)
In medicated diet	
conc. (ppm): 500	100
125	88
By single oral dose	
dose (mg/kg): 200	100
25	88
By subcutaneous injection	
dose (mg/kg): 200	100
50	100

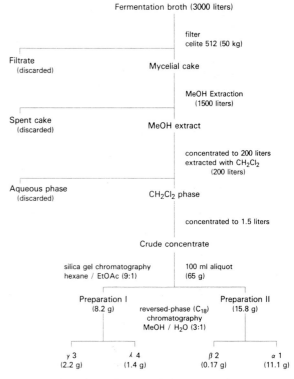

Fig. 1. Isolation and purification scheme for LL-F28249α, β, γ and λ.

nol extract was concentrated to an aqueous suspension and the macrolides extracted into methylene chloride. Evaporation under reduced pressure yielded a crude concentrate, which was first chromatographed on silica gel eluted with hexane/ethyl acetate (9:1). Fractions were pooled to yield two preparations: I containing the less polar 5-*O*-methyl derivatives 3 and 4, and II composed of 5-hydroxy components 1 and 2. Further chromatography on a reversed-phase (C18) column eluted with methanol/water (3:1) was used to resolve the individual compounds in these two preparations.

A summary of selected physico-chemical properties of 1–4 is presented in Table 2. The compounds were generally obtained as white fluffy solids upon freeze-drying from *t*-butanol. These agents are freely soluble in most common organic solvents, soluble in hexane and nearly insoluble in water. The similarity of spectroscopic data to those of the milbemycins [9] suggested a close structural relationship. The electron impact mass spectra (EI-MS), in

Table 2

Selected physico-chemical properties of LL-F28249α, β, γ and λ

	LL-F28249α 1	LL-F28249β 2	LL-F28249γ 3	LL-F28249λ 4
Molecular formula	$C_{36}H_{52}O_8$	$C_{34}H_{48}O_8$	$C_{35}H_{50}O_8$	$C_{37}H_{54}O_8$
M⁺ (HREIMS)	612.3705	584.3388	598.3543	626.3806
$[\alpha]_D^{26}$ (acetone)	+136° (c = 1.04)	+116° (c = 1.02)	+153° (c = 1.06)	+148° (c = 1.18)
UV λ_{max}^{MeOH} nm (ε)	244 (30 500)	244 (26 000)	244 (28 900)	244 (28 400)
IR ν_{max}^{KBr} cm⁻¹	3521 1714 1181 997	3520 1714 1166 995	3528 1712 1168 996	3523 1713 1180 997

HREIMS = high-resolution electron impact mass spectroscopy.

particular, were most useful in the structure assignments. Fig. 2 depicts the major structurally diagnostic EI-MS fragmentation pathways that were employed in the structure determination. Analysis of these data as well as ¹H- and ¹³C-NMR spectra led to the structures 1–4 as shown [3]. The relative stereochemistry was assured by an X-ray crystallographic determination of 3; the resultant three-dimensional representation is shown in Fig. 3. The novel structural feature found in 1–4, which differentiates them from the milbemycins and avermectins, is the unsaturated C-25 side chain. The structure of this side chain reflects a fundamental biosynthetic divergence of the LL-F28249 compounds from milbemycin and avermectin.

Feeding ¹³C-labeled acetate and propionate to growing cultures of *S. cyaneogriseus* ssp. *noncyanogenus* yielded 1 with the labeling pattern indicated in Fig. 4. Excluding the side chain portion, this pattern is identical to that determined for avermectin [1] and milbemycin [10]. The six-carbon unsaturated side chain of 1 is derived from two acyl units linked through the $\triangle^{26}$ double bond. As shown in Fig. 4, C-25 is derived from C-1 of propionate, C-26 and -26a arising from C-2 and -3 of propionate, respectively. The remainder of the side chain is con-

milbemycin D R₁ = H   R₂ = H
avermectin B₂ᵦ R₁ = OH   R₂ = (oleandrose)₂

structed from the condensation of C-1 of an isobutyrate unit with C-26, resulting in the double bond. Position 27 was labeled quite extensively when the fermentation medium was supplemented with [1-¹³C]isobutyrate. These studies reveal that the polyketide precursors of the LL-F28249 macrolides are one unit longer than those attributed to any other member of this class of compounds. The origin of the oxygen atoms of 1 was also determined by growing the culture in the presence of stable isotope-labeled precursors. With the exception of

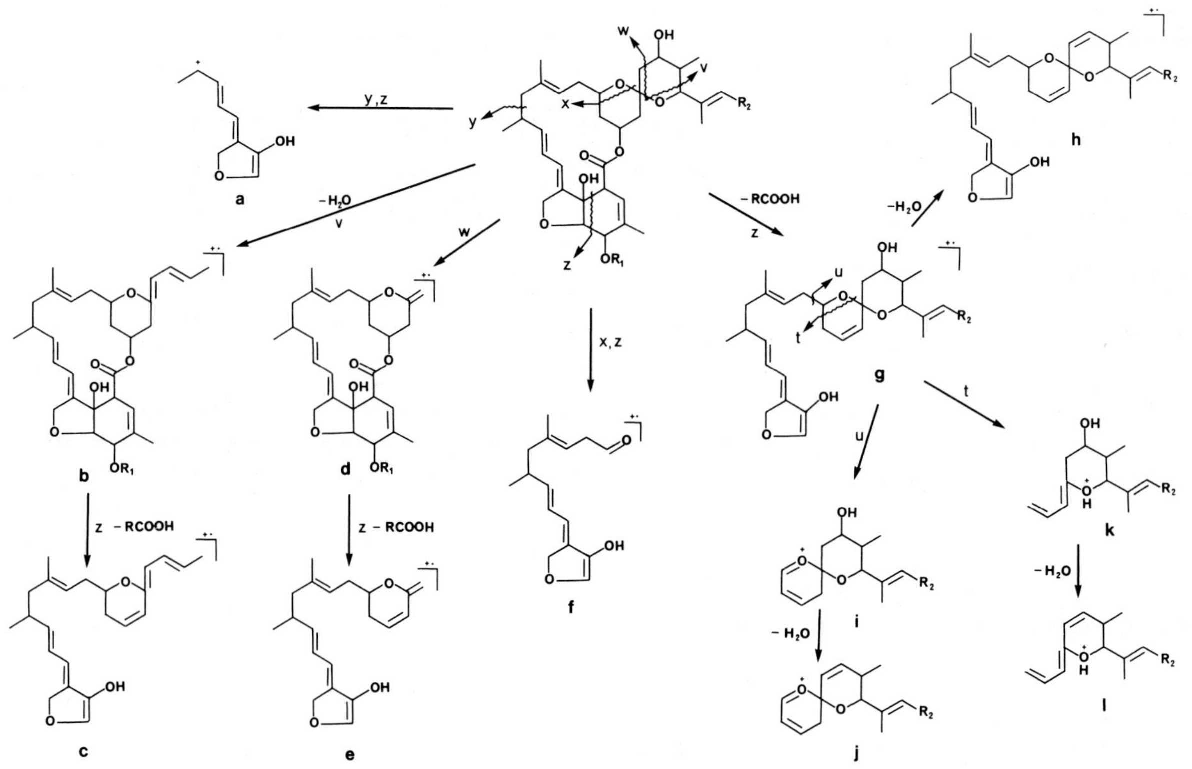

		m/z (relative abundance)						
	1		**2**		**3**		**4**	
a	151.0753	(76)	151	(100)	151	(100)	151	(88)
b	482.2648	(1)	482	(1)	496.2824	(1)	496	(1)
c	354.2818	(9)	354	(12)	354	(27)	354	(14)
d	442.2375	(1)	442	(1)	456.2512	(4)	456	(2)
e	314.1877	(8)	314	(11)	314	(20)	314	(11)
f	248.1405	(4)	248	(7)	248	(4)	248	(7)
g	484.3211	(1)	456.2876	(1)	456.2876	(3)	484	(2)
h	466.3097	(15)	438.2780	(18)	438	(55)	466	(26)
i	265.1786	(3)	237.1491	(8)	237	(6)	265	(4)
j	247.1705	(6)	219.1380	(11)	219	(10)	247	(7)
k	237.1838	(5)	209.1534	(10)	209	(13)	237	(6)
l	219.1740	(6)	191.1427	(13)	191	(14)	219	(8)

Fig. 2. EI-MS fragmentations of the LL-F28249 macrolides 1–4.

the ether oxygen (O-6) between C-6 and -8a, all the oxygen atoms are derived from the carboxyl groups of their respective acyl precursors. An analogous result was previously found in the avermectin series by Cane and coworkers [1]. Experiments with ^{18}O-enriched molecular oxygen in a specially designed fermentor [11] established that O-6 originates from atmospheric O_2.

The anthelmintic efficacy of 1 versus several commercially important nematode parasites of cattle is presented in Table 3 [12]. Excellent control was obtained for all parasites, either by injection or oral administration. Activity has also been demonstrated against various ectoparasites of cattle and sheep including *Psoroptic mange* and sucking lice. LL-F28249α, 1, is effective in controlling certain tissue nematodes (filarids) with a single oral dose. The compound is relatively nontoxic; an oral LD$_{50}$ in the rat was established at 348 mg/kg. No toxic effects were observed in rats fed 45 mg/kg/day for 45

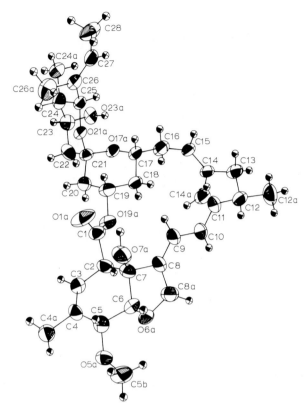

Fig. 3. Three-dimensional representation of LL-F28249γ.

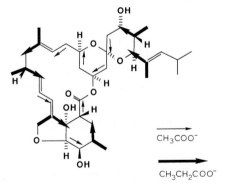

Fig. 4. Incorporation pattern of acetate and propionate in LL-F28249α.

days and no teratogenic abnormalities were detected in rats fed 5, 15, or 45 mg/kg/day for 45 days.

LL-E19020 GROWTH PROMOTANTS

Culture LL-E19020 was initially selected for evalu-

ation of its anticoccidial activity as indicated in our *Eimeria tenella*/chick kidney cell prescreen. *E. tenella* and several other *Eimeria* species are protozoan parasites which infect the digestive tract of chickens. Unchecked, the infestation drastically reduces weight gain and overall quality of the birds, making them unsuitable for market. The *in vitro* prescreen uses a primary chick kidney cell line infected with an invasive form of the parasite. Fermentation broths are added to the system and positives are scored on the basis of a reduction in the number of schizonts and infective forms of *E. tenella* present, in comparison to untreated controls. The second phase of the evaluation involves treating the infected birds with preparations derived from fermentations of the active cultures. Activity in this *in vivo* test is judged on two levels: first, survival from the lethal challenge, and then a decrease in the number of lesions found in the birds upon necropsy.

Broths and extracts of LL-E19020 showed sufficiently good activity in the primary and *in vivo* tests, respectively, that the culture was selected for investigation of the active principles. An isolation and purification scheme is reproduced in Fig. 5. The compounds were recovered from the fermentation broth by extraction with one half-volume of methanol, followed by filtration and concentration under reduced pressure to a highly aqueous suspension. Extraction with ethyl acetate partitioned the antibiotics into the organic phase. Concentration of the extract yielded a thick black syrup which was triturated with hexane to dissolve nonpolar impurities, prior to reversed-phase preparative HPLC. The chromatographic system consisted of a C_{18} column eluted with a gradient of acetonitrile in pH 4.5 0.05 M NH_4OAc. A single pass on this column was adequate to produce material of 85% purity for analysis and efficacy evaluations. Selected physico-chemical properties of the two major components, designated LL-E19020α and β, are presented in Table 4. As the data indicate, the two compounds are isomeric with very similar physico-chemical profiles. Despite these similarities, the compounds are well separated on reversed-phase HPLC, as shown in Fig. 6.

The structures of LL-E19020α, 5, and β, 6, were determined by a combination of chemical and spec-

Table 3

Parenteral (s.c.) and oral efficacy of F-28249 against natural infections in cattle

Nematode	% Efficacy			
	4.17% formulation (s.c.)		1% formulation (oral)	
	2.0 mg/kg	1.0 mg/kg	0.6 mg/kg	0.3 mg/kg
Ostertagi oster-tagi (11,413)	100	99.8	100	99
Trichostrongylus axei (13,877)	100	100	99	99
Trichostrongylus axei (L$_4$) (413)	100	100	100	100
Cooperia spp.[a] (13,252)	99	99	99	99
Oesophagosto-mum radiatum (235)	100	100	100	100
Trichuris ovis (35)	100	99	100	100

Lungworm (*D. viviparus*) was present in 4 of 5 controls; no lungworms were recovered in treated calves. Injection formulation: propylene glycol/Tween 80; 5 cattle per treatment level.

[a] *C. oncophora* (20%), *C. punctata* (80%).

troscopic methods [4]. Two-dimensional NMR techniques were employed in the identification of substructural units which were linked together with the aid of several degradation products. These structures represent highly modified versions of the aurodox family of antibiotics. Recently two other related compounds were reported. Of these, L-681,217 [6] was the first example of this subtype without the pyridone ring characteristic of the other aurodox relatives. L-681,217 is similar to 5 and 6, but lacks the trisaccharide, retaining the C-21 ethyl substituent; also there is no phenyl acetate ester, no oxygen at C-23 and a hydroxyl group in place of one of the *gem*-methyls at C-25. More closely related are phenelfamycins E and F [5], which are isomeric with 5 and 6, having the phenyl acetate ester fixed at the 23-position and the trisaccharide attached to O-24. Phenelfamycins E and F are diastereoisomeric, differing in configuration at C-21.

Testing 5 and 6 in chicks infected with *E. tenella* soon revealed that the compounds were far better growth promoters than anticoccidial agents. Although some degree of protection against *E. tenella* was achieved at relatively high levels in the diet, there was little lesion moderation. Even at subtherapeutic levels, where the birds would eventually die from the infection, their initial growth rates were enhanced by as much as 25% over normal nonmedicated controls. This observation led to their further evaluation as growth-promoting agents and the coining of the name 'BIG BIRD' to describe the compounds. Preliminary results from floor pen studies have shown superior performance in chicks treated with the LL-E19020 compounds in comparison to commercial agents such as virginiamycin and bacitracin. Improvements in weight gain and feed conversion efficiency of between 5 and 6% have been obtained in several trials.

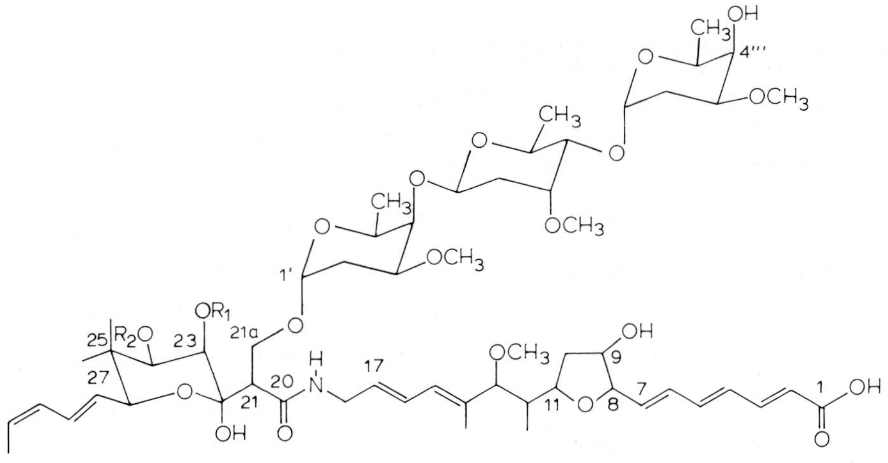

5	E19020 α	R_1 = PhCH$_2$CO	R_2 = H
6	E19020 β	R_1 = H	R_2 = PhCH$_2$CO

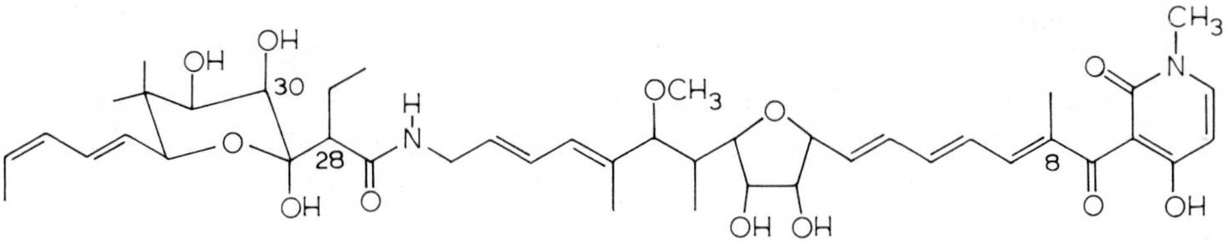

aurodox

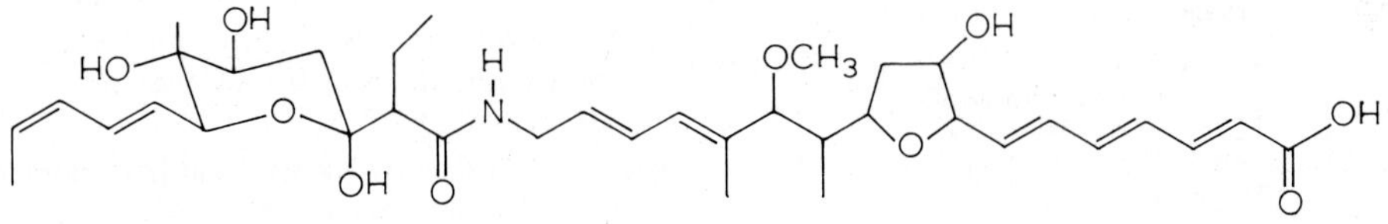

L-681,217

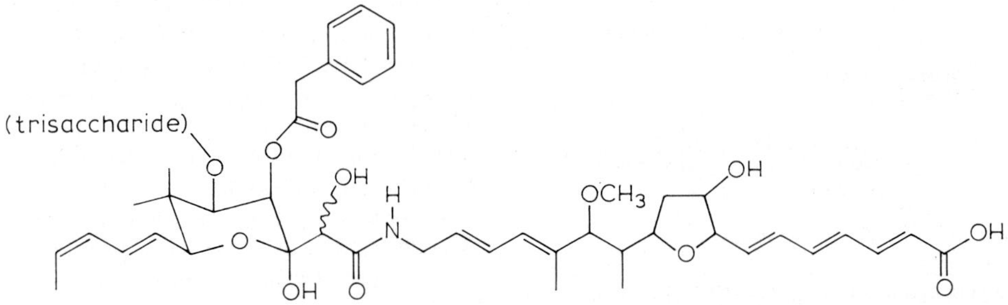

(trisaccharide)

Table 4

Selected physico-chemical properties of LL-E19020α (5) and β(6)

	5	6
Molecular formula	$C_{65}H_{95}NO_{21}$	$C_{65}H_{95}NO_{21}$
Molecular weight	1225	1225
Molecular ion $(M + Na)^+$ HRFABMS	1248.6187	1248.6193
$[\alpha]_D^{26}$ (MeOH)	−8 @ 1.0%	−17 @ 0.46%
UV (MeOH) λ_{max} nm (ε)	233 (49 800) 290 (36 600)	233 (47 000) 290 (34 100)
IR (KBr) cm⁻¹	3420 1617 2970 1525 2925 1445 1717 1365 1695 1092 1647 1018	3430 1543 2970 1454 2930 1367 1712 1265 1648 1098 1620 1020

HRFABMS = high-resolution fast atom bombardment mass spectroscopy.

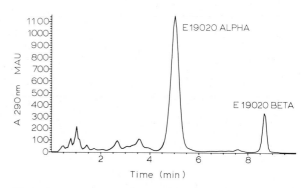

Fig. 6. Reversed-phase HPLC chromatogram of the crude extract from LL-E19020. (Column: 2.1×100 mm 5μ C_{18}, acetonitrile/pH 4.5 0.05 M NH_4OAc gradient.)

LL-E19020α and β have an extremely narrow antimicrobial spectrum, showing activity primarily against various *Streptococcus* species and anaerobes. The compounds are nontoxic, as indicated by an oral LD_{50} of 1368 mg/kg in the rat. These factors, coupled with their effectiveness as growth promoters and divergence in structure from compounds used in human therapy, make the LL-E19020 compounds ideal candidates for use in the livestock industry.

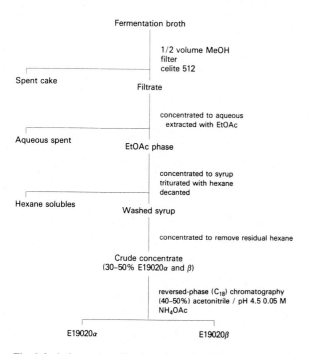

Fig. 5. Isolation and purification scheme for LL-E19020α and β.

REFERENCES

1 Cane, D.E., T.-C. Liang, L. Kaplan, M.K. Nallin, M.D. Schulman, O.D. Hensens, A.W. Douglas and G. Albers-Schonberg. 1983. Biosynthetic origin of the carbon skeleton and oxygen atoms of the avermectins. J. Am. Chem. Soc. 105: 4110-4112.

2 Carter, G.T., J.A. Nietsche and D.B. Borders. 1987. Structure determination of LL-F28249α, β, γ and λ, potent antiparasitic macrolides from *Streptomyces cyaneogriseus* ssp. *noncyanogenus*. J. Chem. Soc. Chem. Commun. 1987: 402–404.

3 Carter, G.T., J.A. Nietsche, M.R. Hertz, D.R. Williams, M.M. Siegel, G.O. Morton, J.C. James and D.B. Borders. 1988. LL-F28249 antibiotic complex: a new family of antiparasitic macrocyclic lactones. Isolation, characterization and structures of LL-F28249α, β, γ, λ. J. Antibiot. 41: 519–529.

4 Carter, G.T., D.W. Phillipson, J.J. Goodman, T.S. Dunne and D.B. Borders. 1988. LL-E19020α and β, novel growth promoting agents: isolation characterization and structures, J. Antibiot. 41: 1511–1514.

5 Hochlowski, J.E., M.H. Buytendorp, D.N. Whittern, A.M. Buko, R.H. Chen and J. McAlpine. 1988. Phenelfamycins, a novel complex of elfamycin-type antibiotics. II. Isolation and

structure determination. J. Antibiot. 41: 1300–1315.

6 Kempf, A.J., K.E. Wilson, O.D. Hensens, R.L. Monaghan, S.B. Zimmerman and E.L. Dulaney. 1986. L-681,217, a new and novel member of the efrotomycin family of antibiotics. J. Antibiot. 39: 1361–1367.

7 Labeda, D.P., J.H. Martin and J.J. Goodman. 1983. Process for producing antibiotic X-14868A. US Patent 4,407,496, October 4, 1983.

8 Lee, T.M., D.B. Borders, G.T. Carter, M. Hertz and J.P. Kirby. 1986. LL-D42067α and β, novel antibacterial and antiprotozoal agents: isolation, characterization and structure determination. Abstract No. 222, 26th Interscience Conference on Antimicrobial Agents and Chemotherapy, New Orleans, LA, October, 1986.

9 Mishima, H., J. Ide, S. Muramatsu and M. Ono. 1983. Milbemycins, a new family of macrolide antibiotics, structure determination of milbemycins D, E, F, G, H, J, and K. J. Antibiot. 36: 980–990.

10 Ono, M., H. Mishima, Y. Takiguchi, M. Terao, H. Kobayashi, S. Iwasaki and S. Okuda. 1983. Milbemycins, a new family of macrolide antibiotics. Studies on the biosynthesis of milbemycins α2, α4, and D, using ^{13}C labeled precursors. J. Antibiot. 36: 991–1000.

11 Tsou, H.-R., Z.H. Ahmed, R.R. Fiala, M.W. Bullock, G.T. Carter, J.J. Goodman and D.B. Borders. 1987. LL-F28249 antibiotic complex, a new family of antiparasitic macrocyclic lactones. IV. Origin of the carbon and oxygen atoms of LL-F28249α. Abstract No. 999, 27th Interscience Conference on Antimicrobial Agents and Chemotherapy, New York, October, 1987.

12 Wood, I.B., J.A. Pankavich and M.E. Doscher. 1987. LL-F28249 antibiotic complex, a new family of antiparasitic macrocyclic lactones. V. Spectrum of antiparasitic activity. Abstract No. 1000, 27th Interscience Conference on Antimicrobial Agents and Chemotherapy, New York, October, 1987.

Novel Microbial Products for Medicine and Agriculture
Editors: A.L. Demain, G.A. Somkuti, J.C. Hunter-Cevera and H.W. Rossmoore
© 1989, Society for Industrial Microbiology

CHAPTER 27

Novel activities from marine-derived microorganisms

David J. Newman[1], Paul R. Jensen[1], Jacob J. Clement[1] and Cristina Acebal[2]

[1]SeaPharm Inc., Fort Pierce, FL, and [2]PharmaMar SA, Madrid, Spain

SUMMARY

The metabolites obtained by fermentation of aerobic microorganisms (bacteria, actinomycetes and fungi) isolated from marine sources have been evaluated for their potential as sources of pharmacologically active agents in a variety of disease states. These microbes have been isolated and purified from microorganisms of many taxa, from sediments and water columns, collected in both shallow and deep water (0–800 m), from various areas of the world, including unique sites of significant environmental stress. Locales include Malaysia, the Galapagos Islands and the Caribbean. Environments include oceanic, lagoonal and intertidal. Screening the metabolites produced by small-scale fermentation of > 500 separate isolates (covering a variety of genera) has shown significant activities in the areas of immunomodulation (both stimulatory and depressor), antiviral (herpes, coronavirus), antitumor (murine and human cell lines), and antibacterial and antifungal activities. Data showing these activities are presented on extracts made from at least six genera other than the common marine genera, _Vibrio_ and _Pseudomonas_.

INTRODUCTION

Although the terrestrial sphere has been searched for many years for microorganisms that produce metabolites that exhibit activities in both pharmacological and nonpharmacological areas, as exemplified by the work of the late Professor Hamao Umezawa and his collaborators at the Institute of Microbial Chemistry, relatively few results utilizing the corresponding marine flora have been reported in the literature (see Hunter _et al._ [1], Nair and Simidu [2] and Okami [3]).

As part of an ongoing study of the potential of marine macroorganisms as sources of bioactive agents, about 18 months ago we began to isolate and study the heterotrophic microorganisms that coexist with these marine flora and fauna. We have deliberately designated such microorganisms as 'marine-derived' rather than become enmeshed in a philosophical discussion as to 'what is a marine microbe?'.

These organisms were collected, isolated, purified, identified where possible and tested under a variety of conditions, in order to produce materials that could be assayed for activity against tumors,

Current addresses:

D.J. Newman, Lederle Laboratories, Pearl River, NY, U.S.A.
P.R. Jensen, Scripps Oceanographic Institution, La Jolla, CA, U.S.A.
J.J. Clement, Abbott Laboratories, North Chicago, IL, U.S.A.

viruses, bacteria, fungi and also as modulators of the immune system.

In the following sections, we will discuss the sources of microorganisms, the production of secondary metabolites, the assays utilized, and results of these assays on a 'pharmacologic area' basis and end with examples of separation and partial purification of multiple activities from selected organisms.

SOURCES OF ORGANISMS

Microorganisms, i.e. bacteria, actinomycetes and fungi, were collected from areas of the Earth that could be classified as 'environmentally stressed'. Such areas are shallow (< 40 m) and deep (40–800 m) oceanic waters, intertidal (i.e., the area exposed between high and low water) zones, lagoons, slow-flowing estuarine zones and salt marshes. Obviously, two or more of the last four areas could coalesce and be treated as one.

In order to isolate microbes from these areas of stress, samples were taken from macroorganisms, marine flora, sediments/muds and water columns by using 'aseptic' techniques. In the case of shallow samples, this was done by means of scuba techniques and suitably prepared collection devices (sterile tubes, whirlpacs, etc.). For deeper samples, which were collected using deep diving submersibles, a trained microbiologist was the first person to meet the vessel on return to the mother ship, and would remove samples from the collection bins using suitable techniques designed to minimize cross-contamination with shipboard microbes.

The samples, once collected and 'tagged', were either held at wet ice temperature for transport back to the laboratory (on shore or on ship) for immediate workup, or were frozen at $-20°C$ for later treatment.

MICROBE ISOLATION, PURIFICATION AND STORAGE

The basic techniques used are variants of those originally used for isolation of microbes from terrestrial sources. The major differences are the choice of media and, because of the desire to minimize the number of actinomycetes isolated, a minimum of heat treatment of samples prior to plating.

In general, samples were treated as follows. The original specimen was ground in a sterile homogenizer with a suitable medium (see later for media composition) at a ratio of 1:10. The homogenate was diluted to 1:100, 1:1000 in the same medium and 'plated' or 'streaked' onto isolation plates. If a liquid sample was used, such as from a 'water column', then the dilutions were made with sterile artificial seawater (ASW).

Occasionally, a form of 'enrichment dilution' was used. In this, the initial sample was either diluted or ground in one of the media referred to below, rather than in sterile ASW. Following incubation at room temperature for up to 4 days, the suspension was then diluted as mentioned above, with all further 'workup' as shown above.

Following incubation at 15–25°C in air for a period that could extend to 30 days, organisms were 'picked' by means of sterile disposable loops (Nunc) and restreaked on a variety of media to check for purity. Once an organism was defined as 'pure' by this technique coupled to light microscopy, then the isolate was transferred to liquid medium (usually, but not always, the same as the isolation medium), at a ratio of ≈ 10 μl to 5 ml, and allowed to grow with shaking at room temperature or slightly above.

In the case of fungi and actinomycetes, sporulation was encouraged when necessary by gentle heat treatment of the agar plates or by partial drying. Spores were recovered by irrigating the growth plates with medium or ASW. Growth in liquid culture was performed using the spores rather than the mycelia as the source of the inocula, and in the case of fungi, by growing both with and without shaking.

Before freezing away as mentioned below, organisms from liquid culture were checked microscopically for initial morphology, color and gram reaction, in order to obtain some preliminary information as to taxonomic diversity.

Initially, all organisms were maintained on agar

slants when adjudged 'pure', transferring as necessary at intervals of about a month. The liquid cultures obtained from these were glycerolized ($\approx 10\%$ v/v) and frozen away at $-76°C$. Viability checks were run (giving 90–95%) after 4–6 months of storage under these conditions, and if the isolate was viable, the slant was discarded. Thus the only organisms in the general collection were those that could be grown under such conditions. There are others that we have not yet succeeded in growing reproducibly in liquid culture, but are stable and pure on agar plates. These are still under investigation.

MEDIA USED

In all cases mentioned below, ASW made according to the Sieburth [4] formulation was used as a proportion of the diluent. The proportion ranged from 50 to 100% depending upon the salinity required. In certain cases, we would supplement the isolation plates with up to 5% of NaCl, but this was not a regular occurrence.

For actinomycetes and fungi we used the media shown in Table 1 for initial isolation.

For subsequent growth both in liquid and on

Table 1

Media used to isolate and purify actinomycetes and fungi

Defined:	arginine-glycerol-ASW
Semidefined:	soluble starch-casein-ASW; Czapek-Dox-yeast Extract-ASW
Undefined:	chitin-ASW; cellulose-ASW

Table 2

Media used for isolation and growth of bacteria

LN1	0.05%	yeast extract	CY	0.1%	yeast extract
	0.05%	peptone		0.3%	casitone
	75%	ASW		0.1%	$CaCl_2$
				0.15%	$MgSO_4 \cdot 7H_2O$
				50%	ASW
M2	0.2%	yeast extract	SP2	0.1%	yeast extract
	0.5%	tryptone		0.1%	casitone
	0.1%	casamino acids		0.002%	NaOAc
	75%	ASW		75%	ASW
PC	1.5%	Pharmamedia	GG	2.5 g	glycine
	3.0%	soluble starch		20 ml	glycerol
	20 g	corn steep liquor		75%	ASW
	1.0%	yeast extract			
	50%	ASW			
P2	0.1%	yeast extract	BMMB	8.0 g	Tris-HCl
	0.2%	peptone		1.03 g	NH_4Cl
	0.05%	casamino acids		0.06 g	K_2HPO_4
	0.5 g	Tris-HCl		0.02 g	$FeSO_4$
	1 ml	metals		50%	ASW
	75%	ASW			
Metals		1.0 mM $ZnSO_4$			
		1.0 mM $MnCl_2$			
		1.0 mM $Fe(NH_4)_2SO_4$			

When necessary, more concentrated media were made by using multiples of the ingredients. Such media would be denoted by a change in the designation; thus LN3 is a 3-fold concentrate of LN1.

agar, a modification of Emerson's YPSS was used. In this, we either removed the phosphate, or reduced it to < 10% of normal, since due to the pH of ASW being > 8.0, precipitation of metal phosphates occurred at 'normal' phosphate levels.

For bacteria, the media shown in Table 2 were used as necessary.

TAXONOMIC IDENTIFICATION

Bacteria

Because of the lack of defined taxonomic descriptions of most marine bacteria (with the exception of genera such as *Vibrio*, *Flexibacter*, *Alteromonas* and some pseudomonads), we used methods analogous to those established by Colwell and her coworkers (Tabor *et al.* [5]) in that we established a series of metabolic tests that permitted us to 'group' isolates and, in certain cases, to assign to genera. Discussions with experts in the field of marine taxonomy confirmed that they too had similar problems, particularly with organisms from deep waters.

Actinomycetes and fungi

We used similar techniques to those used for 'terrestrial' isolates for the actinomycetes, and in the case of those of interest, we arranged for experts in the field of actinomycete taxonomy to identify to at least genus level.

With fungi, we were able to obtain speciated isolates of some slow-growing marine fungi, and are in the process of speciating some of the other fungal isolates that we have collected ourselves.

GROWTH AND EXTRACTION OF METABOLITES

Small-scale and seed growths (10–15 ml)

In order to produce material for initial screening in the four major areas of interest, we modified a shaker platform to hold 320 25 × 150 mm disposable glass tubes. The modifications permitted us to alter the 'shake angle' of tubes in 80 tube increments from vertical to 45° in 5° increments. In general, we used a 60° setting.

Fifteen milliliters of medium were placed in each tube, sealing with a plastic 'Kim Kap' and sterilized. One hundred microliters of thawed glycerolized culture (or washings from a slant) were added to each tube and the suspension shaken in air at 18–25°C for varying time periods. In such an experimental series, we usually kept the number of variables to a maximum of a 4 × 4 matrix (time and medium). Tubes were removed as required and either used as seed cultures or frozen at −20°C, and then lyophilized using a Virtis 15 SRC, endeavoring to treat all tubes from a given matrix at the same time.

The lyophilizates were then extracted by adding 1.5 ml of 95:5 absolute ethanol/HPLC grade dimethyl sulfoxide (DMSO), macerating the dried material with glass rods and recovering the solvent/solute by centrifugation. The ≈ 1 ml of solution recovered was transferred to a suitable vial and held at −20°C until required for assay.

Larger scale (up to 15 liters)

If a particular organism/medium combination was found to be sufficiently active in a given assay then the material was grown on a larger scale as follows.

The 15 ml seed culture was grown in tubes for 24–48 h, transferred to 100 ml of medium in a 500 ml Erlenmeyer flask and grown for 24–72 h at 200–250 rpm in air. This culture was then used as seed for 1 liter of medium in a 2.8 liter Fernbach flask. Once growth had finished and metabolite production reached a maximum, usually 72–96 h, the contents of the flask were recovered by centrifugation, keeping the pellet and broth separate.

The broth and pellet could be extracted in a variety of ways depending upon the particular metabolites of interest (see examples later), but in general, broths were extracted at final pH with ethyl acetate or methylene dichloride, and the lyophilized cell mass was triturated with 80–100% ethanol. On removal of the extraction solvents, the tared residues were dissolved in ethanol/water mixtures (70–100% ethanol), or in ethanol/DMSO (95:5) to a known concentration.

Where more than 1 liter was required, we either grew multiple flasks (< 6 liters), or used an LH 20

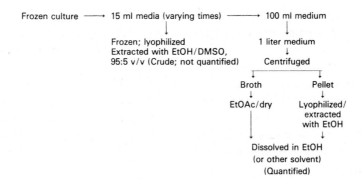

Fig. 1. Growth and isolation for bioactivity studies.

liter fermentor (6–16 liters), with pH, p_{O_2} and temperature probes as the growth vessel. Subsequent workup was similar to that used on a small scale.

A scheme of the process is shown in Fig. 1.

BIOLOGICAL ASSAYS USED

The following are brief descriptions of the assays that we used to quantify the bioactivities of the microbes.

Antitumor assays

P388 (mouse leukemia) assay 1. Cell number reduction, using P388 cells in Dulbecco's minimum essential medium with 10% human serum albumin (HSA). Cell number determination (coulter counter) after 48 h incubation.

P388 (mouse leukemia) assay 2. MTT (3-[4,5-dimethylthiazol-2-yl]-2,5-diphenyltetrazolium bromide) colorimetric assay of viable cells after 48 h incubation in Dulbecco's MEM or RPMI 1640 medium (both 10% HSA). Cells added to extracts in 96-well plates.

HCT-8 (colon), A549 (lung) and T47D (breast), all human cell lines. Cell number reduction: cells grown in 24-well plates (A549, Dulbecco's MEM; HCT-8 and T47D, RPMI 1640; both with 10% fetal calf serum) for 48 h. Extracts added; incubated for a further 120 h. Medium removed, cell sheet stained with either methylene blue (HCT-8) or crystal violet. Cell densities scored versus growth control, in ranges of >90, 75–90, 50–74, 25–49 and <25%. An IC$_{50}$ value of <15 $\mu g \cdot ml^{-1}$, or $I > 75\%$ at 20 $\mu g \cdot ml^{-1}$ is considered active.

Antiviral assays

HSV I. Plaque reduction assay; using CV-1 (monkey kidney) cells, seeded for 24–48 h. Extract adsorbed on sterile (7 mm) disk, placed on 'lawn' of infected cells, incubated for 72 h. Proportion of plaque reduction/cytotoxicity determined after neutral red staining. A score of 10 (diameter in mm of inhibition zone) or less for cytotoxicity coupled to 2+ or 3+ for plaque reduction, considered active.

A59 (coronavirus). Foci of infection assay; using NCTC clone 1469 (mouse liver) cells. Extract placed in sterile dish, cells and virus added, incubated for 12–24 h. Proportion of infection/cytotoxicity determined after methylene blue staining. A score of 0% cytotoxicity coupled to 2+ or 3+ for level of infection, considered active.

PR8 (influenza virus, Type A). Cell survival assay; using MDCK (canine kidney) cells. Extract placed in sterile dish, cells and virus added, incubated for 72 h. Proportion of survivors/cytotoxicity determined after neutral red staining. A score of 0% cytotoxicity coupled to 3+ for level of survival, considered active.

Antimicrobial assays

Conventional disc diffusion or liquid medium minimum inhibitory concentration (MIC) determinations using the following organisms. *Bacillus subtilis, Escherichia coli, Pseudomonas aeruginosa, Candida albicans* and *Aspergillus nidulans*, as the

244

primary screens. Secondary testing utilized mutant/parent combinations with specific resistance patterns.

Immunomodulation assays

Mixed lymphocyte reaction (MLR). Fresh murine lymphocytes from BALB/C and C57 strains are coincubated for 86 h, followed by pulsing with [^{3}H]thymidine for 16 h (or colorimetric for 6 h using the MTT dye reaction).

'B'-cell stimulation. Optimized amounts of lipopolysaccharide and poke weed mitogen are incubated with BALB/C lymphocytes for 72 h. Pulsed with [^{3}H]thymidine for 16 h.

'T'-cell stimulation. As 'B' cells, but using concanavalin A and phytohemagglutinin as mitogens.

Lymphocyte viability (LCV). Resting BALB/C lymphocytes; incubated for same time as MLR. Cell viability using MTT colorimetric assay.

RESULTS OF ANTITUMOR, ANTIVIRAL AND ANTIMICROBIAL STUDIES

In Tables 3 through 5 below, we have summarized the 'hit rates' for antitumor, antiviral and antimicrobial assays. A similar summary for immunomodulation was not made, because of the intrinsic difficulties of deciding on a specific 'cutoff' for activity in these complex systems. Instead, in a later section, we have shown data from selected organisms of various taxonomic groups.

It should be noted that in Tables 3, 4 and 5, the term 'discrete growths' means an organism/medium combination grown for a specific time. Hence one organism/medium combination grown for three different times would be counted as three discrete growths.

GENERAL COMMENTS ON SUMMARY TABLES

Inspection of Tables 3, 4 and 5 indicates that a significant number of active materials are produced in the three areas covered when marine-derived organisms are fermented and extracted.

Table 3

'Hit rates' of marine-derived actinomycetes, bacteria and fungi in antitumor assays (P388 and human cell lines (HCL))

(A) Grown to 1 liter; separated; extracted and extracts quantified

Organism	No.	No. actives ($I > 50\%$ at 20 μg·ml^{-1})	Comments
Actinomycetes/ fungi	79	29	17 P388/HCL 7 HCL, *no* P388 2 HCL > P388 2 P388
Bacteria	160	29	8 P388/HCL 2 HCL > P388 19 P388

(B) Fifteen milliliter growths; lyophilized; extracted with EtOH/DMSO (95:5, v/v), using varied media and times

Organism	No.	No. of discrete growths	No. with > 50% inhibition of P388
Actino mycetes	45	200	28
Bacteria	71	180	5

Table 4

'Hit rates' of marine-derived actinomycetes, bacteria and fungi in antiviral assays

Organism	No.	No. of discrete growths	No. active in:		
			HSVI	A59	PRB
Actinomycetes and fungi	120	300	2	2	NT
Bacteria	231	340	4	2	6[a]

Various growth and extraction conditions, with replicate data removed.
[a] Note: one organism also active *vs.* A59.

We have not attempted to separate or identify activities in more than one test system in these summary tables. However, in later sections of this paper, we will give examples of physico-chemical separation of microorganism extracts in which we

Table 5

'Hit rates' of marine-derived actinomycetes, bacteria and fungi in antimicrobial assays

Organism	No.	No. discrete growths	No. active in:					
			G+	G−	G+G−	G+AF	AF	All
Actinomycetes and fungi	120	300	15	0	4	9	2	20
Bacteria	231	340	24	6	1	12	3	3

Various growth and extraction conditions, with replicate data removed.

have been able to separate one bioactivity from another.

As in the case of terrestrial organisms, a significant number of 'actives' are seen when actinomycetes (and some fungi) are used as the source. However, the 'yield' from bacteria is also significant, particularly when, as shown in the antitumor screening (Table 3), organisms are grown on a larger scale and then chemically extracted and concentrates of the extract are assayed. We should also draw attention to the initial differences seen in the relative activities towards the murine and human cell lines used in this study.

As part of a study funded by the NCI through its SBIR program, selected extracts from the organisms referred to in Table 3 were screened by them in their expanded cell line system.

From preliminary data, one isolate from this series (NSC F090110), a *Streptomyces* sp. (charcoal gray spiral group), collected from the oceanic intertidal zone on South Hutchinson Island, Florida, exhibited an interesting profile in that the material exhibited greater activity against human than against murine cell lines (as we had found in our own limited testing). In particular, in the NCI screen, there was higher activity against the renal tumor line A498, and the ovarian line A2780. Another interesting aspect of this isolate is that it showed effectively the same activity against both P388 and its adriamycin-resistant mutant. This isolate is now in the process of being grown on a larger scale in order to purify the metabolites of interest.

In the area of antiviral testing, much lower 'hit rates' were found, though here bacteria were roughly comparable in 'productivity' to the other

microbes. As will be shown in a later section (see Figs. 3, 4), we were able to physically separate antitumor (P388) from antiviral (A59) activities in the case of a *Cytophaga* sp.

With antimicrobial activities, again roughly comparable productivities were seen with the two groups, though overall a higher number of (probably) cytotoxic agents (the group shown under 'All' in Table 5) were found from actinomycetes and fungi.

MODULATION OF THE IMMUNE SYSTEM

As mentioned earlier, we did not produce a table showing 'productivities' in these assays. In Tables 6 and 7, we have shown some of the data obtained in both the immunostimulatory (IS) and immunodepressive (ID) assays, when we studied extracts from specific microorganisms. In a later section, we have also shown results of immunostimulation assays from metabolites elaborated by an actinomycete.

In these tables, we have shown only the results of the MLR and LCV assays. In our hands, we consider modulation of the 'B' or 'T' cell responses in the absence of a corresponding effect on the MLR to be a 'mitogen-like' effect, and do not score such results as positive. Thus in the cases shown above, there were no significant effects upon 'B' and 'T' cells when compared to controls.

For scoring purposes, in the case of IS, a 3-fold increase in MLR coupled to no significant effect upon lymphocyte viability is adjudged active. Inspection of Table 6 shows that bacteria from deep

Table 6

IS activities of marine-derived bacteria

Organism	Source	Taxonomy	Medium/Time (h)	Diln.	MLR	LCV
SOE103	Sed; Galapagos at ≈ 600 m	?	M2/48	1	1.1	0.14
				10	3.0	1.4[a]
				100	2.0	1.0
				1000	2.0	0.4
			LN3SW/48	1	1.8	0.8
				10	2.1	0.5
				1000	1.8	0.4
SOE122	Sed; San Salvador at > 300 m	?	LN3/120	1	3.4	2.8[a]
				10	2.5	1.3
				100	2.5	1.7
SOE123	Sed; San Salvador at > 300 m (not same as 122)	?	LN3/120	1	3.5	1.6[a]
				10	1.7	1.8
				1000	0.7	1.4

[a] Initially considered as active.

Table 7

ID activities of marine-derived bacteria

Organism	Source	Taxonomy	Medium/Time (h)	Diln.	MLR	LCV
SOC829	Sed; Galapagos at 480 m	coryneform	LN/48	1	0	0.9
				10	0	0.9
				100	0	1.0
				1000	0	1.0[a]
			LN/72	1	0	1.0
				10	0	1.0
				100	0	1.0
				1000	0	1.0[a]
SOC863	Sed; Galapagos at 180 m	?	LN/48	1	0.6	2.1
				10	0	2.1
				100	0.4	1.5
				1000	0	1.1[a]
			LN/72	1	0.9	3.6
				10	0.3	2.1
				100	0	1.4
				1000	0	1.4[a]

[a] Considered as active.

waters produce active materials in this assay, though in at least one case, SOE103, a change in medium appears to eliminate this activity.

With ID, total depression of the MLR with no significant effect on lymphocyte viability is adjudged active. In Table 7, we show the results with extracts of other bacteria isolated from a similar area to those in Table 6. Of interest is the lack of activity against lymphocytes, thus indicating that these are not obvious cytotoxins. Also of interest is that SOE829 has been provisionally identified as a coryneform bacterium. We are also purifying these metabolites in order to obtain an idea as to their chemical novelty.

PHYSICO-CHEMICAL SEPARATION OF ACTIVITIES FROM SELECTED ORGANISMS

As mentioned in an earlier section, we frequently found that a given organism/medium combination would elaborate a metabolite or metabolites that would give significant activities in more than one area of interest. This is a well known phenomenon with terrestrial microbes, but similar information on organisms from marine sources is not freely available in the literature, though may well be in proprietary data collections.

In order to demonstrate some of the potential of such marine-derived organisms, we will show in the following figures (3 and 4) and tables (8 and 9) the results obtained when we began to 'dissect' (using physico-chemical tools) the crude extracts obtained by fermentation of an actinomycete (whose taxonomy is under investigation) (SOB055) and a bacterium (that we have identified as belonging to the genus *Cytophaga* (SOC142)).

SOB055: ANTITUMOR AND IMMUNOMODULATION ACTIVITIES

This actinomycete was isolated by conventional means from a sediment collected at a depth of 20 meters off Conception Island in the Bahamas. It is a 'cream-brown' microorganism, whose taxonomy is currently under investigation.

Initially, this material was found to be active against P388 when grown in a series of shake tubes in YPSS for various periods of time, with maximal activity after 72–84 h (data not shown). This timing also held for larger scale growth. For the experiments shown below, we grew a total of 5 liters of broth using 1 liter of medium in 2.8 liter Fernbach flasks at 250 rpm using a 10% inoculum from the same seed culture for each flask. Subsequent work-up was as shown in Fig. 2.

The biological activities of these fractions in all our assay systems are given in Table 8.

The two fractions from the pellet shown as posi-

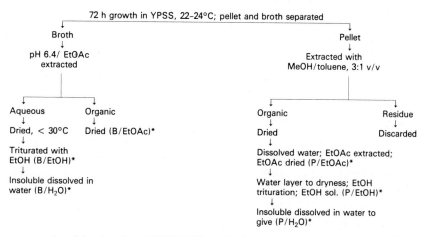

Fig. 2. Preliminary separation of fractions from SOB055. *These fractions were quantitated and assayed for biological activities.

Table 8

SOB055: results of biological activity studies

Fraction	Conc. (mg)	Antitumor P388 (IC$_{50}$, μg)	ID	IS	Antimicrobial		Antiviral A59 (μg/ml)
					BS	CA (MIC, μg)	
B/EtOAc	0.5	<0.63	−	−	22	3.1	O^{+++}(0.2)
B/EtOH	10	0.9	−	−	24	n.d.	O^{++}(200)
B/H$_2$O	10	14	−	−	24	n.d.	O^{+++}(20)
P/EtOAc	1	<0.63	+	(cyto)	22	6.2	O^{++}(20)
P/EtOH	1	14	−	+	12	n.d.	O^{+++}(20)
P/H$_2$O	10	n.d.	−	+	n.d.	n.d.	n.d.

[a] cyto means cytotoxic to lymphocytes during the test.

BS = *B. subtilis*; CA = *C. albicans*; n.d. = not determined.

Table 9

SOB055: IS results with P/EtOH and P/H$_2$O

Fraction	Conc.	Dilution	Stimulation	LCV
P/EtOH	1	1	0.2	0.4
		10	2.0	1.1
		100	3.0	1.0[a]
		1000	3.4	1.2[a]
P/H$_2$O	10	1	0	0.3
		10	1.8	1.5
		100	3.4	1.0[a]
		1000	3.0	1.1[a]

[a] Considered significantly active.

tive in the immunostimulant assays in Table 8 were further assayed and it was demonstrated that, even at a 1:1000 dilution, they still elicited significant effects in an MLR study (Table 9).

In addition to the significant IS activity shown above, we were also interested in the antitumor data of certain of these fractions (cf. Table 8), so proceeded to chemically purify these fractions using the techniques below.

Bioautography of the two fractions against P388 and *B. subtilis* gave similar results, so *B. subtilis* activity was used to follow isolation from regrows. The 'spent broth' (equivalent to B/EtOAc and B/H$_2$O) was extracted with CHCl$_3$/MeOH (13:7:8 (broth)), the lower phase dried and the dried mate-

rial extracted with CHCl$_3$/MeOH (1:1) and chromatographed on LH20 in the same solvent.

These operations yielded material that was judged to be better than 90% pure by ^{1}H- and ^{13}C-NMR, and gave indications that the structure may well be novel.

SOC142: ANTITUMOR AND ANTIVIRAL ACTIVITIES

This organism was isolated from Lake Surprise, a marine lake at the head of the Florida Keys. Following isolation and purification, we identified the organism as belonging to the genus *Cytophaga*. The organism was grown on a variety of scales, culminating in a 16 liter lot using an LH 20 fermentor, with initial antitumor bioactivities of IC$_{50}$ (P388) 15 μg·ml^{-1} and >85% inhibition of the human cell lines HCT8, A549 and T47D when assayed at 20 μg·ml^{-1}.

The subsequent workup of this fermentation beer and separation of the different activities are shown in Figs. 3 and 4 below.

Inspection of the data in Figs. 3 and 4 indicated that we were able to separate at least two antitumor active fractions from the antiviral activity on the basis of intrinsic polarities. Work is now continuing on the further chemical purification and identification of these fractions with the aim of determining their *in vivo* activities in suitable models.

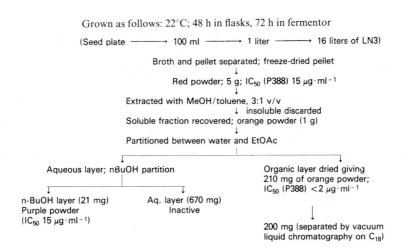

Grown as follows: 22°C; 48 h in flasks, 72 h in fermentor

(Seed plate ——→ 100 ml ——→ 1 liter ——→ 16 liters of LN3)

Broth and pellet separated; freeze-dried pellet
↓
Red powder; 5 g; IC_{50} (P388) 15 $\mu g \cdot ml^{-1}$
↓
Extracted with MeOH/toluene, 3:1 v/v
↓ insoluble discarded
Soluble fraction recovered; orange powder (1 g)
↓
Partitioned between water and EtOAc

Aqueous layer; nBuOH partition

n-BuOH layer (21 mg)
Purple powder
(IC_{50} 15 $\mu g \cdot ml^{-1}$)

Aq. layer (670 mg)
Inactive

Organic layer dried giving
210 mg of orange powder;
IC_{50} (P388) <2 $\mu g \cdot ml^{-1}$
↓
200 mg (separated by vacuum
liquid chromatography on C_{18})

Fig. 3. Growth and Initial Isolation of Activities from SOC142.

Solvent mixture (v/v ratio)
↓

Water	70	50	30	10				
CH_2CN	30	50	70	90	100	100 (wash)		
CH_2Cl_2							100	
n-Pentane								100
Yields (mg)	10	2	2	2	5	41	146	15

Bioactivity
↓

IC_{50} (P388) ($\mu g \cdot ml^{-1}$)	IA	IA	IA	≈15	IA	<1	<1	IA
A59 assayed at 2 $\mu g \cdot ml^{-1}$	IA	3+	3+	IA	IA	IA	cyto	IA

Fig. 4. Vacuum liquid chromatography of SOC142 pellet fraction. Chromatography conditions: C_{18} Amicon; 1 × 30 cm; sequential elution with water/CH_3CN; CH_3CN; CH_2Cl_2; n-pentane; 15–20 ml aliquots of each mixture; 50 ml for wash. IA = inactive at concentration tested; cyto = cytotoxic to virus-containing cells.

SLOW-GROWING MARINE FUNGI

As the last example of activities from marine microbes, we would like to report on the potential of an ill studied group from the aspect of production of novel pharmacophores, the slow-growing marine fungi.

From one of our collaborators, we were able to obtain speciated isolates of a variety of these organisms and, because of the slow reproductive cycle of these organisms, we decided to study the effect of shake cultures *vs.* static cultures in the same medium for a selected group. The source and genus of the isolates used in this study are given in Table 10.

The organisms were inoculated into 1 liter of YPSS medium in 2.8 liter Fernbach flasks from fresh slants of the same medium. One flask of each

set was placed at 20°C in air on the bench, whilst the other was shaken at the same temperature at 200 rpm for a period of 20–30 days. At the end of the growth period, both flasks were treated in the

Table 10

Slow-growing marine fungi: taxonomy and source

SPI No.	Genus	Geographic area isolated
SOB501	*Orbimyces*	Denmark; Baltic Sea
SOB502	*Dendryphiella*	S. West Coast; English Channel
SOB503	*Wilsoniella*	Welsh Coast; Irish Sea
SOB507	*Cirrenalia*	Seychelles Is; Indian Ocean
SOB508	*Varicosporina*	Kuwait; Persian Gulf
SOB509	*Arenariomyces*	Washington; Pacific Ocean
SOB511	*Halosarpheia*	Malaysia; Johore Strait
SOB515	*Biatrospora*	Brunei; South China Sea

Table 11

Slow-growing marine fungi: antitumor, immunomodulation, antimicrobial and antiviral results

Organism	Antitumor[a]					Antimicrobial[b]			Antiviral[c]	
	P388	HCT8	A549	T47D	IM	BS	EC	CA	HSVI[c]	A59
SOB501BSh	24	n.d.	< 50	n.d.		n.d.	n.d.	n.d.	n.d.	n.d.
Static	75	n.d.	n.d.	n.d.		10	n.d.	31.2	n.d.	O++
SOB501PSh	12	n.d.	n.d.	n.d.	ID	n.d.	n.d.	n.d.	n.d.	n.d.
Static	7	n.d.	n.d.	n.d.		n.d.	n.d.	n.d.	n.d.	n.d.
SOB502BSh	55	n.d.	n.d.	n.d.	IS	11	10	n.d.	10+++	n.d.
Static	n.d.	n.d.	n.d.	n.d.		n.d.	n.d.	n.d.	n.d.	n.d.
SOB502PSh	n.d.	n.d.	n.d.	n.d.		n.d.	n.d.	n.d.	n.d.	n.d.
Static	n.d.	n.d.	n.d.	n.d.		n.d.	n.d.	n.d.	n.d.	n.d.
SOB503BSh	n.d.	n.d.	< 50	n.d.	ID	9	n.d.	31.2	n.d.	n.d.
Static	61	n.d.	n.d.	n.d.	ID	n.d.	n.d.	n.d.	n.d.	n.d.
SOB503PSh	n.d.	n.d.	n.d.	n.d.		n.d.	n.d.	n.d.	n.d.	n.d.
Static	n.d.	n.d.	n.d.	n.d.		n.d.	n.d.	n.d.	n.d.	n.d.
SOB507BSh	n.d.	n.d.	n.d.	n.d.		n.d.	n.d.	n.d.	n.d.	n.d.
Static	n.d.	n.d.	n.d.	n.d.		12	n.d.	n.d.	n.d.	n.b.
SOB507PSh	n.d.	n.d.	n.d.	n.d.		n.d.	n.d.	n.d.	n.d.	n.d.
Static	n.d.	n.d.	n.d.	n.d.		n.d.	n.d.	n.d.	n.d.	n.d.
SOB508BSh	66	n.d.	n.d.	n.d.	ID	14	9	250	n.d.	n.d.
Static	74	n.d.	< 75	< 50	ID	16	15	62.5	n.d.	n.d.
SOB508PSh	16	n.d.	n.d.	n.d.	ID	n.d.	n.d.	n.d.	O++	n.d.
Static	n.d.	n.d.	n.d.	n.d.		n.d.	n.d.	n.d.	n.d.	n.d.
SOB509BSh	n.d.	n.d.	n.d.	n.d.		10	n.d.	n.d.	8++	n.d.
Static	41	n.d.	n.d.	n.d.		n.d.	n.d.	n.d.	n.d.	O+++
SOB509PSh	n.d.	n.d.	n.d.	n.d.		n.d.	n.d.	n.d.	n.d.	n.d.
Static	n.d.	n.d.	n.d.	n.d.		n.d.	n.d.	n.d.	n.d.	n.d.
SOB511BSh	79	n.d.	n.d.	n.d.		9	n.d.	31.2	n.d.	n.d.
Static	no growth									
SOB511PSh	n.d.	n.d.	n.d.	n.d.		n.d.	n.d.	n.d.	n.d.	n.d.
Static	no growth									
SOB515BSh	10	> 75	> 75	> 75	ID	9	n.d.	250	O++	O+++
Static	88	n.t.	n.t.	n.t.		8	n.d.	n.d.	O++	cyto
SOB515PSh	70	n.d.	< 25	< 25	ID	n.d.	n.d.	n.d.	n.d.	O+++
Static	n.d.	n.d.	n.d.	n.d.		n.d.	n.d.	n.d.	n.d.	n.d.

[a] % Inhibition at 20 μg·ml^{-1} of extract.

[b] BS and EC zone at 500 μg·disk^{-1}; CA MIC μg·ml^{-1}.

[c] Score at 20 μg·ml^{-1} of extract.

Sh = shake; B = broth extract; P = pellet extract; n.d. = not detected; n.t. = not tested; cyto = cytotoxic; IM = immunomodulation; BS = *B. subtilis*; EC = *E. coli*; CA = *C. albicans*.

following manner. Broth was separated from the mycelium by centrifugation and extracted at broth pH with ethyl acetate. The mycelium was dried by lyophilization, and triturated with ethanol. Following removal of the solvent from both fractions, the residues were dissolved in ethanol at a concentration of 10 mg·ml^{-1} and tested for activity in the four areas of interest. The results are shown in Table 11.

Inspection of Table 11 indicates that, not unexpectedly, growth conditions in these types of organism also cause differences in both the types and quantities of activities seen on assay. Of particular interest are the differences shown in SOB501, SOB508 and SOB515 when shake and static cultures are compared in all of the pharmacologic areas. We are currently investigating the chemical nature of these metabolites when produced in larger scale cultures.

CLOSING COMMENTS

In this paper, we have demonstrated that marine-derived microorganisms isolated from intertidal slopes, or lagoonal, shallow and deep waters can be fermented under relatively simple conditions.

These fermentation beers contain secondary metabolites (in some cases of potentially novel chemistry) that exhibit activities of interest in the antitumor, antiviral, immunomodulatory and (perhaps) antimicrobial areas.

We are currently continuing these studies, using microbes isolated from a variety of areas of the globe as a source of novel pharmacophores.

ACKNOWLEDGEMENTS

We would like to thank the members of the scientific staff of SeaPharm Inc., and of the Harbor Branch/Seapharm Project, whose efforts allowed the completion of this paper.

REFERENCES

1 Hunter, J.C., M. Fonda, L. Sotos, B. Toso and A. Belt. 1984. Ecological approaches to isolation. Dev. Ind. Microbiol. 25: 247–266.

2 Nair, S. and U. Simidu. 1987. Distribution and significance of heterotrophic marine bacteria with antimicrobial activity. Appl. Environ. Microbiol. 53: 2957–2962.

3 Okami, Y. 1986. Marine microorganisms as a source of bioactive agents. Microb. Ecol. 12: 65–78.

4 Sieburth, J. 1979. Sea Microbes, p. 123, Oxford University Press, New York.

5 Tabor, P.S., K. Ohwanda and R.R. Colwell. 1981. Filterable marine bacteria found in the deep sea: distribution, taxonomy and response to starvation. Microb. Ecol. 7: 67–83.

Novel Microbial Products for Medicine and Agriculture
Editors: A.L. Demain, G.A. Somkuti, J.C. Hunter-Cevera and H.W. Rossmoore
© 1989, Society for Industrial Microbiology

CHAPTER 28

Eicosapentaenoic acid from microalgae

Paul W. Behrens, Scot D. Hoeksema, Kathy L. Arnett, Melissa S. Cole, Tara A. Heubner,
John M. Rutten and David J. Kyle*

Martek Corporation, Columbia, MD, U.S.A.

SUMMARY

The ω-3 polyunsaturated fatty acid (PUFA), eicosapentaenoic acid (EPA), is thought to be the active ingredient in fish oil which results in reduced serum triglycerides and cholesterol in human populations whose diets consist primarily of oily fish. Cold water marine fish are rich in both EPA and docosahexaenoic acid (DHA), although it is unclear whether the fish themselves have the capability of synthesizing either of these PUFAs. The phytoplankton in the food chain, however, are well known to be primary producers of ω-3 fatty acids. We have screened and selected a strain of microalgae (MK8620) which produces an oil containing EPA as its primary PUFA. This offers the advantage of simplifying the purification steps required for the preparation of pure EPA, and it represents a unique source of a PUFA-based oil which contains EPA only (i.e., no DHA). Through manipulations of the cultural parameters, we have improved the oil content of MK8620 to 30–40% of its biomass and the overall EPA content is 50–60 mg/g dry weight. This strain has been scaled up to a 500-liter pilot plant photobioreactor and produces about 2 kg of oil-rich dry biomass in a 2-week batch run. Further cultural and strain improvements are planned which should lead to the production of an EPA-containing oil at the industrial level using these microorganisms.

INTRODUCTION

Recent epidemiological data and clinical investigations have indicated a significant correlation between dietary supplements of ω-3 polyunsaturated fatty acids (PUFAs), especially eicosapentaenoic acid (EPA), and reduced incidence of coronary heart disease [1, 10, 13, 18], selective killing of human cancer cells [2, 3, 11, 15], and relief of symptoms of rheumatoid arthritis [12, 22]. At present, the only source of ω-3 PUFAs is the oil expressed from certain marine fish. However, many diverse

marine microalgae also contain large quantities of PUFAs and the relative abundance of each fatty acid can be considered a fingerprint of a particular species [5, 16]. For example, species in the Class Bacillarophyceae (diatoms) contain large amounts of EPA and essentially no docosahexaenoic acid (DHA), whereas those in the Dinophyceae (dinoflagellates) contain predominantly DHA (Table 1). Since many of these species also sequester triglyceride oil as a storage product [5, 14], they can be considered natural overproducers of ω-3 PUFAs.

We have pursued a strategy of screening and optimization of EPA production from microalgae cultured in enclosed photobioreactors since offshore

---

* To whom correspondence should be addressed.

Table 1

EPA and DHA content of several microalgal species

Microalgal species	EPA[a]	DHA[a]	Ref.
Chlorophyceae			
Dunaliella tertiolecta	10	0	21
Bacillarophyceae			
Skelotonema costatum	30	0	12
Phaeodactylum tricorna-			
tum	26	1	12
Nitzschia angularis	21	0	12
Haptophyceae			
Hymenomonas carterae	0	16	22
Imantonia rotunda	31	0	22
Dinophyceae			
Cryptocodinium cohnii	0	30	11
Prorocentrum minimum	0	25	11
Gonyaulax cattenella	11	34	11
Cryptophyceae			
Cryptomonas sp.	16	10	23
Rhodophyceae			
Porphrydium cruentum	17	0	11

[a] All values are presented as % of total fatty acids.

fish have the potential for contamination by coastal pollution and the harvest is unpredictable. As microorganisms in culture, the microalgae may not only represent a reliable source of EPA, but they have a great potential for enhancing the productivity of ω-3 PUFAs through genetic modification and selection.

MATERIALS AND METHODS

Cyclotella cryptica (UTEX 1269), *Cylindrotheca fusiformis* (UTEX 2083), *Navicula pelliculosa* (UTEX 2030), *Nitzschia angularis* (UTEX 2037), *Phaeodactylum tricornatum* (UTEX 640), *Porphyridium cruentum* (UTEX 161), *Pavlova gyrans* (UTEX 992), and *Prymnesium parvum* (UTEX 995) were obtained from the University of Texas Culture Collection. Shake flask cultures were grown autotrophically at 20°C using the medium suggested for each species by the UTEX Culture Collection. MK8620 is a proprietary diatom strain previously selected for high EPA productivity. The various fish used for lipid

analyses were obtained fresh from a local market and lyophilized before analysis.

Temperature optimization studies were carried out in a closed cylindrical photobioreactor (*ca.* 1 liter) operated in continuous mode with a turbidostat control as described by Radmer *et al.* [19]. Once the culture attained a stable productivity at a given temperature, the overflow rate was measured and a sample of biomass was removed and lyophilized prior to lipid analysis. The temperature was then adjusted to a new level and the experiment repeated.

Medium component optimization experiments were carried out in 7-liter flat plate photobioreactors with illumination provided by fluorescent lights (300 μE/m^2/s). Temperature was controlled in these tanks by internally positioned stainless steel cooling coils fed by a temperature-regulated water bath. Both cylindrical and flat plate photobioreactor geometries operate on air-lift circulation and the air was enriched with 2% CO_2 to ensure carbon saturation.

A rapid microanalytical procedure was developed for the determination of total cellular fatty acid and EPA (as their methyl esters) using 5–50 mg of dried algal cells. Sampling of a culture involved harvesting an aliquot of cells by centrifugation, followed by washing the sample with an isotonic solution before lyophilization. To each lyophilized algal sample (50 mg), 100 μl of an internal standard (methyl pentadecanoate; 10 mg/ml) was added, followed by 2.0 ml of commercially available methanolic base reagent (Supelco Inc., Bellefonte, PA). The tubes were then flushed with nitrogen, sealed and heated to 70°C for 15 min for simultaneous extraction from the cell biomass and transesterification. When cooled, 2.0 ml of water was added and the fatty acid methyl esters were extracted with 2.0 ml hexane. Hexane extracts were injected directly into a gas chromatograph equipped with an SP2330 packed column (He flow at 30 ml/min; 210°C column temperature; FID detection). The peak areas corresponding to individual fatty acids were integrated by computer using commercially available chromatography software. The total extractable fatty acid was then calculated based on the ratio of the internal standard peak area to the total fatty acid area.

For the separation of complex lipids, the lyophilized cell biomass was extracted four times with chloroform/methanol (1:1). The extract was concentrated to dryness under a stream of nitrogen, resuspended in a small volume of hexane and applied to a solid phase disposable silica column (SEP-PAK, Waters Inc., Milford, MA). The complex lipid fractions were then serially eluted from the column using solvents of increasing polarity (hexane, benzene, chloroform, acetone, and methanol). The eluants were dried under a stream of nitrogen and their fatty acid methyl esters were prepared as above.

RESULTS

The microalgal species screened exhibited considerable variability in both the total amount of extractable fatty acid and their EPA content (Table 2). Even within a species, different culture conditions (i.e., nitrogen-sufficient *vs.* nitrogen-starved) resulted in significant changes in the fatty acid profile. In most cases, however, the screened algal strains contained significantly more EPA on a dry weight basis than the oily fish.

Some of the algal species indicated in Table 2 contained a high percentage of EPA in their lipids but had a low oil content (e.g., *N. angularis* and *Prym. parvum*), whilst others produced large amounts of oil but had a low percentage of EPA in the lipid (e.g., *C. fusiformis* and *Nav. pelliculosa*). In the case of both *Cyc. cryptica* and *P. tricornatum*, nitrogen-sufficient cultures had low oil content and a high percentage of EPA in the lipid, whereas nitrogen-deficient cultures had elevated oil levels but depressed EPA levels. These results suggest that EPA may be preferentially associated with membrane lipids in these species, and when triglyceride production is stimulated by nitrogen deficiency, the EPA is diluted out by the accumulation of triglyceride-associated fatty acids.

It has been well established that medium nutrient depletion (especially nitrogen) generally increases

Table 2

Fatty acid and EPA contents of microalgal species growing in shake flasks compared to oily fish obtained from a local market

Species	% Fatty acid in biomass	% EPA	
		in lipid	in biomass
Microalgae			
Cyclotella cryptica	10.6	23.8	2.5
Cyclotella cryptica[a]	29.6	10.0	3.0
Cylindrotheca fusiformis	24.4	7.2	1.8
Navicula pelliculosa	25.4	9.0	2.3
Nitzschia angularis	7.7	24.7	2.2
Phaeodactylum tricornatum[a]	9.2	26.9	2.5
Phaeodactylum tricornatum	21.3	11.4	2.4
Porphyridium cruentum	6.8	3.7	0.3
Pavlova gyrans	21.0	8.3	1.7
Prymnesium parvum	12.0	23.3	2.8
MK8620[a]	40.1	12.6	5.1
Fish			
bluefish	3.9	3.4	0.1
haddock	1.8	11.0	0.2
monkfish	3.8	3.8	0.1
seatrout	9.1	4.3	0.4
salmon	19.0	9.6	1.8
sheepshead	6.9	4.7	0.3

[a] Nitrogen-deficient culture.

the production of storage oils in oleagenous microorganisms [20, 23]. The effect of nitrogen depletion was studied in more detail with *P. tricornatum* and MK8620. Batch cultures were set up using a flat plate photobioreactor geometry, and experiments were designed to monitor the accumulation of biomass, total lipid and EPA. Based on the elemental analysis of the organisms, a medium composition was designed to limit growth at a density of *ca.* 4 g dry weight/l, at which time the selected nutrient would be exhausted and further growth would be in a nutrient-deficient medium. The data in Fig. 1 indicate that nitrogen limitation had a greater effect on lipid accumulation in MK8620 than in *P. tricornatum*. The production of specific lipids was also affected by nutrient limitation. The percentage of EPA in the lipid of *P. tricornatum* dropped as the

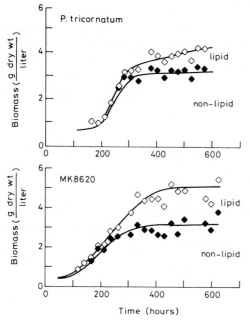

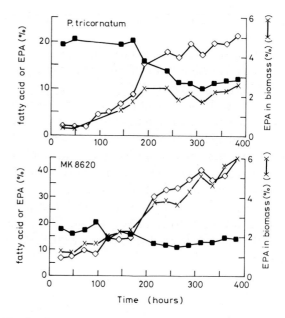

Fig. 1. Biomass accumulation in *P. tricornatum* and MK8620 in a flat plate photobioreactor under conditions that lead to nitrogen depletion at biomass densities of *ca.* 3–4 g dry weight/l. ◇ = total biomass; ◆ = delipidated biomass (i.e., total biomass − extracted fatty acids).

Fig. 2. EPA and fatty acid contents of *P. tricornatum* and MK8620 grown in flat plate photobioreactors under conditions that lead to nitrogen depletion. In both cases the cultures became nitrogen-limited between 150 and 200 h. Fatty acid values (◇) are presented as percent of total biomass. EPA values are represented both as percent EPA in the lipid (■) and as percent EPA in the biomass (X).

overall fat levels increased in response to nitrogen depletion. This had the net effect that the overall EPA in the biomass remained at *ca.* 2–3% (Fig. 2). The EPA level in the lipid of MK8620, on the other hand, did not appear to drop as dramatically even though the bio-oil accumulated to a greater extent during the oil production stage. Consequently, the EPA content in MK8620 increased to levels of 5–6% of the dry biomass in parallel with the oil accumulation. This observation suggests that there may be a significant amount of EPA in the triglyceride oil of MK8620.

Determination of the EPA content in the triglyceride fraction as well as other complex lipid fractions of MK8620 required total lipid extraction from the biomass. A crude complex lipid fraction prepared by chloroform/methanol extraction contained pigments, polar and nonpolar complex lipids, sterols, and free fatty acids. These components were applied to SEP-PAK columns so that individual lipid fractions could be eluted. The triglyceride

fraction (eluted with hexane and benzene) accounted for about 90% of the total lipid in nitrogen-depleted MK8620 cells. This was not unexpected because microscopic examination of these cells revealed the appearance of large oil droplets. Analysis of the fatty acids of each of the eluted fractions indicated that although higher levels of PUFAs were found in the polar (membrane) lipid fractions, the triglyceride components contained 10–14% EPA. Thus, the EPA profile in the nitrogen-stressed MK8620 indicates that the majority of the EPA in the cell is associated with the nonpolar triglycerides (Fig. 3).

The literature is replete with data indicating that most organisms respond to decreasing temperatures by increasing the degree of unsaturation in their fatty acids [8, 21]. Such a response in membrane lipids has the effect of maintaining their relative fluidity (therefore functionality) at low temperatures. The effects of temperature on the fatty acid composition of *P. tricornatum* and MK8620 were

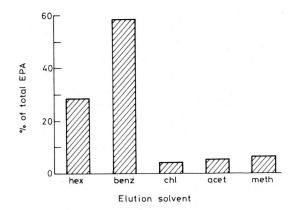

Fig. 3. EPA profile of the complex lipid fractions of nitrogen-deficient MK8620 cells. With this separation procedure triglycerides are eluted with hexane (hex) and benzene (benz); free fatty acids with chloroform (chl); and the polar membrane lipids with acetone (acet) and methanol (meth).

determined using a cylindrical continuous culture photobioreactor described previously [19]. The overflow rates from the reactor reflect the culture productivity, and the data in Table 3 indicate that decreasing temperatures significantly lowered the biomass production rate in both *P. tricornatum* and MK8620. The lipid compositions of the cells at the same growth stage were also compared in these continuous cultures under different temperature conditions. Contrary to our prediction, however, the EPA levels showed little correlation with temperature under the conditions studied (Table 3). The major change in the fatty acid composition in both of these organisms was an increase in the C16:1/C16:0 ratio with decreasing temperature. This would be consistent with the rationale of increasing levels of unsaturation with lower temperatures, but in these two species this generalization did not appear to apply to polyunsaturated fatty acids such as EPA.

A larger scale production process was studied using MK8620 cultivated in a 500-liter photobioreactor designed and constructed in-house. Four-liter cultures were used to inoculate a 25-liter flat plate photobioreactor which, in turn was used to inoculate the 500-liter pilot plant. Under the growth conditions established by the previous studies this bioreactor exhibited maximum biomass production

Table 3

The effect of temperature on the productivity and fatty acid composition of *P. tricornatum* and MK8620 growing in continuous culture

	P. tricornatum			MK8620		
	10°C	15°C	20°C	10°C	15°C	20°C
Productivity overflow (mg/l/h)	25	40	50	< 5	40	70
Fatty acid (%)						
14:0	6	5	6	3	3	4
16:0	16	22	23	17	18	18
16:1	36	28	19	31	28	26
16:2	7	5	4	10	10	5
18:1	4	3	5	8	7	7
18:2	10	13	9	7	4	3
18:3	3	7	9	–	–	–
18:4	–	–	–	3	2	10
20:4	1	1	1	2	2	2
20:5	17	14	17	19	22	22
16:1/16:0	2.3	1.3	0.8	1.8	1.6	1.4

rates of 0.6–0.8 g dry weight/l/day. Batch cultures with the medium nitrogen levels adjusted to allow efficient production of EpA-containing oil, produce about 2 kg biomass (700 g oil) in a 2-week batching time.

DISCUSSION

The industrial-scale microalgal production of EPA-containing bio-oil for food and/or pharmaceutical applications requires controlled cultivation of the selected organism. Open pond cultivation is not likely to be feasible in this application due to rigorous purity demands on the product, the possibility of contamination by weed organisms, and the inability to control the culture conditions to provide high biomass densities and EPA productivity. We have cultivated a proprietary microalgal strain (MK8620) which is capable of producing EPA at levels greater than 6% of its dry weight at the bench scale (25-liter reactors) and this has been successfully scaled up to a 500-liter pilot photobioreactor. In

258

order to improve the production economics and make this process a commercially attractive one, the EPA content of MK8620 needs to be further improved. This may be accomplished by conventional microbiological selection techniques for producing overproducers, as well as further optimization of culture parameters.

Another advantage to the production of EPA by photosynthetic microorganisms in enclosed photobioreactors is that it offers the possibility of producing isotopically labeled EPA for metabolic studies. The only carbon source for these organisms is CO_2, which is the least costly form of ^{13}C or ^{14}C. Furthermore, if MK8620 can be grown in medium containing heavy water (as has been demonstrated for other algal species [7, 9]) then the production of deuterated EPA would be possible. Judicious choices of the microalgal species growing in these enclosed photobioreactor geometries should allow for the production of the labeled fatty acids of interest.

ACKNOWLEDGEMENT

This work has been supported in part by a grant from the National Heart, Blood and Lung Institute (R43-HL38547) to D.J.K.

REFERENCES

1 Bang, H.O. and J. Dyerberg. 1972. Plasma lipids and lipoproteins in Greenlandic west coast Eskimos. Acta Med. Scand. 192: 85–94.

2 Begin, M.E., U.N. Das, G. Ells and D.F. Horrobin. 1985. Selective killing of human cancer cells by polyunsaturated fatty acids. Prostaglandins Leukot. Med. 19: 177–186.

3 Booyens, J., P. Engelbrecht, S. LeRoux, C.C. Louwrens, VanderMerwe and I.E. Katzeff. 1984. Some effects of the essential fatty acids linolenic acid and alpha linolenic acid and of their metabolites gamma linolenic acid, arachidonic acid, eicosapentaenoic acid, docosahexaenoic acid, and of prostaglandins A1 and E1 on the proliferation of human osteogenic sarcoma cells in culture. Prostaglandins Leukot. Med. 15: 15–33.

4 Chapman, A.R.O. 1978. Chlorophyta. In: CRC Handbook of Microbiology (Laskin, A.I. and H.A. Lechevalier, eds.), pp. 425–450, CRC Press Inc., West Palm Beach, FL.

5 Cohen, Z. 1986. Products from microalgae. In: Handbook of Microalgal Mass Culture (Richmond, A., ed.), pp. 421–454, CRC Press Inc., Boca Raton, FL.

6 Cox, E.R. 1978. Dinoflagellates. In: CRC Handbook of Microbiology (Laskin, A.I. and H.A. Lechevalier, eds.), pp. 425–450, CRC Press Inc., West Palm Beach, FL.

7 Delente, J. 1987. Perdeuterated chemicals from D_2O-grown microalgae. Trends Biotechnol. 5: 159–160.

8 Erwin, J., D. Hulinicka and K. Bloch. 1964. Comparative aspects of unsaturated fatty acid synthesis. Comp. Biochem. Physiol. 12: 191–207.

9 Graff, G., P. Szczepanik, P.D. Klein, J.R. Chipault and R.T. Holman. 1970. Identification and characterization of fully deuterated fatty acids from Scenedesmus obliquus cultured in deuterium oxide. Lipids 5: 786–792.

10 Hirai, A., T. Terano, H. Saito, Y. Tamura and S. Yoshida. 1987. Clinical and epidemiological studies of eicosapentaenoic acid in Japan. In: Polyunsaturated Fatty Acids and Eicosanoids (Lands, W.E.M., ed.), pp. 9–24, American Oil Chemists Society Publications, Champaign, IL.

11 Karmali, R.A., 1987. Omega-3 fatty acids and cancer. In: Polyunsaturated Fatty Acids and Eicosanoids (Lands, W.E.M., ed.), pp. 222–232, American Oil Chemists Society Publications, Champaign, IL.

12 Kremer, J.M. and W. Jubitz. 1987. Fish oil supplementation in active rheumatoid arthritis: a double blinded, controlled, crossover study. In: Polyunsaturated Fatty Acids and Eicosanoids (Lands, W.E.M., ed.), pp. 148–153, American Oil Chemists Society Publications, Champaign, IL.

13 Kromhout, D., E.B. Bosschieter and C. Coulander. 1985. Inverse relationship between fish consumption and 20-year mortality from coronary heart disease. N. Engl. J. Med. 312: 1205–1209.

14 Kyle, D.J., P. Behrens, S. Bingham, K. Arnett and D. Lieberman. 1988. Microalgae as a source of EPA-containing oils. J. Am. Oil Chem. Soc., in press.

15 Lee, T.H., R.L. Hoover, J.D. Williams, R.I. Sperling, J. Ravalese, B.W. Spur, D.R. Robinson, E.J. Corey, R.A. Lewis and K.F. Austen. 1985. Effect of dietary enrichment with eicosapentaenoic and docosahexaenoic acids on in vitro neutrophil and monocyte leukotriene generation and neutrophil function. N. Engl. J. Med. 312: 1217–1224.

16 Loeblich, A.R. and L.A. Loeblich. 1978. Division Bacillariophyta. In: CRC Handbook of Microbiology (Laskin, A.I. and H.A. Lechevalier, eds.), pp. 425–450, CRC Press Inc., West Palm Beach, FL.

17 Loeblich, A.R. and L.A. Loeblich. 1978. Division Haptophyta. In: CRC Handbook of Microbiology (Laskin, A.I. and H.A. Lechevalier, eds.), pp. 425–450, CRC Press Inc., West Palm Beach, FL.

18 Phillipson, B.E., D.W. Rothrock, W.E. Connor, W.S. Harris and D.R. Illingworth. 1985. Reduction of plasma lipids, lipoproteins, and apoproteins by dietary fish oils in patients with hypertriglyceridemia. N. Engl. J. Med. 312: 1210–1216.

19 Radmer, R., P. Behrens and K. Arnett. 1987. An analysis of

the productivity of a continuous algal culture system. Biotechnol. Bioeng. 24: 488–492.

20 Ratledge, C. 1987. Lipid biotechnology: a wonderland for the microbial physiologist. J. Am. Oil Chem. Soc. 64: 1647–1656.

21 Shaw, R. 1966. Polyunsaturated fatty acids of micro-organisms. Adv. Lipid Res. 4: 107–174.

22 Sperling, R.I., M. Weinblatt, J.L. Robin, J. Ravalese, R.L. Hoover, F. House, J.S. Coblyn, P.A. Fraser, B.W. Spur, D.R. Robinson, R.A. Lewis and K.F. Austen. 1987. Effects of dietary supplementation with marine fish oil on leucocyte lipid mediator generation and function in rheumatoid arthritis. Arthritis Rheum. 30: 988–997.

23 Wheeler, W.N. 1982. Response of microalgae to light quality, light intensity, temperature, CO_2, HCO_3, O_2, mineral nutrients and pH. In: Handbook of Biosolar Resources (Zaborsky, O., A. Mitsui and C.C. Black, eds.), pp. 157–184, CRC Press, Boca Raton, FL.

Novel Microbial Products for Medicine and Agriculture
Editors: A.L. Demain, G.A. Somkuti, J.C. Hunter-Cevera and H.W. Rossmoore

CHAPTER 29

Use of a double-sided plate to screen for microorganisms producing methionine

Hazel G. Aranha* and Lewis R. Brown

Department of Biological Sciences, Mississippi State University, Mississippi State, MS, U.S.A.

SUMMARY

This paper describes an improved method of screening for microorganisms producing growth-promoting chemicals. The technique employs a double-sided plate wherein the production of a desired chemical by a microbial colony on one side of the plate is indicated by the growth of a microorganism requiring that chemical on the second side of the plate. The isolation of methionine-producing cultures from soil is given for illustrative purposes.

INTRODUCTION

A prerequisite for microbiologically based industrial processes is the use of microorganism(s) with a superior ability to elaborate the primary metabolite or idiolite in question. Consequently, microbial culture selection assumes prime importance. Regardless of the origin of the potential producers, i.e., whether the organism has been obtained following tedious primary screening techniques or whether it is a product of elaborate strain improvement procedures or genetic engineering, large numbers of cultures have to be evaluated prior to obtaining a microorganism with potential industrial application.

The routine primary screening procedure for isolation of organisms producing growth-promoting substances involves the agar overlay method. Basi-cally the technique involves growth of potential producers on the surface of agar plates followed by overlay with an indicator organism, usually an auxotroph requiring the growth-promoting substance in question [5]. Replicate plates must be made prior to overlay with the bioassay organism because the plates are exposed to lethal doses of ultraviolet radiation prior to being overlaid to prevent interference with the assay.

In addition to the considerable expenditure of time, effort, and laboratory supplies, the conventional agar-overlay method for primary screening has several limitations, especially when dealing with diverse colonial and morphological types of microorganisms. Using screening for methionine-producing organisms as an example, this paper describes a novel inexpensive technique employing a double-sided plate to screen for organisms producing growth-promoting substances.

---

*Present address: see List of Contributors.

MATERIALS AND METHODS

The cultures employed in this investigation were: *Lactobacillus plantarum* (ATCC 8014), an auxotrophic methionine-requiring mutant; *Corynebacterium glutamicum* (ATCC 21608), a methionine-producing bacterium; and an aqueous soil suspension. For routine maintenance, brain heart infusion (Difco) and Lactobacillus MRS broth (Difco) were employed for *C. glutamicum* and *L. plantarum*, respectively. Incubation temperatures were 25°C, 30°C, and 35°C for soil, *C. glutamicum*, and *L. plantarum*, respectively.

To test the response of *L. plantarum* to methionine concentration, 10 ml of Bacto-methionine assay medium (Difco) solidified with 1.5% Bacto-agar (Difco) and containing 0.1 ml of a *L. plantarum* cul-

ture (approximately 3×10^9 cfu/ml) was poured into each of a number of standard petri dishes. After the agar had solidified, one-quarter inch Bacto-concentration disks impregnated with various concentrations of DL-methionine were placed on the surface of the agar and the plates incubated at 35°C. Beginning at 18 h, the diameter of the zones of growth of the *L. plantarum* were measured.

The ability of *L. plantarum* to respond to the quantity of methionine produced by *C. glutamicum* was determined as follows. Methionine assay agar was poured into compartment A of a Lutri Plate® (Lutri Plate Inc., Starkville, MS) (see Fig. 1), allowed to solidify, and spot-inoculated with *C. glutamicum*. After incubation at 30°C for 48 h, the Lutri Plate® was inverted, the retaining disc removed and 10 ml of methionine assay agar contain-

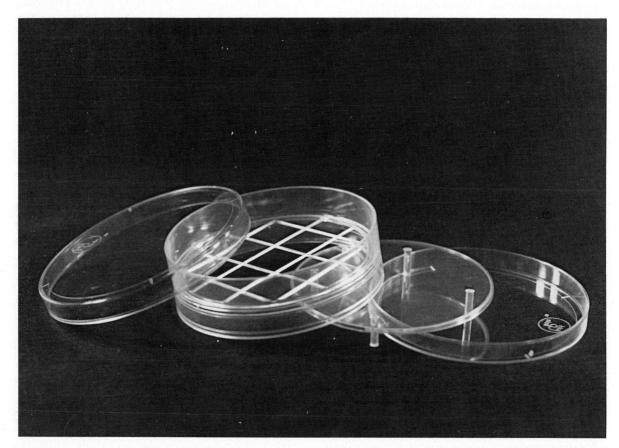

Fig. 1. Photograph of a Lutri Plate®. From left to right the components are (1) lid for compartment A, (2) a cylindrical body with a support grid perpendicular to the sides of the cylinder dividing it into two halves (compartment A and compartment B), (3) a retaining disc in compartment B separating it from compartment A, and (4) a lid for compartment B [1].

ing 0.1 ml of *L. plantarum* cells (approximately 3×10^9 cfu/ml) was poured into compartment B of the Lutri Plate®. The plates then were incubated at 35°C for 72 h.

The technique employed for screening soil samples for methionine-producing microorganisms was: 0.1 ml of an appropriate dilution of the soil sample was surface-seeded onto 30 ml of previously poured methionine assay agar contained in compartment A of a Lutri Plate® (see Fig. 1). The plates were incubated at 25°C until a sizeable number of colonies was evident on the surface (usually 48–72 h). The plates were inverted, the retaining disc removed from each, and 10 ml of methionine assay agar containing 0.1 ml of *L. plantarum* (approximately 3×10^9 cfu/ml) was poured into compartment B of each Lutri Plate®. Following in-

cubation at 35°C for 72 h, the plates were examined for growth of the methionine-requiring auxotroph, *L. plantarum*.

RESULTS

The growth of the bioassay organism, *L. plantarum*, was directly proportional to the quantity of methionine employed. Under the conditions of the test, the diameter of the zones of growth beneath the methionine-impregnated disks varied from 13 mm for a methionine concentration of 0.3 μg to 36 mm for a methionine concentration of 2.4 μg.

The ability of *C. glutamicum* to produce a sufficient quantity of methionine to support the growth of the *L. plantarum* is illustrated in Fig. 2. As may

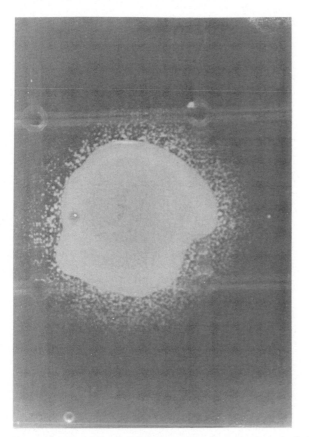 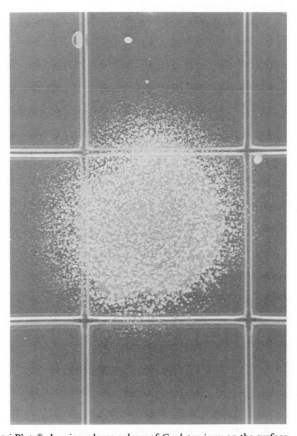

Fig. 2. Photograph on the left is a top view of compartment A of a Lutri Plate® showing a large colony of *C. glutamicum* on the surface of methionine assay agar. Photograph on the right is a view of the Lutri Plate® showing growth of *L. plantarum* in the agar of the methionine assay agar in compartment B directly beneath the *C. glutamicum* colony, which indicates the production of methionine by the *C. glutamicum*.

be observed, the only growth of the *L. plantarum* in compartment B is directly beneath the growth of *C. glutamicum*.

Figs. 3 and 4 show typical results obtained using soil as the source of methionine-producing microorganisms. The one colony in compartment A producing methionine is clearly visible in Fig. 3 while in Fig. 4 the bacterial methionine-producing colony in compartment A is nearly obscured by two actinomycete colonies.

Pure cultures of the organisms from each of the two colonies shown in Fig. 3 and 4 were obtained and retested for their ability to produce methionine as demonstrated by their ability to support the growth of *L. plantarum* in Lutri Plates®. Both isolates produced zones of growth of *L. plantarum*

which were considerably larger than the zone produced by *C. glutamicum* tested under similar conditions.

This technique has been employed successfully using a number of other types of isolation agar in compartment A. Obviously the isolation agar did not contain methionine or any material inhibitory to the *L. plantarum* culture.

DISCUSSION

The conventional methodology employed for primary screening of microorganisms producing growth-promoting substances leaves a lot to be desired. Due to inactivation of the cells by exposure

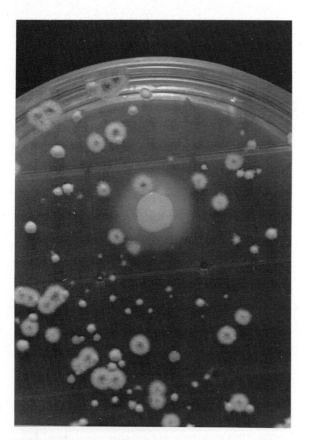
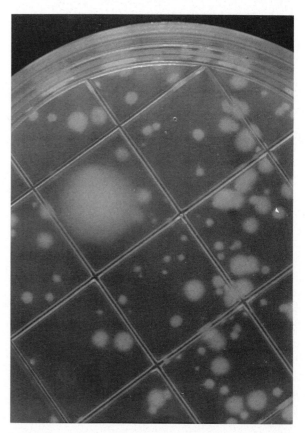

Fig. 3. Photograph on the left is a top view of compartment A of a Lutri Plate® showing numerous colonies from a soil inoculum growing on the agar surface. Photograph on the right shows a hazy area near the center indicating growth of *L. plantarum* in the methionine assay agar in compartment B in response to the production of methionine by one colony in compartment A directly opposite the growth in compartment B.

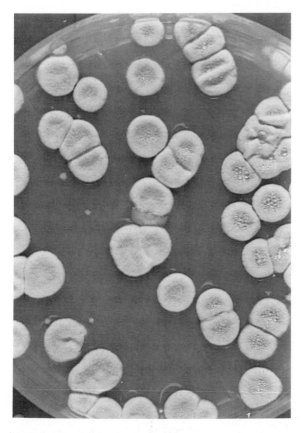
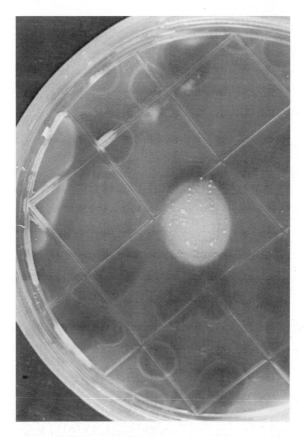

Fig. 4. Photograph on the left is a top view of compartment A of a Lutri Plate® showing numerous colonies from a soil inoculum growing on the agar surface. Note the one bacterial colony sandwiched between two actinomycete colonies in the center of the plate. Photograph on the right shows a hazy area in the center of compartment B indicating growth of *L. plantarum* in the methionine assay agar in compartment B in response to the production of methionine by the bacterial colony growing in compartment A directly opposite the growth in compartment B.

to ultraviolet radiation prior to overlay with the indicator organisms, accurate replication becomes the crucial step in the process. The replica plating technique using velveteen or filter paper, introduced by Lederberg and Lederberg [4], has proven to be invaluable especially in studies involving pure cultures of certain microbial species or alternatively mixed cultures of cooperative types of microorganisms. However, natural materials from which isolation is to be attempted, as, for example, soil, contain a myriad of microbial species with diverse colonial characteristics. Consequently, the conventional replica plating technique is unsuitable. This is especially true for certain colonial types, such as the actinomycetes. Some investigators have sought to utilize a multipoint inoculation

technique (e.g., the device described by Haque and Baldwin [2] and Roberts [6] to decrease smearing of colonies and to facilitate the process of replication [3]) to circumvent this problem. An alternative to the replica-plating technique would involve picking each individual colony prior to ultraviolet inactivation and overlay with the bioassay organism. These techniques, especially the latter, tend to become cost-prohibitive from a labor standpoint when large numbers of samples are involved.

Studies in our laboratory yielded unsatisfactory results with the conventional agar-overlay method. Replicability of plates was affected by several factors including colonial consistency, elevation, etc. Furthermore, actinomycetes, due to their elevation and consistency, are not readily replicable. Attempts to replicate the plate in Fig. 4A were unsuccessful; use of the conventional agar-overlay method only would have resulted in loss of the methionine-producing bacterial colony wedged between two actinomycete colonies. Use of the Lutri Plate® technique obviates limitations posed by the conventional agar-overlay method by circumventing the necessity for replication.

Another important advantage of the isolation technique described herein concerns the nature of secondary metabolites. In the agar-overlay technique, all of the potential metabolite producers are killed at a given time and some slower-growing colonies may not have started or may have just begun elaborating the sought-after metabolite. With the double-sided plate technique, the potential producer colonies are viable throughout the bioassay phase of the method, although admittedly the conditions of incubation during this phase may be slightly different from the original conditions employed. In some instances this difference may accelerate production of the desired substance.

Aside from simplifying primary screening procedures, the double-sided plate technique is readily applicable to optimization and strain improvement.

REFERENCES

1 Brown, L.R. 1982. Antibiotic Testing Vessel. U.S. Patent No. 4,326,028.
2 Haque, R. and J.N. Baldwin. 1964. Types of hemolysins produced by *Staphylococcus aureus*, as determined by the replica plating technique. J. Bacteriol. 88: 1422–1447.
3 Hartman, P.A. 1968. Miniaturized microbiological methods. Adv. Appl. Microbiol. 1 (Suppl.): 85–100.
4 Lederberg, J. and E.J. Lederberg. 1952. Replica plating and indirect selection of bacterial mutants. J. Bacteriol. 63: 399–406.
5 Miller, B.M. and W. Litsky. 1976. Industrial Microbiology, pp. 110–111, McGraw-Hill, Inc., New York.
6 Roberts, C.F. 1959. A replica plating technique for the isolation of nutritionally exacting mutants of a filamentous fungus (*Aspergillus nidulans*). J. Gen. Microbiol. 20: 540–548.